A handbook of
dementia care

A handbook of dementia care

Edited by
CAROLINE CANTLEY

Open University Press
Buckingham • Philadelphia

Open University Press
Celtic Court
22 Ballmoor
Buckingham
MK18 1XW

email: enquiries@openup.co.uk
world wide web: www.openup.co.uk

and
325 Chestnut Street
Philadelphia, PA 19106, USA

First Published 2001

A catalogue record of this book is available from the British Library

ISBN   0 335 20383 3 (pb)   0 335 20384 1 (hb)

Library of Congress Cataloging-in-Publication Data
A handbook of dementia care / edited by Caroline Cantley.
     p. cm.
  Includes bibliographical references and index.
  ISBN 0–335–20384–1 (hbk.) – ISBN 0–335–20383–3 (pbk.)
    1. Dementia–Patients–Care–Handbooks, manuals, etc.   2.
Dementia–Patients–Services for–Handbooks, manuals, etc.   I. Cantley, Caroline.
RC521.H352 2001
616.8′3–dc21   2001021077

Typeset in 10/12pt Sabon by Graphicraft Limited, Hong Kong
Printed in Great Britain by Biddles, Limited, Guildford and King's Lynn

Contents

List of figures and tables

Notes on contributors

John Bond is a sociologist and Professor of Health Services Research. He has written widely on ageing and health. His research interests include: epidemiology and sociology of dementia, quality of life, the management of the diagnosis, insight and risk, and methods of researching dementia and dementia care.

Dawn Brooker is a clinical psychologist with many years experience in dementia care. She has served as Director of the Oxford Dementia Services Development Centre and has broad interests in practice, training and research.

Andrea Capstick is a member of Bradford Dementia Group, University of Bradford. She has played a key role in the development of open and distance learning programmes for care workers that have a particular emphasis on the role of interpersonal communication in maintaining the personhood and well-being of those with dementia.

Charlotte Clarke is Professor of Nursing Practice Development at the University of Northumbria where, since the mid-1990s, she has developed the Practice Development Research Programme which has a particular interest in supporting practitioners to use and create knowledge. She has had a long-standing interest in dementia care research.

Peter Coleman is a Professor of Psychogerontology at the University of Southampton, a joint appointment between Geriatric Medicine in the Medical School and the Department of Psychology. He also holds a Diploma in Religious Studies from the University of Southampton.

Sylvia Cox is a qualified social worker with many years' experience as a practitioner and senior manager. Since 1995 she has been Planning Consultant at the Dementia Services Development Centre, Stirling University, where she is involved in development consultancy and evaluative research. She is also a member of the review panel of the Scottish Health Advisory Service.

Andrew Fairbairn is a consultant in Old Age Psychiatry in Newcastle upon Tyne. He is chair of the Faculty for the Psychiatry of Old Age, Royal College of Psychiatry.

Jane Gilliard has worked as a social worker with carers of people with dementia. She was involved with John Keady in one of the first major studies to consider the perspective of the person with dementia. She is Director of Dementia Voice, the dementia services development centre for south west England.

Valerie Good has spent most of her career working in services for older people as a social worker, service manager and strategic development manager in both statutory agencies and the 'not for profit' sector.

Anthea Innes works for the Centre for Social Research at the University of Stirling. Previously she worked at the Bradford Dementia Group. Her work centres around improving care for people with dementia by understanding the influence of cultures of care on this process and the influence of ethnicity on care provision.

John Keady worked as a community psychiatric nurse in a dementia team for several years before entering the University of Wales, Bangor in July 1993 to facilitate a post-graduate gerontology course. Working with others, John has helped to develop a number of assessment instruments for use with carers and people with dementia.

Jan Killeen has extensive experience of working with disadvantaged communities and groups first through community development and later through specific campaigns to improve the legal rights and quality of life of people with dementia and their carers.

Christina Maciejewski works as a clinical psychologist in Cardiff and is co-director of the Dementia Services Development Centre – Wales. Her particular areas of interest are the neuropsychology of dementia and the needs of younger people with dementia.

Ian McKeith is Professor of Old Age Psychiatry at the Institute for the Health of the Elderly, University of Newcastle upon Tyne. His research interests include the diagnosis and treatment of dementia.

Jill Manthorpe is senior lecturer in community care at the University of Hull where she teaches and researches mainly on ageing and welfare. Recent publications include jointly edited books on risk, institutional abuse, health-related social work and community care, as well as studies of local government, carers, dementia services and mental health inquiries.

Mary Marshall has worked with and for older people for over 25 years as a social worker, lecturer, researcher and voluntary sector manager. She is currently director of the Dementia Services Development Centre at the University of Stirling.

Marie Mills is a psychologist and counsellor who has many years of experience in working with older people.

Mike Nolan has been undertaking research on family care for 15 years. Together with colleagues he has devised a range of assessment instruments that have been translated into a number of foreign languages and have been widely adopted in both research and practice.

Maria Parsons has worked as a social worker with older people with mental health needs in Lambeth and Oxford, and has subsequently trained and lectured in social work. More recently, Maria helped establish the Dementia Services Development Centre at Oxford Brookes University and she is currently Assistant Director of the centre.

Gilbert Smith has held teaching and research posts in the Universities of Aberdeen, Glasgow and Hull. He has been chairman of a health authority, editor of the *Journal of Social Policy*, Deputy Director of Research and Development for the National Health Service and Vice-Chancellor of the University of Northumbria.

David Stanley is head of the Division of Primary Care and Adult and Community Studies, and co-director of the Centre for Care of Older People in the Faculty of Health, Social Work and Education at the University of Northumbria. He has a practice background in social work.

Acknowledgements

We are grateful to the publishers for permission to reproduce in adapted form a figure from Gaster, L. (1995) *Quality in Public Services: Managers' Choices*. Buckingham: Open University Press.

CAROLINE CANTLEY

Introduction

It has become a truism to say that interest in dementia care has grown enormously in recent years. In the past dementia services were without doubt 'Cinderella' services that had low professional and organizational status. Recently, however, we have seen growth in professional enthusiasm for practice development in dementia care. We have also seen increasing policy and managerial concern to develop and improve dementia services. All of this has happened at a time when there have been significant challenges in the way that we think about dementia. It is important to document the change that has taken place. Although there have been very significant changes we still have a long way to go in understanding how best to provide dementia services. Thus practitioners and managers need to know much more about what constitutes 'good practice'. They also need to know more about the range of approaches to practice and service development that are available to help them. This book seeks to make a significant contribution to the further development of dementia services.

The number of people with dementia is substantial and is growing in line with the overall ageing of the population (see for example Hofman *et al.* 1991; Melzer *et al.* 1992; Melzer *et al.* 1997; Harvey 1998). But it is not just the growth in numbers of people with dementia that presents the challenges to health and social services. It is also the complexity of their needs. This complexity means that dementia care involves many different professions and organizations. As a result of this, practitioners and managers need to understand a range of theoretical perspectives that underpin their own, and other people's, practice. They also need to be able to draw upon our growing knowledge about how to develop and implement change in different policy and organizational contexts.

Readers of this book will come from a variety of professional and other backgrounds. They are therefore likely to find some ideas in this book that are familiar to them and some that are very new. Each of the chapters is written with the aim of making the key concepts and findings accessible to non-specialists in that field. This book presents a picture of the richness and complexity of ideas that can contribute to dementia services development. It is not a 'how to do it' handbook. Instead it provides readers with a resource to draw upon in understanding and developing their own practice and in working in partnerships with other professions and organizations.

The three sections of this book each address one broad question: what is the nature of dementia and how can we better understand it? What do we know about what constitutes good practice in dementia care? How does the policy, organizational and research context of dementia care affect service development?

In Section 1 we review a number of theoretical frameworks to show how they can each contribute to our understanding of dementia. We begin with the biomedical perspective. This perspective no longer dominates our thinking about dementia care but there are important scientific advances of which we should be aware. The next chapter is concerned with psychological perspectives. It includes a discussion of the social psychological ideas that have been so influential in recent thinking about dementia care. The chapter that follows is about sociological perspectives. It introduces a range of ideas that are much less commonly used in thinking about dementia care. Similarly the chapter on philosophical and spiritual perspectives provides a range of ideas that can help extend the ways in which we conceptualize dementia care. Section 1 concludes with a chapter on what we know about how people with dementia, their families and carers experience the condition. Throughout this book we shall see how these different perspectives, to varying degrees, inform our thinking about good practice and service development.

In Section 2 we focus on practice in dementia care, taking as a starting point the need for a knowledge-based approach. The section thus begins with a chapter on the creation and use of knowledge in practice and on the processes by which practice can be changed and developed. The chapters that follow provide an overview of current knowledge and highlight key issues in different areas of practice. The areas covered include: assessment and care management, communication, therapeutic activity and working with carers. In this second section of the book we also look at the different practice issues that arise in working with people with dementia in their own homes and in group care settings. This section ends with a discussion of the values and ethics that are central to much dementia care practice.

In Section 3 we explore the context in which dementia care practice and service development takes place. It is not at all unusual for service development in dementia care to involve a number of professions and organizations. This means that the environment for service development is complex. If practitioners and managers do not understand this complexity it is unlikely that their efforts to develop services will succeed fully. So, in this section, we aim to develop a better understanding of the context of service development.

We begin with an overview of policy development and some of the policy themes that are currently shaping dementia care. In the next chapter we outline some key concepts that can help us to understand how professions and organizations operate. We then turn to more practical approaches to service development including organizational development and quality management. Towards the end of the section we develop a theme that is highlighted in earlier chapters: the importance of involving people with dementia and their carers in service development. These earlier chapters show how a range of policy, professional and organizational factors can serve to limit this involvement. But here we see examples of initiatives that demonstrate just how much good practice is possible. The final chapter in Section 3 examines some of the key issues for research in dementia care. It shows how a range of research methodologies is relevant to dementia services development. It also argues that for research to have an impact on services we need to understand the part that it plays in the broader processes of policy making and implementation.

This book concludes by looking at some of the factors that will influence dementia care in the future. We need to make the most of the rich diversity of ideas available to us if we are to ensure optimal development of dementia services in a complex technical, social, moral, organizational and political world.

Understanding dementia

1

IAN MCKEITH AND ANDREW FAIRBAIRN

Biomedical and clinical perspectives

KEY POINTS

- Dementia is the most common serious mental illness affecting older people.
- Scientific knowledge about the dementias has expanded enormously in the last 20 years.
- There are different types of dementia, the most common causes being Alzheimer's disease, dementia with Lewy bodies and vascular dementia.
- Technological advances include the development of earlier diagnosis and drug treatments for Alzheimer's Disease.
- Changes in scientific knowledge and medical treatments have profound implications for clinical practice and care provision.

INTRODUCTION

The objectives of this chapter are to provide an overview of scientific and clinical developments in the **biomedical** aspects of dementia and to consider how these impact on the clinical practice of specialists and non-specialists caring for people with dementia. Topics to be covered include:

- a brief history of our understanding of dementia as a brain disease;
- current definitions of dementia;
- different types of dementia – clinical features, therapeutic potential and pathological basis;
- diagnosis of dementia;

- treatment for dementia; and
- typical service arrangements.

A BRIEF HISTORY OF DEMENTIA

The word dementia is derived from the Latin *demens*, meaning 'without mind'. It has been in common use since the early eighteenth century, implying a lack of competence to manage one's own affairs. It assumed a legal status around the time of the French Revolution and was enshrined in Article 10 of the Napoleonic Code: 'There is no crime when the accused is in a state of dementia at the time of the alleged act' (Code Napoleon 1808).

Medical usage of the word dementia evolved slowly from the early nineteenth century. The term dementia was used to describe patients whose mental disability was secondary to some form of acquired brain damage – usually degenerative and occurring in old age, but not necessarily so. Dementia was thus distinguished from other mental disorders such as schizophrenia, mania or depression and the central importance of cognitive (intellectual) failure began to be recognized. By the beginning of the twentieth century, clinical scientists had started to examine brain tissue of demented patients at post-mortem and to describe specific changes which were not seen in non-demented people. The first important study was that of Marcé in 1863, who described cortical atrophy (shrinkage of the brain), enlarged ventricles (the fluid filled spaces within the brain) and 'softening' of brain tissue. It was initially thought that such softening was due to disorders of blood supply to the brain, but by the latter half of the nineteenth century, scientists had identified more subtle, degenerative changes associated with neuronal (nerve cell) death. In 1907 this culminated in Dr Alois Alzheimer reporting abnormal lesions (**senile plaques** and **neurofibrillary tangles**) in the brain of a female patient who had been admitted to a mental hospital in Frankfurt with dementia. This lady, who was called Auguste D., developed progressive memory failure, language difficulties (she called a cup a 'milk pourer') and agitated, aggressive behaviour when she was only 51 years old. We now know **Alzheimer's disease (AD)** to be the commonest cause of dementia, not only in **early onset dementia** patients like Auguste D., but also in old age.

CURRENT DEFINITIONS OF DEMENTIA

Over the last 15–20 years, definitions of dementia have become much more precise about the clinical features by which it should be identified. Deterioration in intellectual performance from a previous level must be accompanied by a significant decline in personal and social function. Other causes for these impairments must be excluded, e.g. general medical illness or drug toxicity. Different dementia subtypes can often be recognized by their mode of onset, presence of particular psychiatric or neurological features, and the course which the illness takes. The criteria most commonly used in the UK for diagnosing dementia due to Alzheimer's disease are listed in the tenth revision of the International Classification of Diseases (ICD 10–1992). These are broadly

Table 1.1 Comparison of two commonly used criteria for the diagnosis of dementia due to Alzheimer's disease

Characteristics	ICD 10	DSM IV
Memory decline	+	−
Thinking impairment	+	−
Dysphasia, dyspraxia, agnosia or impaired executive function	−	+
Impairment of at least one non-memory intellectual function	+	+
Impairment in activities of daily living	+	−
Social or occupational impairment	−	+
Decline from previous level	+	+
Insidious onset	+	+
Slow deterioration	+	−
Continuing deterioration	−	+
Absence of sudden onset	+	−
Absence of focal neurological signs	+	−
Deficits not limited to a delirious period	+	+
Absence of another major mental disorder	−	+

Note: ICD 10 – International Classification of Diseases, 10th revision.
DSM IV – Diagnostic and Statistical Manual of Mental Disorders, 4th edition.

similar to those in the fourth edition of the USA Diagnostic and Statistical Manual of Mental Disorders (DSM IV – 1994). The common elements of the two definitions are compared in Table 1. 1.

THE NORMAL BRAIN AND AGEING

The human brain is an enormously complex structure that consists of two basic components – grey matter and white matter. Grey matter is composed of neurones (nerve cells) that communicate with each other by releasing a variety of chemical transmitters onto the surface of other neurones, where specifically sensitive receptor sites are located. Important **neurotransmitters** include acetylcholine, glutamate, dopamine, serotonin and noradrenaline – involved in the regulation of memory, mood, sleep, appetite, and behaviour. The supporting grey matter (glial cells) which supplies nutrients to the **neurones** and repairs damage is critically important because, unlike other body cells, neurones are generally incapable of reduplicating themselves and need to be carefully maintained throughout a person's entire lifespan.

The white matter of the brain consists of fibres that connect neurones in different parts of the brain to one another, allowing rapid communication between distant structures. Complex networks of these fibres enable neurones to influence the activity of many hundreds or thousands of other neurones. Anatomically the grey and white matter is organized into four major regions (lobes) collectively referred to as the **cerebral cortex**. The **temporal lobes** regulate memory and mood, a structure on the inner (medial) surface called the **hippocampus** (after the Latin for seahorse which it resembles in shape!) being of particular importance in the learning of new information. The front (anterior) part of the temporal lobe controls the understanding of language and meaning. The **frontal lobes** influence the production of speech, personality traits, decision making, complex behaviours and judgement. The **parietal lobes**, which are set further back, are involved in tactile and **visuospatial** perception of the individual self (for example body image) and of the outside world (for example awareness of location and direction). They are also involved in the execution of complex motor tasks such as cooking a meal or dressing. At the back of the brain are the **occipital lobes** that process incoming visual stimuli. Underneath the cortical lobes sit the **cerebellum**, involved in coordination of balance, posture and movement, and the **mid-brain** and **brain stem** which regulate more basic biological functions such as sleep, appetite and sexual function. Although this is an extensively oversimplified account of brain organization, it serves to illustrate that the type of dysfunction experienced when neurones become damaged depends to some extent upon their location in the brain. For example, damage to, or loss of, neurones in the parietal lobe may cause people to become unable to find their way around their own house. A similar loss in the anterior temporal lobe will not affect this ability but may cause a profound loss of the ability to understand the spoken or written word. Also in the frontal lobe it might cause profound apathy and lack of initiative.

The brain develops through childhood to reach its maximum size, typically 1500–2000 grams by late adolescence. The numbers of connections between neurones continues to increase through adult life and probably forms the basis for the establishment of patterns of behaviour and the acquisition of knowledge. Research studies suggest that mental abilities are related to the extent of 'connectivity' rather than brain size, and that a stimulating environment enhances the tendency of neurones to make, and make use of, these connections. From the fifth decade onwards, grey matter begins to slowly diminish in volume, but since the brain has a considerable 'reserve capacity' the effects upon mental function are generally negligible. A healthy 70-year-old may have lost up to 10–15 per cent of brain mass due to normal ageing, with a minor impact upon the ability to learn new information, e.g. names of new acquaintances, but with no decrement in previous knowledge or 'wisdom'. Dementia occurs when disease processes lead to a greater degree of neuronal damage or loss, when white matter connections are severely disrupted, or due to a combination of these events.

DEMENTIA AND DEMENTIA SUBTYPES

We now understand that dementia can be associated with a wide variety of changes within the brain – all of which contribute in some way to accelerated cell death and impaired function of the remaining cells. Dementia is predominantly a disorder of the very elderly. At age 75 the point **prevalence** (proportion of all people of that age who are affected) is approximately 10 per cent. The prevalence doubles with every five years of increasing age – therefore one can

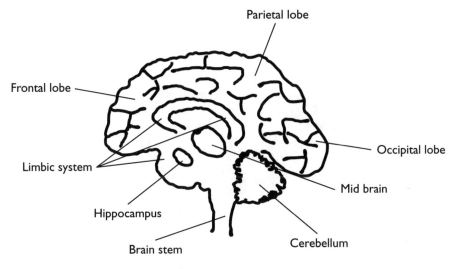

Figure 1.1(a) Section through midline of brain showing structures seen centrally

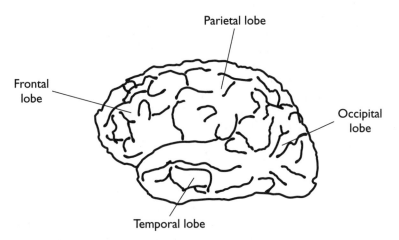

Figure 1.1(b) Brain surface seen from the lateral side showing areas of the cerebral cortex

calculate that by age 85 an extraordinary 40 per cent of the total population has dementia, whereas at age 65 the risk is low at only 2.5 per cent. Although increasing age is the most important known risk factor for developing a dementing illness, dementia is not generally held to be part of the normal ageing process. The normal ageing brain does accumulate some degenerative and vascular changes over the years, and these probably account in part for the small decrements in short-term memory and new learning ability that are common in older people. These mild brain changes and memory symptoms which are sometimes referred to as CIND (cognitive impairment, no dementia) or MCI (minimal cognitive impairment) may represent the very earliest stages

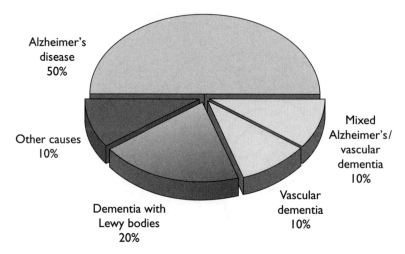

Figure 1.2   Pathological causes of dementia in people over 70 years of age

of dementia in a minority of people but are non-progressive in most cases. There is some **epidemiological** evidence to suggest that in people surviving beyond the age of 90 the risk of developing dementia begins to level off. If this is true dementia may be viewed as a condition for which there is a 'window of risk' in the eighth and ninth decades (70–90 years), presentation outside of this age range being less common.

The different brain diseases that are commonly associated with dementia are illustrated in Figure 1.2, which shows the typical post-mortem findings in brain tissue from elderly patients diagnosed with dementia during lifetime.

Alzheimer's disease is the most common cause of dementia in old age accounting for 50–60 per cent of cases. **Dementia with Lewy** bodies (DLB) which accounts for 15–20 per cent of cases, making it the second most common subtype, has only recently been described. **Vascular dementia** (VaD), that is dementia due to stroke disease or poor cerebral circulation, is a relatively uncommon single cause of dementia but frequently coexists with other pathologies, for example mixed with Alzheimer or Lewy body disease. 10–15 per cent of all cases of dementia have causes which can be considered relatively uncommon. Some of these less common causes are listed in Table 1.2.

Alzheimer's disease

Clinical features

Memory disorder is the most striking feature in the majority of cases of AD, reflecting the fact that the characteristic pathological changes and neurone loss occur first in the medial temporal lobe and hippocampus, structures which are intimately involved in memory function. The disease also involves the more posterior parts of the brain (parietal lobes), producing abnormalities of language skills (dysphasia) and visuospatial and practical abilities (dyspraxia).

Table 1.2 Possible causes of dementia

Degenerative	**Toxic**
Alzheimer's disease	Alcohol-related dementia
Dementia with Lewy bodies	Carbon monoxide poisoning
Frontal lobe dementia	
Huntingdon's disease	**Space-occupying lesions**
Multiple sclerosis	Chronic subdural haematoma
	Primary or secondary brain tumour
Vascular	
(Previously called multi-infarct dementia)	**Metabolic**
	Hypothyroidism
Traumatic	
Following head injury	**Other causes**
Cerebral anoxia, e.g. post-anaesthetic	Normal pressure hydrocephalus
Transmissible	
AIDS – dementia complex	
Creutzfeldt–Jacob disease	
Neurosyphilis	

Note: This list is not exhaustive and does not include very rare causes of the dementia syndrome.

Involvement of the frontal lobe of the brain may lead to profound alterations in personality and behaviour, social judgement and insight frequently being very substantially impaired. The diffuse nature of cerebral involvement in Alzheimer's disease explains why there is usually a global and relentlessly progressive accumulation of symptoms. Mood disorders, predominantly depression and anxiety, occur in 15–40 per cent of patients, usually early in the course of illness – most reactions being self-limiting and reactive to the realization of failing intellect and **functional ability**. A small proportion of patients develop severe symptoms which may be secondary to reductions in central neurotransmitters which regulate mood, for example noradrenaline. Psychotic features (**hallucinations** and **delusions**) are more common in the middle stage of AD (20–40 per cent of cases), and agitation, aggression, and vegetative problems (sleeping, eating and continence) generally occur late. The disease is slightly more prevalent in women and increasing age is the most important risk factor. The rate of progression is very variable. On average an AD patient's performance on cognitive testing will deteriorate by about 10 per cent per year and life expectancy from onset of symptoms varies from two to twenty years with an average of about 10 years. At any given stage in an individual case, predictions of progression and survival are probably best based upon the observed pattern of illness up to that point.

Therapeutic potential

The loss of neurones in AD is selective rather than random. One group of cells particularly affected is in the basal forebrain which projects to most regions of the cerebral cortex using a neurotransmitter called acetylcholine (ACh). ACh levels in the cerebral cortex are reduced by 60 per cent or more in AD and these reductions correlate with the severity of cognitive impairment as measured on cognitive tests. Inhibition of acetylcholinesterase, the enzyme that normally breaks down ACh, results in increased ACh availability, which theoretically should improve cognitive function. Several compounds (donepezil, rivastigmine, and galanthamine) have been developed for this purpose and extensive trials have shown them to have modest, symptomatic effects in AD. Cholinesterase inhibitors would not be expected, however, to have any effect upon the processes underlying neuronal degeneration. Disease slowing strategies that have been suggested in AD include the use of anti-inflammatory drugs, antioxidants such as vitamin E, and hormone replacement therapy (HRT). Although preliminary clinical trials have suggested benefits from each of these treatments, further studies are required before they can be confidently recommended for routine use in the clinic. Rationally designed treatments would reduce the production of senile plaques or the formation of neurofibrillary tangles (see pathology section below). Although such developments are being attempted in animals it remains to be seen whether they can safely be administered to humans and, if so, whether they will be clinically effective.

Pathology

Externally the brain is atrophied (shrunken) with extensive loss of the grey matter and dilatation of the fluid-filled cavities (ventricles). A definite diagnosis of AD can only be made, however, by identifying the two core **lesions** of the disease under the microscope at post-mortem. The first of these is the senile plaque (SP) which is a structure largely composed of a protein called beta-amyloid that is abnormally deposited into insoluble fibrils which then aggregate to form the SP. As the plaque develops it engulfs neighbouring neurones and their connecting fibres. The presence of beta-amyloid triggers an inflammatory response in the brain, mediated by cells called microglia. Paradoxically the products of the activated microglia may induce further beta amyloid production via a positive feedback loop. AD can therefore be conceived as a chronic brain inflammation. It has recently been observed in epidemiological studies that people who have taken anti-inflammatory drugs for long periods, usually because of chronic arthritis, appear to be at less risk of later developing AD. Trials of such drugs, for example ibuprofen, are currently in progress to see if they can delay the progression of dementia.

The other key lesion in AD is the neurofibrillary tangle (NFT). This differs from the SP in that it develops within, rather than outside, the nerve cell and it is composed of a different set of abnormal proteins. NFTs appear under the microscope as paired helical filaments, which are a distortion of the microtubular system, part of the internal skeleton which supports the neurone and which facilitates transport of material from the nerve cell body to its extremities. The chemical composition of the NFT is not fully understood but an abnormal form of a protein called **tau** appears to be present from an early stage. Tau has an important role in the assembly of microtubules and the abnormal form possibly leads to the production of distorted (tangled) microtubules that are non-functional.

Why SP and NFT develop in AD is unclear, as is their relationship to one another. In 1991 a **mutation** was described in a gene, the amyloid precursor protein (APP) gene, on chromosome 21 in a family with early-onset familial AD. This mutation caused production of an abnormal form of beta amyloid, which was more likely to form insoluble deposits. An 'amyloid cascade hypothesis' of AD was developed suggesting that excessive or abnormal deposition of beta amyloid was the primary event in AD. APP gene mutations are however extraordinarily rare and other, as yet unknown, reasons for abnormal beta amyloid deposition must operate in the vast majority of cases. It is likely that these will be at least in part genetically determined. In **Down's syndrome** an extra copy of the APP gene is present which probably explains why AD pathology occurs very frequently in people with Down's syndrome in their fourth and fifth decades.

The most important known genetic factor operating in the general population controls the presence of a circulating blood protein (apolipoprotein E or apoE) which is normally present to regulate cholesterol levels. Three genetically determined variants of apoE exist and it has been repeatedly shown that individuals carrying genes for a variant of the gene called E4 have a two- to five-fold risk of developing AD. It was initially thought that apolipoprotein E4 bound more readily to beta-amyloid than the other forms, increasing the likelihood of SP formation. It has been alternatively suggested that apolipoprotein E4 may have a destabilizing effect upon microtubule assembly, thereby increasing the chances of NFT formation. A coherent model of the events leading to AD remains elusive. A single, unifying theory may not be forthcoming and AD may prove to have several causative mechanisms. Certainly, two additional genes capable of causing AD have recently been identified, both of which appear relevant only for small numbers of early onset familial disease. The presenilin genes on chromosome 14 (PS1) and chromosome 1 (PS2) are structurally similar to one another and have as yet unknown modes of action but possibly exert some of their effects via beta amyloid.

Dementia with Lewy bodies

Clinical features

The central characteristic of dementia with Lewy bodies (DLB) is fluctuating cognitive impairment with periods of increased confusion and windows of relative lucidity. In the early stages this may appear as a series of apparent acute confusional (delirious) episodes in an otherwise normal individual, leading to extensive medical investigations trying to establish a physical or pharmacological cause. As the disease progresses more persistent cognitive impairment and neuropsychiatric features become apparent. Recent memory function is not so severely impaired as in Alzheimer's disease, probably because the pathological changes are not so focused upon the hippocampus. Deficits in attention and alertness are prominent and may manifest in many ways. Daytime somnolence and apathy are common consequences, the patient often appearing glazed or switched off. Three core features of DLB have been described, any two of which are sufficient to make a clinical diagnosis.

Fluctuation, present in up to 90 per cent of cases, is probably based in minute to minute variations in attentional level, only the more extreme of which are apparent to the external observer. Prominent, recurrent visual hallucinations, for example of animals and people in the patient's home, are present in about 80 per cent of cases and frequently precipitate referral for treatment. The third core feature of DLB is the disorder of movement characteristic of **Parkinson's disease**, specifically slowness to initiate movement, muscle rigidity and, less frequently, resting tremor. These abnormal signs are seen in up to 75 per cent of cases but are often only very mild and easily overlooked in an older person. It was initially thought that DLB had a significantly worse prognosis than AD – recent studies suggest, however, that the mean survival time is seven to eight years, similar to AD. A few DLB cases may deteriorate very rapidly, dying within one to two years of presentation.

Therapeutic potential

The most significant management issue in treating DLB is the need to be cautious in the use of **neuroleptic** medications (major tranquillizers), for example thioridazine, haloperidol, risperidone, and olanzapine. These are usually the first-line treatment for **psychotic** symptoms such as hallucinations and delusions and are frequently given to demented patients for aggression, agitation, insomnia and other behavioural disturbances. Their pharmacological action is to block the receptors which are stimulated by the neurotransmitter dopamine. The dopamine system is already compromised in DLB patients who therefore experience acute Parkinsonian side effects. Mortality rates are increased two- to three-fold by these neuroleptic sensitivity reactions. DLB patients have deficits in acetylcholine in the cerebral cortex that are more profound even than those of AD, and which are correlated with symptoms such as hallucinations and cognitive impairment. Trials are in progress to determine whether cholinesterase inhibitor drugs (see section on AD) will be effective and safe treatments for DLB.

Pathology

Although DLB has only recently been recognized as a common cause of dementia in old age (15–30 per cent of all cases) this is simply because the hallmark lesions (Lewy bodies – LB) were difficult to see under the microscope until new methods of staining brain sections made them more readily visible. Review of autopsy material collected in the 1960s reveals that 17 per cent of dementia cases had DLB, which was simply overlooked at that time. DLB is therefore not a new disease, just a newly recognized one. LB are composed of abnormally processed neurofilament proteins, a fundamentally different part of the neuronal structure than that affected in AD. LB represent an attempt by dying nerve cells to protect themselves and as such are simply a marker that cell death is imminent. The underlying process remains unknown although recent work suggests that there is abnormal regulation of a neuronal protein called α-synuclein which is involved in neuronal repair and learning. Senile plaques similar to those of AD are also seen in DLB but NFT are rare or absent.

LB were first described in Parkinson's disease (PD) in which they mainly occur in the brain stem and mid-brain leading to the motor disorder that characterizes this disease. Some but not all DLB patients share the physical characteristics of Parkinson's disease. Cognitive failure and psychiatric features in DLB appear to be associated with α-synuclein-related neuronal loss (see above) and LB formation in the cerebral cortex. Little is as yet known about risk factors for DLB, genetic or environmental, although the apolipoprotein E4 gene does appear to confer increased risk in the same way as for AD (see section on AD). DLB tends to be slightly more prevalent in men (1.5:1), the converse of AD.

Vascular dementia

Clinical features

Symptoms often have a sudden and dramatic onset and may be relatively focal, for example with almost complete loss of language skills but sparing memory, reasoning and visuospatial abilities. Whether or not such individuals should be deemed as demented is a moot point. A history of a stepwise deterioration in cognitive impairment may correspond to repeated episodes of stroke and be associated with evidence on physical examination of focal neurological signs such as unilateral limb weakness or exaggerated tendon reflexes. The prevalence of dementia after stroke is tenfold higher than in a general population of similar age distribution. In addition to those who develop dementia immediately after the event, a further 30 per cent go on to develop dementia over a period of several months and the risk period extends out at least five years.

Therapeutic potential

Theoretically, vascular dementia should be the most amenable of all dementia syndromes to treatments aimed at reducing recognized risk factors. In reality, no **interventions** have been reliably demonstrated to be effective although some large-scale trials of blood pressure lowering agents have suggested a 50 per cent reduction in rates of dementia over a two-year follow up period. Aspirin may be of therapeutic benefit in stroke disease although a recent publication has not confirmed the protective value of aspirin in vascular dementia.

Pathology

Concepts about the pathological basis of vascular dementia are currently changing very rapidly. Vascular dementia is a term used to gather together a variety of conditions which share a basis in impaired brain blood flow. Patients who have had a stroke in a strategically important location, or who have had multiple small strokes, may develop cognitive impairment and behavioural change sufficient to warrant a diagnosis of dementia. The term **multi-infarct** dementia (MID) was originally coined for this syndrome and is often still used by clinicians. Often the stroke lesions can be seen by structural brain imaging such as **Computerised Tomography (CT)** or **Magnetic Resonance Imaging (MRI)**. Increasingly recognized is a more insidious type of dementia which is related to a slow 'furring up' of small blood vessels penetrating the deepest parts of the brain, typically the white matter which constitutes the bundles of nerve fibres relaying messages from one anatomical location to another. White matter lesions are poorly understood, and although they are frequently reported as present on brain imaging, especially MRI, it is not known to what extent they truly represent vascular lesions. Finally, it is becoming more apparent that vascular disease frequently coexists with degenerative pathologies such as AD or DLB. Pure vascular dementia is probably uncommon and a diagnosis of mixed dementia may be more appropriate in many cases with evidence of cerebrovascular disease or stroke. Risk factors for vascular mediated dementia are thought to be the same as for **cerebrovascular** disease in general – age, race, male sex, **hypertension** and diabetes.

Frontal lobe dementia

Clinical features

Two separate clinical syndromes, or sets of symptoms, have been described. The frontal type is characterized by personality change, usually apathy and inertia but occasionally disinhibition, over-activity, poor social judgement and recklessness. Memory, language and visuospatial skills are well preserved initially. In the other variant, affecting the anterior temporal lobe, there is an early loss of language ability and knowledge of meaning of verbal and visual information. Other aspects of intellect and behaviour may be well preserved. Frontal lobe dementia tends to be more common in younger individuals, women in their fifties and sixties being particularly at risk. Survival is again very variable, the average being five to ten years. Prognostic factors separating fast from slow declines are unknown.

Therapeutic potential

Little is understood about the mechanisms leading to degeneration of the frontal lobes and no specific treatments exist. Patients do not have a deficit in acetylcholine and use of cholinesterase inhibitors (see section on AD) may increase agitation, insomnia and disinhibition.

Pathology

Frontal lobe dementia (FLD) is a less common degenerative disease in which neurones are selectively lost from the frontal lobes and the anterior part of the temporal lobes. There are a variety of typical inclusions in the neurones which differ from those in AD and DLB. About 50 per cent have so-called 'Pick bodies' associated with neuronal loss, gliosis (scarring) and spongiform change. Some forms of frontal dementia are associated with motor neurone disease and others with a Parkinsonian syndrome. A chromosomal abnormality has been described in this latter (rare) disorder and may be closely linked with one of the genes regulating tau protein (see section on AD). In a significant proportion of cases no specific pathology is seen apart from the localized neuronal loss.

Other dementias

A full description of other dementia subtypes is outside the scope of this brief chapter, which concentrates on a brief description of alcohol-related dementia, **Creutzfeldt–Jacob** disease, and **Huntington's disease**.

Alcohol-related dementia usually affects short-term memory, and other cognitive functions may be relatively preserved. It is thought to occur because of a nutritional deficiency in vitamin B1 (thiamine) caused by heavy sustained drinking. In the early stages it may be reversible by appropriate vitamin supplementation.

Creutzfeldt–Jacob disease (CJD) is a rare and rapidly progressive dementia, often progressing to death within a year. Dementia is associated with muscle rigidity, difficulty with speech (**dysarthria**) and jerking movements (myoclonus). CJD is caused by a brain protein called prion protein becoming folded into a lethal configuration. Prion disease may occur due to inherited or spontaneous mutations in the gene that carries the code for the protein. It may also be transmitted by transfer of infected material from one individual to another. Human to human transmission has been reported following infected corneal grafts, injection of human growth hormone and from contaminated neurosurgical instruments. Prion disease in cattle produces bovine spongiform encephalopathy (BSE). Transmission to humans by eating infected material appears possible in genetically susceptible individuals, causing 'new variant' CJD, which presents between the ages of 20 and 50, often with psychiatric features such as anxiety and depression, progressing to dementia and neurological disability over a slightly longer course of 1–2 years.

Huntington's disease (HD) is an inherited form of dementia, associated with abnormal, writhing movements of the trunk and limbs (chorea). It usually begins in mid-life and has a protracted course of 15–20 years. Fifty per cent of HD family members are at risk of developing the disease. A genetic test is available to identify those who have inherited the affected gene on chromosome 4, but since there is no specific treatment currently available, the uptake of the test is relatively low and should only be offered after appropriate genetic counselling.

ISSUES IN DIAGNOSIS

Differentiating between delirium and dementia and between depression and dementia

The **differential diagnosis** of 'confusion' is that of the three 'Ds' – depression, **delirium** and dementia. Depression can mimic an apparent confusion and this is described as depressive pseudo-dementia. Patients will often have a past history of depressive illness. There may be an apparent inconsistency to the clinical picture. For example, the degree of confusion may seem to be profound yet other aspects of the individual's daily functioning may remain relatively spared. The person with depression will be inclined to answer formal memory tests with 'don't know' answers whereas the person with dementia is often inclined to have a go at answering questions no matter how inaccurately. The difference between delirium and dementia is primarily that of speed of onset. Delirium is the onset of acute confusion due to an underlying physical cause whereas dementia is a slowly progressive degenerative brain disorder. Therefore, history taking, typically from a carer, will help differentiate. Typically, the carer will describe an individual who is suffering from delirium as being perfectly fit until a very clear-cut off point when they became suddenly confused. In contrast, the carer of a person with dementia will describe a gradual downhill deterioration with the exact starting point being unclear. The importance in the differential diagnosis is that in older people as well as in younger people, depressive illness is a highly treatable disorder. Also, delirium may typically be highly treatable, the prognosis depending entirely on the underlying physical condition.

Coexisting physical problems

The approach to diagnosis described above suggests a relatively straightforward process. But people, and older people in particular, are inevitably more complex than that. It is very rare to get one single diagnosis and most older people will present with both mental and physical health problems. This also means that delirium can be superimposed upon dementia. In these circumstances a reliable witness may be able to inform the clinician that the person with dementia had been slowly declining but that there was a more dramatic event in the recent past which had caused a superimposed additional confusion. As with everything, 'common things occur commonly' so the underlying cause of a superimposed delirium is likely to be a common condition such as an infection. As a principle any coexisting physical condition should be actively treated in order to optimize the individual's health and well-being. Quite often polypharmacy, the prescribing of multiple drugs, can be a problem and it is a good premise of geriatric medicine that, when in doubt, medication should be stopped as it can always be restarted.

Diagnosis in special groups

People from ethnic minority communities

People from ethnic minority communities are particularly disadvantaged. This can be because clinicians have limited understanding of cultural expectations in their communities but it can also be because of language problems. There is increasing awareness of the particular needs of people with dementia from ethnic minority groups. It is most important to make an accurate diagnosis in the first place and this will frequently require good translation skills. Translation services are increasingly available in health and social services and they can be of immense value in helping to diagnose dementia in people from ethnic minority communities.

People with learning disabilities

People with learning disabilities are particularly vulnerable to dementia (Holland 1997). There is an association between Down's Syndrome and Alzheimer's disease (see above) but also other people with learning disabilities can be vulnerable. Diagnosis will often rely on the concept of 'change'. An informant will be able to say that an individual with learning disabilities had been functioning at a certain level but has now deteriorated. For example, language skills, which were previously present, may be lost or a particular level of day-to-day functioning may start to deteriorate.

Younger people with dementia

Dementia is rare under the age of 65 therefore any suspicion of dementia should be intensively assessed. The diagnosis initially can be quite difficult to make on the basis that the individual might be suffering from some other kind of mental health problem such as an atypical presentation of schizophrenia, anxiety or depression.

The diagnostic process

It is relatively rare for the patient to present complaining of a poor memory. Indeed, worrying about memory problems can be a sign that the individual is depressed rather than demented. Most patients are presented by their families or other carers. Home care workers have been described as the eyes and ears of the specialist services. They usually know their clients well and often are the first to flag up problems. Similarly, informal carers are frequently the experts in recognizing new problems because they literally live with the problem. The important history will often come from the carer. The interview with the patient is much more likely to concentrate on level of severity rather than providing history. Many dementia patients will already have lack of **insight** in the early stages of the disease process and therefore will be unaware of problems and indeed resistant to the idea that there might be any problems (Fairbairn 1997).

The purpose in making any diagnosis is to inform the patient accurately about what is wrong with them, what can be done about it and what the future holds. In the UK first contact tends to be with general practitioners (GPs) and their **primary care** team colleagues, although this contact may often have been initiated by social services. The role of primary care in the initial assessment of dementia is seen as particularly problematic by carers (Audit Commission 2000). There is evidence that general practitioners tend not to recognize dementia until late and that even when they do recognize it they are slow to involve **secondary** specialist services or social services (Audit Commission 2000). It is regrettable that the over-75s' health check, a general health screening check to be undertaken by general practices, has not generally been used in primary care as this might have been an opportunity for routine screening of a vulnerable population group for cognitive impairment.

General practitioners should be able to differentiate between delirium and dementia. They should be aware that dementia is more than simply memory impairment and that people can present with behaviour problems or indeed basic difficulties with daily living. In making a diagnosis in general practice, a full history and physical examination will be necessary. This will assist in identifying potentially treatable causes of an apparent dementia or indeed possibly identifying superimposed delirium (see above).

Simple, remediable conditions such as hypertension will often only be picked up as part of routine examination. Routine investigations would probably include an **ECG**, chest X-ray and a number of blood investigations including full blood count and tests of liver, renal (kidney) and thyroid function. Clinical guidelines are now available to assist the primary care team in assessing and treating people with dementia (Eccles *et al.* 1998).

Referral to the specialist secondary services, mainly old age psychiatry, is to be encouraged. However, because of the high prevalence of dementia, most specialist old age psychiatry services find it impossible to make a comprehensive medical assessment of every case of dementia in the community. Therefore some filtering and prioritizing of cases needs to take place. Before specialist old age psychiatry services are involved alongside primary care and social services, there is likely to be at least one additional or complicating factor. Examples might be: the need for advice on **anti-dementia drugs**; some atypical element to the presentation, for example a relatively rapid deterioration; obvious **carer stress**; significant behaviour problems; the use of medical services as an introduction to later social care packages.

It is likely that the specialist service will make use of a variety of scales to assess the patient. For example, the severity and progression of memory loss might be assessed by the **Mini-mental State Examination MMSE** (Folstein *et al.* 1975), behaviour might be assessed by the MOUSEPAD (Allen *et al.* 1996), and activities of daily living might be assessed by the progressive deterioration scale (DeJong *et al.* 1989). However, a word of caution about all scales. They should only be used in the context of the total picture and they are not diagnostic in their own right.

The routine use of brain scanning remains controversial. It is reasonable to say that an American audience might well expect routine CT scanning but British old age psychiatry services have always been cautious over making such a routine recommendation. Perhaps the middle route is that CT scanning should be available to the clinician but that each case should be considered on its individual merits.

Even with all the comprehensive detailed investigations that are now possible, including brain scanning, there can still be diagnostic uncertainty. In these circumstances it may be necessary to review in six months to a year and again observe for potential deterioration. Living with this uncertainty can be difficult for both the patient and the clinician but occasionally it is necessary.

Views about disclosing information about diagnosis have changed significantly in recent years. There is now an increasing expectation that people with dementia are entitled to know about their diagnosis. This is partially a cultural change but it is also reasonable to inform people of the diagnosis when there may be some potential to treat the disease – in this case with anti-Alzheimer medication (see section on AD above). Despite this, there is often family ambivalence about telling the person with dementia the diagnosis. As a result of this ambivalence the apparently simple process of 'telling' can often involve sensitive three-way negotiations between the professionals, the family and the person with dementia.

Accurate diagnosis is a prerequisite for appropriate treatment and care. Ideally medical diagnosis is part of a broad multidisciplinary **assessment** which forms the basis of ongoing care planning and provision (see Chapter 7).

ISSUES IN TREATMENT

Anti-dementia drugs

Recent licensing of anti-cholinesterase treatments such as donepezil and rivastigmine (see section on AD above) has increased the importance of accurate diagnosis of Alzheimer's disease in particular. When initiated these medications need to be monitored by an appropriate specialist (old age psychiatrist, geriatrician or neurologist) in order to review the efficacy of the drug. Assessing efficacy in a progressively deteriorating condition is particularly problematic as the index of success may not simply be improvement, nor indeed stabilization, but could be the slowing of deterioration. There are recommendations (Fairbairn 2000) that this type of medication should be reviewed after approximately three months when decisions about long-term treatment can be made. Recent guidelines issued by the National Institute for Clinical Excellence (NICE 2001) have substantially confirmed these views in relation to three anticholinesterase drugs. However, often three months can be a rather short length of time in which to gauge the value of the treatment. There is evidence now accumulating that 50–60 per cent of patients are continuing on anti-Alzheimer medication after the three months when original predictions were that only a third were likely to remain on medication beyond this time. There is no clear view on when long-term medication should be stopped, although 'drug holidays' have been described as potentially useful. If there has been any value in the medication, drug holidays should allow the clinician to observe the deterioration in mental state upon cessation of medication. It is reported that the mental state generally recovers once the medication is started again. Although originally licensed for Alzheimer's disease it is likely that these anti-cholinesterase drugs will have a role in the therapy of dementia with Lewy bodies.

The management of non-cognitive problems

There is a tendency to concentrate on the memory problems of dementia. Yet men are reportedly more likely to present with behaviour problems rather than memory difficulties. Carers and care staff will often report that they find non-cognitive aspects of dementia the most difficult and frustrating to manage (Levin 1997). These non-cognitive features might include psychotic phenomena such as delusions or hallucinations. Non-cognitive problems might also involve significant personality change, which can be a complete change of personality and not simply exaggeration of previous personality features. For example, dynamic individuals can become slothful and apathetic and, paradoxically, some difficult and aggressive individuals can become easier to live with. In other cases, easygoing individuals can become awkward. Other non-cognitive problems are persistent wandering, which can be deemed to be purposeful or purposeless, and sexually inappropriate behaviour.

In all these examples of non-cognitive difficulties, it may be legitimate to consider the use of medication. However, it needs to be emphasized that non-medical management must be the first line. Skilled non-medical management will inevitably involve the education and training of carers and care staff.

The use of medication in behaviour management is a controversial area. On the one hand there are concerns that doctors inappropriately use anti-psychotic medication to act as a chemical straightjacket to control people with dementia who are behaviourally disturbed. On the other hand, judiciously reviewed prescriptions of anti-psychotic medication may allow individuals to be supported in a particular setting, such as their own home, for longer than might otherwise have been the case. For example, nocturnal wandering can be particularly wearing for carers. In such cases it would not seem inappropriate to use judicious prescription of hypnotic medication for the person with dementia to allow the carer to get a good night's sleep.

Modern anti-psychotics are tolerated much better than the older anti-psychotics, with less likelihood of side effects and sedation. Therefore, increasingly old age psychiatry services are using drugs such as risperidone rather than older drugs such as haloperidol when it is felt that medication is necessary. Of course, it is most important to register that anti-psychotic medication should not be used to compensate for inadequate nurse staffing or poor quality of care.

Symptoms of anxiety and depression are common in the early stages of dementia and are often highly amenable to treatment with anti-depressants. Once again, the more modern anti-depressants (selective serotonin reuptake inhibitors (SSRIs) such as paroxetine) are better tolerated, with lower side effects than older drugs (tricyclics such as amitriptyline).

The diagnosis of dementia inevitably creates problems in relation to informed **consent** for any treatment intervention, be it psychiatric or physical (see Chapter 13). Nevertheless, there should be a constant professional duty to optimize both the mental and physical health of people with dementia.

The management of coexisting medical problems

We noted above that people with dementia commonly have other medical conditions. They are therefore significant users of acute medical care. The problems of providing good care for people with dementia in acute hospital settings have been recognized and the specialist old age psychiatry team has an important liaison role with acute medical, geriatric and orthopaedic wards (Anderson and Philpott 1991). It is important to recognize that acute confusion, that is delirium, is a symptom of physical illness and therefore best assessed and managed in a medical rather than a psychiatric setting.

The future

Future generations will insist on accurate timely diagnosis, and differential diagnosis, of confusion. The diagnosis of a particular kind of dementia will need to be given directly to the patient as well as to the family. This will allow informed judgements, hopefully at a reasonably early stage, about life choices and so allow individuals to put their affairs in order. It could be envisaged that, as part of a comprehensive diagnostic, treatment and care package, the person with dementia and their family would be able to be involved in comprehensive and appropriate educational programmes. These might operate along similar lines to other 'life change' programmes such as the parenthood classes associated with antenatal care.

Traditionally specialist old age psychiatry services have undertaken the first contact visit at the patient's home. This allows an initial diagnosis to be made and information about social circumstances to be acquired without major intrusion. Also, in familiar surroundings people with dementia can be expected to reveal themselves at their best. That said, changes are under way that may lead to a different approach in future. The requirements for early and accurate diagnosis and the need to keep complex drug therapies under constant review may well lead to increasing use of 'memory clinics' where people attend as outpatients for diagnosis and review. It is unlikely that there will be a single service model for assessment and review. It may well be that periodic hospital contact for a medically orientated review will take place in conjunction with a community-orientated service where other professionals maintain regular contacts to support people with dementia and their carers.

FURTHER READING

Harvey, R.J., Fox, N.C. and Rossbor, M.N. (1999) *Dementia Handbook*. London: Martin Dunitz. A straightforward, up-to-date guide to the investigation of suspected dementia with practical advice about the management of different subtypes and of behavioural problems.

Howard, R. (1999) *Everything You Need to Know about Old Age Psychiatry*. London: Wrightson. A review of old age psychiatry as currently practised in the UK, including detailed information about the common forms of dementia, risk factors and approaches to treatment.

Maurer, K., Volk, S. and Gerbaldo, H. (1997) Auguste D. and Alzheimer's disease, *Lancet*, 349:1546–9. A fascinating account of the first reported case of Alzheimer's disease.

2   **CHRISTINA MACIEJEWSKI**

Psychological perspectives

KEY POINTS

- The psychological perspective on dementia has undergone a radical shift in emphasis and approach over the last 20 years.
- The concept of personhood and the accompanying theory of dementia have had a profound influence on the psychological perspective of dementia.
- Personhood has provided us with a philosophical base against which we can assess our current work and around which future therapeutic approaches can be developed.
- The key challenge for the future is communication: to communicate the value of psychological perspectives in dementia care, but above all to communicate with people with dementia.

INTRODUCTION

In common with many other approaches the psychological perspective on dementia has undergone a radical shift in emphasis and approach over the last 20 years. The shift in culture proposed by Kitwood (1993) is as relevant to psychology as to any other discipline. Psychological approaches to therapy are undergoing a shift away from an emphasis on the problem of dementia and a focus on behaviour that must be managed, and wherever possible normalized. They are moving towards acceptance of the person with dementia as, first and foremost, an individual person who has the same needs as any other human being. The key task is to seek to understand the person with dementia and to respect his or her individuality. Where there are difficulties and fears the task is to help identify the problems and to work with the person with dementia, his or her family and other caregivers to find solutions which are acceptable to them.

Dementia is multi-factorial and there are many possible perspectives one can adopt to seek to understand the condition and how it affects individuals and those who care for them. This chapter will describe a number of conceptual frameworks that have been developed by psychologists to aid our understanding of dementia, and will outline the therapeutic approaches based on them. Many of the therapeutic approaches described can be used by all who work with people with dementia. In addition, this chapter will also outline some of the specialist approaches that require training in clinical psychology. The value in these various perspectives lies in the different contributions that they make to the understanding of dementia. The challenge for clinical psychology lies in developing appropriate assessments, formulations and interventions which draw on the varied perspectives, and in promoting their use in combination as well as individually to assist the person with dementia.

THE NEUROPSYCHOLOGICAL PERSPECTIVE

Historically, psychologists working with people with dementia were not concerned with delineating the various problems that those people might have. The major emphasis was in terms of aiding the diagnosis and dementia was seen as total brain failure. Research papers characteristically referred to samples of 'dements' and no attempt was made to differentiate between individuals. However, just as in other areas, neuropsychologists have begun to study the different patterns of deficits that people can present with, and to relate these to theories of cognitive function and to the physical changes occurring in the brain (see Chapter 1 for description of brain structure and functioning). For detailed consideration of this work see for example Miller and Morris (1993), Morris (1996), and Butters *et al.* (1997). We can develop a better understanding of the person with dementia if we have an understanding of the nature of his or her cognitive difficulties.

Memory

Dementia is characteristically seen as affecting a person's memory. In Alzheimer's disease it is common for the temporal lobes and the subcortical structures which lie below to be affected. Neuropsychologists tend to conceptualize memory in terms of two components: short-term memory and long-term memory. Short-term memory has a very short duration and then the new information is coded and entered into long-term memory. It is also common to distinguish episodic memory (memory for events) from semantic memory (knowledge about the world, meaning and facts). The principal memory deficit in Alzheimer's disease is thought to be an inability to store new information. It is difficult for people who are affected by Alzheimer's disease to add any new information into long-term memory and new information which is stored is also more likely to be lost more quickly. The normal pattern is for the short-term memory to be affected first and then longer term memory. In dementia episodic memory is impaired as a consequence of this difficulty in retaining new information (Morris and McKiernan 1994). Clinical psychologists seek to describe the deficit and then to quantify the degree of deficit. They will typically use a range of assessment materials that employ different measures of memory, for instance by using recognition as well as recall tasks and by introducing a delay between the presentation of the material and the testing. However, as Morris (1996) stresses, the problems with memory seen in a person with dementia should not be considered in isolation and can be composed of problems with language and with meaning of words. In addition to this, new information may not be registered because of difficulties in attention and concentration rather than a 'pure' memory difficulty.

An understanding of the neuropsychology of memory can contribute to therapeutic work. For example, simple external aids such as the use of calendars and reality orientation boards are well-recognized tools to help those with a memory problem. More sophisticated individualized memory training (Backman 1992) and use of modern technology such as pagers is still very much in its infancy and is an exciting area of development.

Language

Language function involves the temporal and frontal areas of the dominant hemisphere of the brain, which for most people is the left hemisphere. As with many other aspects of dementia, specific language disorders in relation to dementia have only been studied closely in recent years. Skelton-Robinson and Jones (1984) have reviewed a number of studies which indicate that patients with various degrees of dementia show significantly greater expressive difficulties than age-matched controls. Expressive problems, especially in naming, can be detected at an early stage of the illness. In comparison, receptive problems are more likely to occur at a later stage. By assessing expressive language the clinical psychologist can determine the extent of a person's difficulties and also suggest ways to minimize the difficulties. For example, if a person is repeatedly frustrated by not being able to come up with the names of objects they can be encouraged to use circumlocution if friends and family understand that this is a useful strategy. It can also help carers to understand that problems like perseveration, where the person 'gets stuck' on a word or phrase, are a result of damage to the frontal lobes of the brain and are not within the control of the person with dementia.

Perception

An area of cognitive function that is not considered as frequently as that of memory and language is perception, that is how the brain interprets messages from our senses. However, difficulties in perceptual abilities can have dramatic consequences. Damage to the right parietal lobe and its connections is associated with difficulties in visual perceptual abilities. This kind of damage can be seen in people with Alzheimer's disease and is also sometimes a feature of a vascular dementia. Many screening instruments include a component that examines perceptual abilities. For example the Middlesex Elderly Assessment of Mental State (MEAMS) (Golding 1991) includes a test where the person has to identify a series of letters of the alphabet which appear incomplete and also a series of photographs taken from unusual angles. If the clinical psychologist suspects a problem in this area, they will consider using more detailed testing, for example the Visual Object and Space Perception Battery (VOSP) (Warrington and James 1991). This includes a range of assessments that look at basic perception, for example discriminating a figure from its background, before proceeding to more integrated perceptual tasks such as identifying a photograph of an object taken from an unusual view. As with all neuropsychological assessments, the value of detecting a perceptual problem lies in the potential for identifying solutions. In some cases this will involve advice to the carer, for example to turn round the plate of a person who has a limited visual field, and in others it will involve modifications to the environment.

Motivation and planning

Some dementias particularly affect the frontal lobes of the brain. These are described in Chapter 1. The best researched of these conditions is **Pick's disease**. However, there are other conditions, such as frontal–temporal dementias, which can present with a pattern of frontal impairment. In addition a vascular dementia and Alzheimer's disease can be characterized by damage to the frontal lobes.

Some people with frontal damage have difficulty planning and organizing their lives. The clinical psychologist will assess this using paper and pencil tests or the newly developed computerized tests such as the Cambridge Neuropsychological Test Automated Battery (CANTAB) (Robbins et al. 1994). Examples of tests include asking a person to think of as many items as they can from within a specific category in a limited amount of time or asking them to rearrange a series of pictures so that they tell a story.

Sometimes the person with dementia will appear to get stuck on a particular idea or response and will perseverate. This can be formally assessed by asking the person to follow a particular rule which requires them to change their response under certain conditions. The person with a perseverative difficulty will continue to respond in the same way while, very often, being able to tell you verbally the correct details of the rule they are meant to be following.

The neuropsychological assessment

In many cases a person with a suspected dementia will be referred to a clinical psychologist for a neuropsychological assessment. This is routine practice in the majority of memory clinics and the information obtained from the assessment is used to aid in the differential diagnosis of dementia and to help distinguish between, for example, depression and dementia. In some cases a more detailed assessment will be required and a referral may be made to a specialist neuropsychologist.

The main purpose of the neuropsychological assessment is to build up a comprehensive picture of the person's cognitive strengths and weaknesses, and ascertain whether there has been any deterioration in these. Often the clinical psychologist will try to obtain an estimate of a person's previous level of cognitive functioning to see if any change has occurred. Estimates of intellectual functioning based on a person's employment history are particularly unreliable for the current cohort of older people. They did not have the same opportunities for education as are available today, and they were sometimes prevented from pursuing education or gaining employment because of the need to support other family members or because of the disruption of the Second World War. Employment history is also of little value for a female cohort who often stayed at home to care for their family. However, there is an alternative means available in the form of the National Adult Reading Test (NART)(Nelson 1982). The test requires the person to read a list of 50 words which it is not possible to pronounce correctly without knowledge of the word (e.g. chord, syncope). Nelson found that the results of this test correlated very well with a person's intelligence level. O'Caroll *et al.* (1987) **validated** the test longitudinally with a group of people affected by dementia and found no decline in performance on the NART over a year compared with a significant decline on other tests of neuropsychological functioning. Therefore, at least in the early stages of the illness, the NART can be used as a predictor of **pre-morbid** intelligence levels. Obviously the test cannot be used with people who have language problems to the extent that they are no longer able to read or for those whose first language is not English.

Having obtained an estimate of level of pre-morbid functioning, the clinical psychologist will then proceed to carry out a screening of core areas of functioning, for example language, memory and perception. There are a number of screening assessments, such as the Mini-mental State Examination (Folstein *et al.* 1975), which assess a broad range of cognitive abilities. Normal adults would be expected to score in the 27–30 range out of a possible 30. However, older and poorly educated individuals often score below the cut-off of 23. Thus it can be difficult to determine whether a person has a difficulty on this test because of dementia or some other cause. The clinical psychologist is more likely to use a more detailed screening assessment such as the CAMCOG which is part of the Cambridge Mental Disorders of the Elderly Examination (CAMDEX)(Roth *et al.* 1986). This assessment covers all the key areas of cognitive functioning but in greater detail than brief screening tools. When

---

Case study 2.1 Using a neuropsychological assessment in practice

The daughter of a lady suffering with a vascular dementia reported that her mother was often incontinent and did not seem to recognize the toilet when taken to the bathroom. An assessment revealed that this lady had some difficulty distinguishing figure from ground and discriminating an object from its surroundings. Her problem was compounded by the fact that her daughter, with whom she lived, had a rather trendy purple bathroom suite. Thus it was difficult for the lady to recognize the function of the purple toilet and to discriminate the seat from the remainder of the toilet. Her daughter was advised to change the colour of the toilet seat to a white one so that this could easily be distinguished. This made a considerable improvement to the situation and the frequency of times that the lady failed to recognize the toilet decreased. Her daughter also reported that she felt she had a better understanding of her mother's difficulties.

---

completed it provides the clinical psychologist with a cognitive profile which can be compared with norms for the age group. A less demanding screening instrument which can be used with people who have difficulty concentrating for any length of time is the MEAMS (Golding 1991). It may be more appropriate for the clinical psychologist to use the Wechsler Adult Intelligence Scale – Revised (WAIS – R) (Wechsler 1982), or the newly developed WAIS III, as a screening tool for a younger person with suspected dementia as this has a wide range of age-specific norms.

Following on from this initial screening, if there are identified areas of difficulty or uncertainty the clinical psychologist may carry out further more detailed assessment. This may involve assessments of memory, expressive and receptive language, visual perception, orientation, ability to carry out action, and ability to plan and organize. Once the assessment is complete it can aid in the diagnosis and can also form the basis for a therapeutic programme aimed at maximizing the person's potential. It is also common for an assessment to be carried out as a baseline against which future assessments can be compared. This is particularly useful where there is initial uncertainty about the diagnosis and where repeated testing over time is required in order to identify a pattern of deterioration in certain areas of cognitive functioning. Repeated assessment is also becoming particularly relevant to assess the benefits of the cognitive enhancing drugs such as donepezil. Case Study 2.1 demonstrates how a neuropsychological assessment might be used in practice.

THE BEHAVIOURAL PERSPECTIVE

One of the commonest reasons that a clinical psychologist may be asked to see or advise about a person with dementia is because the person is described as having a behaviour problem or **challenging behaviour**. In such cases the clinical psychologist may use a behavioural perspective to consider how a person with dementia responds to others and to their environment. Such a perspective considers any behaviour to be a response to stimuli in the environment and considers whether the behaviour is reinforced and, therefore, likely to increase in frequency. Positive reinforcement describes the situation where a behaviour occurs more frequently because it is followed by positive consequences (for example, a person gets attention when they call out). Negative reinforcement describes the situation where the frequency of a behaviour increases because it is followed by the omission of an anticipated aversive event (e.g. if a child cries the food it does not like will be taken away). An initial difficulty may be encountered in ascertaining details of the nature of the behaviour and for whom it is a problem. Stokes (1996) suggests a tripartite model of assessment of challenging behaviour. This starts with the presenting problem, such as 'aggression', and then attempts to draw up an **operational definition**. For example, in a residential home this may involve staff in describing episodes of a person's behaviour that they have considered 'aggressive' and then coming to a consensus about a description of the behaviour. This in turn is used to draw up a list of the behaviour characteristics, such as shouting at other residents, which define the behaviour and descriptions of behaviours that can be observed. This will then form the basis for an assessment of the problem using direct observations, wherever possible, and including recording of what was happening before the behaviour took place, what behaviour characteristics were observed, and what happened immediately afterwards.

It is important to remember that any behaviour needs to be seen as an interaction between the neuropathological changes of dementia, how this impacts on the person and their **personality** and life history, and the environment in which they find themselves. Stokes (1996: 608) argues that 'environmental and psychological factors do not cause dementia, but they provide explanations for the individual behaviour consequences of the presumptive disease'. Similarly Kitwood (1990) reminds us of the power of **malignant social psychology** where it can come to be assumed that challenging behaviour is solely resultant from neuropathological changes.

Therapeutic approaches

Therapeutic approaches based on a behavioural perspective consider how behaviour can be modified. Typically this involves close observation of the behaviour, and what happened immediately before and after it, in order to undertake a functional analysis. Stokes (1986a, b, 1987a, b) applies this to the sometimes-challenging behaviour of people with dementia. He includes in his analysis consideration of other background factors such as whether the behaviour pattern fits in with a person's previous occupation: for example, the person who repeatedly piles furniture in the middle of the room may have been a furniture remover or have worked assembling large structures. This work has been extended by Moniz-Cook (1999) who considers how any challenging behaviour can be seen as an interaction between the person's physical environment, their

---

Case Study 2.2 Using a behavioural perspective in practice

Miss M. had recently been admitted to the residential home. Little was known about her other than that she had previously lived alone in a flat and had shown increasing levels of self-neglect as her dementia progressed. She had been admitted to the home because she was considered to be at **risk** in the community. Miss M. had some insight into this and staff reported that she had told them that she felt safe in the home. However, they were concerned by her frequent urinary and faecal incontinence. This happened despite the fact that she had an en-suite toilet in her room. She was beginning to be labelled as 'difficult' by the staff and some of the other residents found her incontinence distressing.

The staff were asked to keep detailed records of episodes of incontinence for a one-week period, recording wherever possible what had happened prior to the incontinence and the consequences. This recording revealed that Miss M. was not using the toilet in her room. She would sometimes wander out into the corridor or leave the dayroom and go towards her room but frequently failed to find the toilet. She never asked staff to direct her to a toilet. Her only relative, a niece, reported that her family had always considered Miss M. a very private and retiring lady. When in her room staff observed that Miss M. would sometimes open the door to her toilet and appeared surprised and pleased that she found a toilet in the 'cupboard'.

Thus it became clear that Miss M.'s difficulties appeared not to be related to an incontinence problem *per se* but were more likely to be due to difficulties in finding and identifying appropriate toilets and a reluctance to ask others to direct her to them.

The intervention involved a number of modifications to the environment. It was noticed that although all the toilets were labelled, the signs were above the toilet doors, and as Miss M. was a little over four feet tall she probably could not see the signs. All toilets in the home were labelled with clearer signs on the doors at eye level. This included the en-suite in Miss M.'s room. In addition, some towels and bathroom fixtures from Miss M.'s flat were brought into her toilet to aid her recognition of this as her bathroom. Staff began gently prompting her to use the toilet after meals and at regular intervals throughout the day. Monitoring of the frequency of episodes of incontinence over the following weeks revealed a marked drop in instances of incontinence.

---

social environment, and both physical and psychological aspects of their self. Thus when a person repeatedly calls out for help this may be an interaction of their need for security with an environment in which their room door is closed. Another person's calls may be a result of totally different interactions. Case Study 2.2 describes the application of a behavioural approach.

THE COGNITIVE BEHAVIOURAL PERSPECTIVE

Cognitive behaviour therapy is a well-recognized therapy which was originally developed to help people who were suffering from depression (Beck 1976; Beck *et al.* 1979) and was later expanded to cover other difficulties such as anxiety. The application to people suffering from depression is based on the theoretical perspective that depression is the result of the interaction of behaviour, cognitions, emotions and physiological factors. It has been identified that when people are suffering from depression they tend to think the worst of any situation and express a range of negative thoughts. For example, when friends do not acknowledge them when crossing the street they assume that the friends are ignoring them rather than that they did not see them. Depression is manifested as a continuous feedback loop of negative thoughts that result in negative moods and behaviours. These in turn feed back to create more negative thoughts. Cognitive behavioural therapy aims to provide sufferers of depression with strategies to identify and challenge their negative thought patterns and to motivate them to perform activities in order to increase their positive mood. The underlying principle is that people with depression can learn to evaluate and test their own hypotheses about any situation, such as friends who ignore them, and then learn that they can make a significant contribution to their own outcomes and subsequent mood (Beck *et al.* 1979).

Therapeutic approaches

Working with people with dementia

Gallagher-Thompson and Thompson (1992) have expanded the cognitive behavioural perspective to work with older people. They recommend some simple alterations to the therapeutic method to assist older adults. These include the need to consider that the current cohort of older adults may not have experienced any form of **psychotherapy** before and may equate the need for therapy as a sign that they are 'going mad' and consequently may be very fearful. The use of cognitive therapy has only just begun to extend to work including older people in the early stages of dementia. Teri and Gallagher-Thompson (1991) describe a cognitive approach to treat depression in people with a mild dementia coupled with a more behavioural emphasis to an approach for those with moderate and severe dementia. There is considerable scope for the use of these techniques in work with people who have a depressive illness secondary to a dementia and also to help the person with dementia adjust to the changing world in which they find themselves. Many of the practical modifications suggested for older people will apply equally to those with dementia. For example Dick *et al.* (1996) describe the use of notebooks for the client to record homework to be undertaken between sessions, and the provision of a work book and therapy notes to facilitate memory of what has happened in an individual session. They also advocate a slower approach to therapy in which the client is encouraged to summarize what has been covered and suggest that audio and video tapes can be used to enable clients to maximize their understanding and memory of sessional material.

Working with carers

A cognitive behavioural approach has also proved to be of value in both individual and group work with carers of people with dementia. It is well recognized that care giving is associated with stresses to family carers and can lead to depression and other mental health difficulties (see Zarit and Edwards 1996). DeVries and Gallagher-Thompson (1993) describe a group treatment approach for anger in caregivers that uses a cognitive approach focusing on identifying negative thoughts and challenging and replacing them with more adaptive cognitions accompanied by relaxation and assertion training strategies. It is also common for a cognitive behavioural perspective to be used in helping carers understand the behaviour of the person they are caring for. An example would be helping a carer understand that when the person with dementia appears not to recognize them at some times but does so at others this is not because they are 'being awkward'. It would encourage carers to seek out alternative explanations and to reframe the behaviour.

THE PSYCHODYNAMIC PERSPECTIVE

As there are a number of different schools of **psychodynamic** psychotherapy an introduction to the key theoretical stances and therapeutic methods is beyond the scope of this chapter. However, a very readable introduction is provided in Nelson-Jones (1982). Freud (1924) considered that psychodynamic psychotherapy was inappropriate for older people and hence this area of psychotherapy was neglected for some time. It was assumed that older people did not possess the prerequisites for dynamic therapy. These were considered to be a high level of cognitive resources, psychological sophistication, a capacity for introspection and the ability to develop a therapeutic alliance (Cath 1982). This has been challenged by a number of therapists who have worked successfully with older people and the work is beginning to be extended to include people who have dementia. Hausman (1992) suggests that the aims of psychotherapy can be met in many cases of a person with dementia. She argues that the key components of establishing a relationship in which the person feels cared about and has an emotional outlet can almost always be met to some extent, and that their self-esteem is enhanced. Diminution of verbal communication skills can make it difficult to work psychotherapeutically with people with dementia. The most difficult challenge is that of the development of insight in the person with dementia. Hausman suggests that it is impossible to know whether or not insight has actually taken place when the patient can no longer verbalize. Cheston and Bender (1999) argue that insight should not be seen as something that the person with dementia either has or does not have. Both insight and denial should be seen as **coping** mechanisms that are used in relation to the level of support in the environment around the person and his or her own personal resources.

Case study 2.3 Using a psychodynamic perspective in practice

Miss L. was referred to a psychology service for help in coping with her dementia. She had recently been diagnosed as suffering from a vascular dementia and depression. An aspect of the illness which was particularly distressing for her was that she was experiencing visual hallucinations. The psychologist was asked to become involved with Miss L. after she had had a disagreement with her social worker who felt that Miss L. had become too dependent on her. After a number of sessions Miss L. began to talk to the psychologist about the difference between her world and that of the social worker. She could not understand the latter, did not wish to, and was very angry that she was being asked to. She recounted to the psychologist the 'rules' of her world, which centred on her life as a senior teacher and the respect she had enjoyed from fellow staff and pupils. She had had no private life as such and now had few friends. Following this the psychologist was able to explore with her the difficulties with her social worker. She perceived this woman as her friend and found it difficult to accept the role of the social worker. There was clearly a conflict between her world and that of the social worker and the health care system. This had resulted in misunderstandings and misinterpretations. Miss L. was also expressing her anger at her illness by directing it at the social worker. She did not wish to accept the world of the social worker because she did not wish to accept her illness. By accepting her illness she felt threatened and isolated from all previous coping mechanisms.

Together, the psychologist and Miss L. were able to explore the difference between the two worlds and also to consider the difference between her old understood world of teacher and her new frightening world of 'person with dementia'. There was considerable opportunity for both transference of emotions from Miss L. to the therapist and countertransference from the therapist to Miss L. as Miss L. expressed her desperation and fear of failure and the psychologist in turn felt that she might not be able to help her.

Therapeutic approaches

Direct therapeutic work with people with dementia is often concerned with the secondary problems of anxiety and depression. The work is aimed at helping the person with dementia examine his or her coping skills and reflect on the process of their illness. In many cases it is also concerned with grieving over losses, either directly through the illness or as a consequence of other losses throughout life.

Cheston and Bender (1999) consider the potential for exploratory psycho-therapy with people with dementia where the therapist's aim is to help the person with dementia explore what is happening to him or her and gain their own understanding. They suggest that this approach needs to provide an environment in which the person with dementia can grieve for their losses and accept the pain of these losses.

Sutton and Cheston (1997) emphasize what can be achieved by listening to a person with dementia tell his or her story. They believe that by providing opportunities for people with dementia to tell their stories and to be listened to in psychotherapy, they are providing them with an opportunity to make sense of the world in which they live, and to grieve the losses they have suffered. Through the stories that people with dementia tell can be seen echoes of losses and threats that they have experienced in the past. Thus, psychotherapy can be seen as a way of helping the person with dementia have an understanding of the present and explore it using his or her previous life experiences. Sutton and Cheston (1997) also highlight the fact that the stories told often include reference to previously valued **roles** within society such as a teacher or a nurse. This emphasizes the importance to us of our identity and the contrast there may be for the person with dementia between their previously valued and respected identity and their new identity of a 'patient' who has to be 'cared for' and is 'dependent on others'. Many of the issues raised by Sutton and Cheston are featured in Case Study 2.3.

Kaplan (1990) suggests that one of the reasons why therapists find it hard to work with people with dementia, and sometimes seek to ignore what they say, is that the issues raised link too closely to the therapist's own unresolved fears about the potential for the illness to affect them.

THE SYSTEMIC PERSPECTIVE

One way of thinking about any perceived problem is to consider its relation to the wider family, organization or **system** of care, rather than relating it solely to any one individual such as the identified person with dementia. Within psychology there are a number of different schools of family or **systems therapy** (see for example Minuchin 1974; Bowen 1978; Selvini Palazzoli *et al.* 1978). Historically the main concern of psychologists who work systemically has been with problems presented by younger families where the identified person with the problem is often a child within the family. Older people have been included in the systemic perspective in their roles as grandparents who are sometimes involved in childcare. In comparison with the work with children there has been relatively little work with families where the older person is the identified person with the problem. However, it has been recognized that a systemic perspective can be very useful in work with families with older members (Walsh 1982; Neidhardt and Allen 1993). Most family therapy teams working with older adults do not restrict themselves to one school of therapy but instead draw from earlier work and employ a variety of techniques. Zarit and Zarit (1983) aim by their family meetings to bring the family's level of information up to that of the primary supporter, identifying the primary supporter's greatest needs and problem solving with the family to recruit more support if necessary.

Many of the methodologies used with younger families transfer directly to work involving older people, in particular the concepts of roles within the family and transitions. However, with an older family we may be talking of changes in role such as the transition from employment to retirement rather than the changes when an adolescent leaves home. There are additional issues to consider when working with older people. This kind of therapy may be quite alien to the older person, and thus a clear explanation of what is involved and what the older person can expect to happen as a result of therapy is needed. Traditional family therapists work using a two-way mirror where the therapist sits with the family on one side of the screen and consults with other members of the therapy team who observe the interactions from behind the screen. Thus the therapist does not work alone but as part of the team often tailoring interventions on the basis of the observations of those behind the screen. It may be impossible for some older people to get to therapy sessions and the therapist may have to travel to them. This requires modifications to the process with the therapist working alone or perhaps with one other co-worker. However, there are also additional benefits in seeing the older person in his or her own environment with other family members.

Family therapy and dementia

There are a number of issues to be considered when family therapy involves an older person with dementia and Roper-Hall (1987) discusses some of the potential difficulties. One of the major concerns for therapists and for other family members is often the desire to protect the person with dementia. Thus other family members may be unwilling to talk in front of the person about the difficulties caused by the illness. Alternatively, the therapist may be fearful that an angry family will direct their anger on to the person with dementia and scapegoat them for all the difficulties involved. In such a situation the therapist might then find him or herself seeking to protect the person with dementia and hence abandoning the principle of neutrality in which the therapist should not be seen as allied to any one family member. Others would argue that very often what will be discussed by the family are the issues arising out of the dementia and therefore the person who has the illness has a right to be part of the discussions. There is no clear answer as to whether the person should be involved. However, perhaps the question should be framed in terms of examining the justification for not involving the person. Benbow et al. (1993) reported on a study that examined the content and techniques employed in family therapy sessions involving older people. In 16 of the families the identified client suffered from a dementia and in the remaining 17 families the identified client had some other mental health problem. They found that the techniques used and the content of the sessions was very similar between the two groups. The only differences were that more time was spent discussing issues of forgetfulness in the dementia group and there were also fewer issues concerning changes in the amount of time spent together in this group. Case Study 2.4 is an example of family therapy involving someone with dementia.

Case study 2.4   Using a systemic perspective in practice

Mrs W. was a 75-year-old lady who was diagnosed as suffering from vascular dementia. She had considerable insight into her condition and was particularly concerned that she should not be a burden on her two daughters. Both daughters were worried about their mother but disagreed as to what was the best way forward. It was decided that it would be helpful to convene a family meeting and Mrs W. was asked to invite anyone she considered important in helping her. She invited her two daughters and her next door neighbour. During the course of the family session led by a social worker trained in family therapy a genogram was constructed. A genogram, or family map, provides a graphic summary of a family's current composition and relationships. This showed clearly that the key people within the family were female. Mrs W.'s husband had died when her two daughters were quite small and she had brought them up single-handed. Both daughters admired her considerably. One daughter was married with three children and the other was unmarried with one child. This second daughter still relied heavily on her mother, for example regularly asking her to mind her daughter. Mrs W. did not invite her son-in-law to this meeting, as she did not consider that it was his role to help her and she did not wish him to be involved. By questioning each member of the family in turn the therapist was able to ascertain that there was a close bond between Mrs W. and her two daughters. The bond between the two daughters was not as strong as those with the mother. The elder daughter felt responsible for her younger unmarried sister. The younger daughter in turn looked to her mother for support. During the session the three women and Mrs W.'s neighbour were able to talk about their concerns about her illness. It emerged that the younger daughter wanted her mother to be cared for and thought that this would best be achieved if she went into residential care. However, she was still very confused by the diagnosis and, for example, could not understand why her mother found it difficult, and was worried about, caring for her granddaughter. This daughter was able to say that she knew that her elder sister and her mother felt that Mrs W. should remain at home for as long as possible. However, she felt that this would put undue stress on her elder sister. This sister in turn identified that she was fearful of putting stress on her younger sister. The session concluded with all present agreeing that no major decisions had to be made yet. Mrs W.'s neighbour and her elder daughter agreed to communicate regularly so that the daughters could be alerted to any concerns that the neighbour had. Mrs W. was happy with this as it fitted with her schema of not wishing to burden anyone. Her younger daughter agreed not to ask Mrs W. to look after her young daughter for her but instead to bring her to visit each week. This would be arranged including the elder daughter so that she knew she did not have to visit on that day. It was agreed that further sessions could be convened at the request of any of those present.

Systemic interventions in care organizations

It can also be of great value to consider a systemic perspective when examining the impact of dementia on an organization or system of care. For example, when working with staff in a residential home it can be of considerable value to work with the whole staff group and consider their relationships with an individual client. Thus one carer may have a positive relationship with the client and not be aware of any difficulties while another carer may be frightened by that client's aggressive behaviour. Consideration of the whole system may reveal that the behaviour only occurs when the client is asked to bathe. Staff may then be encouraged to work systemically and think what it must feel like to be the client and may then come up with alternative strategies for handling difficult self-care tasks. Similarly a systemic perspective can be of value if considering change within an organization. For example, Garland (1996) refers to the concept of 'working myths' within a residential home or care setting which are a set of assumptions by staff about the residents of the home and the care practices employed. Work with the staff may involve exploration of these 'myths' to examine which are useful for the work of the home and which serve to prevent change and **person-centred** care.

PERSONHOOD AND DEMENTIA CARE

The concept of **personhood** and the accompanying theory of dementia care as developed by Kitwood (1990, 1993, 1996) have had a profound influence on the psychological perspective of dementia. As Kitwood (1996) explains, the history of psychological approaches, as of those of other specialties, had tended to focus on the individual and to consider that person from the perspective of their cognitive deficits. While many psychologists strove to value the person with dementia as an individual with unique rights and needs, the study of dementia lacked an overarching theoretical stance and philosophy.

Kitwood (1996) has presented us with a formulation of dementia (D) as having five key factors as exemplified by the equation

$$D = P + B + H + NI + SP$$

where P stands for the person's personality or resources for action, B their biography, H their physical health, NI the neurological impairment and SP the **social psychology** that surrounds the person with dementia from day to day. Thus, Kitwood argues that the experience of dementia is unique to the individual and will depend on the interaction of the various components as depicted in the equation. Whereas, at one time, the neurological impairment (NI) was seen as the most important influence on the dementing process Kitwood considers it as but one component. Kitwood (1993) also considers the importance of the social psychology of the environment with which the person with dementia interacts. That environment can promote interactions that either maintain or destroy the personhood of the individual. Kitwood introduces the concept of 'malignant social psychology' to refer to an environment of care which would serve to disempower, invalidate and devalue the person with dementia. He stresses that this does not imply malice on behalf of the care workers but rather that they were working in a culture of dementia care which served to create an environment which destroyed the personhood of the person with dementia. In contrast, Kitwood and Benson (1995) describe 'a new culture of care' which serves to promote the personhood of the person with dementia. In this new culture care involves caring for the needs of the whole person and recognizing that those who have dementia are equal members of the human race. A basis for this is a clear and accurate understanding of a person's abilities, tastes, interests, **values** and forms of spirituality. It also requires a willingness for carers to 'put themselves in the shoes' of the person with dementia and consider their perspective.

Cultural and ethnic diversity

A key element of maintaining the personhood of the person with dementia lies in respect for their cultural and ethnic origins. This needs to begin as early as their first assessment when dementia may only be suspected. The majority of neuropsychological tests do not have **normative** data for people from ethnic minorities, are not culturally appropriate and hence do not produce valid results. Lowenstein *et al.* (1994) discuss the cross-cultural issues involved in neuropsychological assessment. Similarly, there are dangers in adopting what may be very inaccurate cultural stereotypes for the person with dementia and those providing care for him or her. As with any family there will need to be a careful assessment of need taking into account both the needs of the person with dementia and his or her carer. Efforts to maintain the personhood of the individual should then be directed at providing culturally appropriate and acceptable support.

Psychological therapies that promote personhood

In Chapter 10 of this book Brooker provides an extensive review of the various psychological 'therapeutic approaches' which have been used with people with dementia. Here we examine three approaches from the perspective of personhood and, more specifically, we assess how much these therapeutic approaches serve to maintain the personhood of people with dementia.

  Reality orientation (RO) therapy is clearly one therapy which can be used or abused. Within the classroom setting there is clearly scope for the development of a 'malignant social psychology' where the people with dementia are treated as distinct from the staff and are infantilized. Twenty-four-hour RO encourages interaction between staff and the person with dementia throughout the day. There is potential for this to encourage the development of a close relationship in which staff members come to know more about the person with dementia as a unique person. However, an over-simplistic interpretation of the therapy would limit interactions to the provision of orientating information and could once again serve to infantilize and stigmatize the person with dementia and discourage an appreciation of personhood.

Reminiscence therapy is widely used in hospitals and residential care settings to promote communication in people with dementia. Coleman (1986b) emphasized that there are individual differences in older people's attitudes to reminiscence and identified a subgroup of older people in his study who did not wish to reminisce. Thus, any reminiscence work with people with dementia needs to be very carefully planned in order first to gauge an individual's feelings about reminiscence and to ascertain if there are any painful topics from their life history which they may not wish to share in a group setting. With careful planning and an individualized approach much can be gained from reminiscence work with people with dementia. It can enable staff to find out more about the life of the person with dementia and to value that person as an individual. It can also help the person with dementia preserve their individuality and emphasize their self-worth.

On first inspection **validation therapy** as developed by Feil (1993) would appear to describe an approach which values the personhood of the person with dementia and recognizes their individuality. The central approach is to consider any communication from a person with dementia in terms of the feeling being communicated rather than the words used. Thus when a person with dementia says that they are looking for their mother and appears distressed the response would be aimed at acknowledging their distress rather than any attempt to address the reality of the fact that their mother died some years ago. However, there is little support for Feil's ideas that the person with dementia has unfinished business from earlier in their life and that he or she will progress through the four stages that Feil terms malorientation, time confusion, repetitive motion and vegetation. The suggestion that a carer can prevent deterioration by the use of validation is also without foundation and could be particularly damaging to a carer who finds him or herself caring for someone in the terminal stages of the illness. In addition the use of the term vegetation is far removed from respect for the personhood of the individual with advanced dementia.

The concept of personhood has provided us with a philosophical base against which we can assess our current work and around which future therapeutic approaches can be developed.

NEW CHALLENGES FOR PSYCHOLOGICAL PERSPECTIVES

From a psychological perspective there are a number of challenges in the field of dementia care. The most important challenge relates to truly respecting the personhood of people with dementia. One particular issue is communication with people with dementia (see Chapter 9) and the need to develop ways to ascertain their wishes and consent to psychological and other interventions. In practice psychologists have often operated on a principal of **beneficence**, doing what was considered best for the person with dementia at that time. This is no longer good enough.

On a therapeutic level working with individuals there are a number of exciting developments in psychological therapies for both younger and older people. The challenge is to integrate these approaches and modify them appropriately so that they can be used with people with dementia. These approaches need to be carefully researched, evaluated and communicated to others.

Psychology also has a role to play in developing environments and particularly in developing a social psychology that supports people with dementia and their carers. This role ranges from the experimental investigation of technological innovations for dementia care, to developing the philosophy of a home for life, and to campaigning politically for equal recognition of the needs of people with dementia and their carers alongside other citizens.

At the core of all these challenges is one key word: communication.

FURTHER READING

Butters, M.A., Salmon, D.P. and Butters, N. (1997) Neuropsychological assessment of dementia, in M. Storandt and G.R.VandenBos (eds) *Neuropsychological Assessment of Dementia and Depression in Older Adults: A Clinician's Guide*. Washington, DC: American Psychological Association. A detailed consideration of the neuropsychology of dementia.

Cheston, R. and Bender, M. (1999) *Understanding Dementia: The Man with the Worried Eyes*. London: Jessica Kingsley. Challenges the medical model of dementia and discusses psychotherapeutic work with people with dementia.

Neidhardt, E.R. and Allen, J.A. (1993) *Family Therapy with the Elderly*. Newbury Park, CA: Sage. Introduces family and systemic work with older people.

Woods, R.T. (ed.) (1996) *Handbook of the Psychology of Ageing*. Chichester: Wiley. For more information on therapeutic approaches, the neuropsychology of dementia and an introduction to the work of Kitwood.

Zarit, S.H. and Knight, B.G. (1996) *A Guide to Psychotherapy and Aging: Effective Clinical Interventions in a Life-stage Context*. Washington, DC: American Psychological Association. For consideration of the potential of psychotherapy for people with dementia and a discussion of ethical issues.

3

JOHN BOND

Sociological perspectives

KEY POINTS

- Sociology and biomedicine conceive dementia in very different ways.
- Sociological theory draws on a variety of philosophical and ideological perspectives.
- As a social phenomenon dementia can be understood within a range of sociological perspectives.
- The choice of perspective determines the way we view dementia and dementia care and our policy response to it.

INTRODUCTION

The purpose of this chapter is to introduce the reader to a number of sociological ideas and concepts and highlight their significance to our understanding of dementia and dementia care. The chapter will map the social theory that underpins these and locate and describe the sociological perspectives responsible for them.

We begin our overview of sociological perspectives and dementia by discussing three contrasting models for investigating dementia: the traditional biomedical model; a psychological model which focuses on the concept of personhood; and a social or sociological model which focuses on the meaning of the disease to the person with dementia.

PERSPECTIVES ON DEMENTIA

Biomedical model

The biomedical model is a product of the Enlightenment; an eighteenth-century movement based on notions of human progress through the application of reason and **rationality**. The Enlightenment philosophy created the belief that through science and technology all human life will be improved. The science and humanism of medicine is therefore perceived as largely beneficial and progressive in understanding and responding to illness and disease. The biomedical model is based on six assumptions. First, that mind and body can be treated separately. Second, that the body is rather like a machine and can be repaired when it breaks down, although biomedicine has not yet perfected techniques for every breakdown. Third, by implication medicine should develop a technological solution for everything, even when other responses might be more appropriate. Fourth, biomedicine is **reductionist**, explaining disease in biological terms while ignoring psychological and social factors. Fifth, it is assumed that every disease has a specific aetiology (cause). Finally, biomedicine claims to be an objective science and therefore medicine is the only valid perspective for understanding disease and illness (Atkinson 1988; Nettleton 1995).

A key feature of the biomedical approach is the way in which disease is seen as the loss of 'normality'. From a biomedical perspective dementia and the impact of the condition on family caregivers can be best understood in terms of 'personal tragedy theory' (Oliver 1986), with the associated labelling of people with dementia as 'victims' or 'sufferers'. We explore the sociological insight into this process below when discussing **labelling** theory. Other consequences of this approach for people with dementia has been the individualization and medicalization of the illness (Lyman 1989; Bond 1992a), processes which lead to the blaming of the individual and loss of personhood (Kitwood and Bredin 1992c).

Medicalization of dementia

One of the processes inherent in the biomedical model is the **medicalization** of disease (Conrad 1975; Freidson 1975; Estes and Binney 1989). By medicalization is meant defining behaviour as a medical problem and mandating the medical profession to find some form of treatment for it. There are a number of aspects to the medicalization of dementia:

- *Expert control.* The medical profession comprises experts who have a monopoly over knowledge about anything relating to disease or illness (Freidson 1975). Diagnosis and treatment is controlled by the medical profession. Although there was limited improvement in the last decade of the twentieth century, it is still the case that the medical profession controls much social knowledge through domination of grant-awarding bodies for research on dementia.

- *Social control.* In its role as arbiter of social values medicine acts as an institution of social control and doctors as agents of **social control** (Zola 1972). Medicine has the power to legitimize and confer a social status and incorporates procedures by which the status of ill or well are judged by the doctor. Only psychiatrists have the authority to give a person the diagnosis of dementia.
- *Individualization of behaviour.* Medicalization supports the individualization of behaviour. Society thus seeks explanations and solutions for complex social problems in the individual rather than the social structure. In general terms the biomedical model focuses on the individual and the diagnosis and treatment of the illness, rather than seeing an individual's illness in the context of the social system. In the same way the effect of dementia on the caregiver is individualized and not related to the social structure of the caring unit and caring relationship. It is, for example, the personalities of the person with dementia and of the caregiver which are highlighted rather than material conditions or other structural characteristics.
- *Depoliticization of behaviour.* By defining the behaviour and cognitive problems of dementia the biomedical model ignores the meaning of the individual's behaviour in the context of the social system. The perspectives of the person with dementia and of his or her caregiver are ignored. Thus when people in long-term institutional care exhibit behaviour characteristics similar to those diagnosed with dementia there is little attempt to seek an explanation within the context of the loss of power of a person in a **total institution** (Goffman 1961) rather than a neurological disorder.

Medicalization through expert control, social control and individualization of behaviour justifies control as the appropriate treatment for the 'good of the patient'. The biomedical model, however, does not consider the ways in which the caregiving relationship and conditions of the caregiving context affect both individuals with dementia and their caregivers. If dementia is viewed only as a medical condition then the behaviour of people with dementia is individualized and relationships between people with dementia and their caregivers is perceived as unimportant. But from a public policy perspective the 'burden' experienced by formal and informal caregivers (Aneshensel *et al.* 1995) is a key issue since if the burden can be minimized people with dementia can be maintained in the community. The biomedical model offers a solution to such policy issues by the medicalization of the caregiving role (Bond 1992b).

It is worth noting that the medicalization of dementia and caregiving is not just a matter of the power and authority of doctors to control the social lives of people with dementia. Long before dementia was recognized as a disease, people with dementia were seen as problematic. Families would seek advice from doctors because they had no other form of advice and they demanded assistance. Dementia may have become a medical responsibility because the other social supports and agents of social control, particularly the Church, were unable to respond. Thus medical responsibility for dementia was progressively legitimated and confirmed by its recognition as a disease (Hamilton-Smith *et al.* 1992).

Psychological model

Traditional psychological approaches to dementia have adhered to the dominant biomedical model. An important and distinctive contribution has emerged from the work of Kitwood and colleagues in the Bradford Dementia Group (Kitwood 1997b). This new way of thinking about dementia and the new culture of dementia care (Kitwood and Benson 1995) reflects the view that people with dementia are *people* foremost and that there is much that can be done to improve the **quality of life** for people with dementia while waiting for the 'magic bullets' of new biomedical advances. By focusing on personhood the paradigm reminds us that all individuals are unique and have an absolute value. But individuals do not function in isolation, they also have relations with others; all human life is interdependent and interconnected.

Traditional concepts of personhood embody a number of principles. Individuals require a consciousness of self; a capacity for abstract thinking; the ability to act with intention, to live life according to a set of moral principles and be accountable for their actions; and the capacity to form and manage relationships with others (Quinton 1973). In biomedical models which focus on individuals as objects, psychiatric patients in general and people with dementia in particular are excluded from the categories of normal personhood defined by traditional principles. Challenges to traditional concepts of personhood argue against rationality and **autonomy** as necessary features of personhood (Post 1995). In contrast, personhood should be defined by feelings, emotion and the ability to live in relationships. Kitwood (1997b) reflects that people with dementia are often highly competent in these areas, sometimes more so than their informal caregivers.

Through the recognition of personhood in dementia care, the new psychological **paradigm** addresses a number of the shortcomings of the biomedical approach. However, it continues to categorize dementia in terms of **disability**, and is therefore concerned with the social psychological adjustment by people with dementia and their informal caregivers to the condition. Thus, like social adjustment to physical impairment theories (Oliver 1996), the new psychological paradigm can be criticized for being too focused on the individual's behaviour, for ignoring the external economic, political and social worlds, and for undermining the meaning and subjective interpretations of dementia to people with dementia and their informal caregivers.

Sociological model

A sociological model of dementia which adopts the social model of disability (Oliver 1990) would focus on the way that people with dementia and their informal caregivers interpret their own experiences of living with dementia and the meaning that their situation has for them. The onset of dementia is a significant life event for the individual and close family members but is only the beginning of a new trajectory within the life course and the starting point for understanding the practical and personal consequences of dementia. The political and social environment, material resources and, critically, the meanings which individuals attach to situations and events in their lives are key factors in the development of a social model of dementia. Changes in the underlying pathological and psychological features of the disease as well as in the material and social circumstances of people with dementia and their informal caregivers mean that the experience of dementia has a temporal or time dimension.

The personal responses of individuals to dementia and its consequences are central to a social model. Personal responses cannot be understood as merely a reaction to the condition or as a response to the oppression by the social structure (Foucault 1973). An understanding of dementia has to be located within a framework which takes account of the life histories of people with dementia and their informal caregivers, their material circumstances, the meaning dementia has for the individuals and the struggle they experience to be included as citizens of their societies.

The social model described above is somewhat different to that described in earlier texts on the sociology of health and illness which reflected mainstream sociological theories. The emphasis of earlier 'social models' was on a model which 'would illuminate how social process worked in defining illness, understanding the causes of illness and promotion of health or in interpreting the organizational structures within the health care system' (Bond and Bond 1994: 8). Partial acceptance of this model by the medical profession, particularly public health medicine, and evaluation from critical sociological perspectives have generated a sociological model which focuses more on the meaning that the disease has for the individual and **social constructionist** ideas. We return to these ideas later in the chapter.

MAPPING SOCIOLOGICAL PERSPECTIVES

In order to understand the often conflicting ways that sociology has theorized about society it is helpful to categorize different sociological perspectives. This is an intellectually dangerous exercise given the enormous variation of ideas present within any one school of sociology. It is not within the remit of this chapter to attempt to summarize even the key ideas of these different perspectives; these are provided by some of the texts listed as recommended further reading. Rather we will examine those theoretical ideas which have had greatest impact on the sociological investigations of chronic illness. Because of both implicit and explicit links between different perspectives we structure our discussion chronologically starting with the mainstream perspectives which had so much influence on the development of 'medical sociology' in Britain during the 1970s and 1980s. We will then examine challenges to this orthodoxy from **postmodernism** and **feminism**.

STRUCTURAL FUNCTIONALISM

When medicine first became a topic of sociological interest **structural functionalism** was the dominant perspective taken by sociologists investigating the professions of medical and health care and the individual's experience of health and illness. A key assumption of structural functionalism is that all our social behaviour is the result of the organization and structure of society in which we live. A particular feature of all societies is their ordered nature and a belief that in most social situations the range of possible actions is fairly limited. For structural functionalists societies are regarded as stable and generally integrated wholes which differ by their **cultural** and social structural arrangements. This perspective in sociology grew out of the Enlightenment philosophy and shares the same scientific paradigm as many of the natural and biomedical sciences. As in the biomedical model, structural functionalists often claimed that they were scientifically neutral. Yet it is clear from the basic tenets of structural functionalist theory that this was not the case and that they provided an **ethnocentric** and male-oriented view of the world.

Health and illness

A basic contribution of structural functionalism was the distinction made between medically defined disease and socially constructed illness. Disease refers to a medical concept of pathology, which is indicated by signs and symptoms. From a medical perspective dementia is characterized by a loss of intellectual power, which can lead to difficulties in remembering, making decisions, thinking through complex ideas, carrying out practical tasks, retaining information and acquiring new skills. Psychiatrists using a common body of knowledge make the decision as to whether or not a person has the disease. In contrast, illness is usually defined by the person who has the signs and symptoms of the disease. It refers primarily to a person's subjective experience of 'health' and 'ill health' and is indicated by the person's reaction to the symptoms. Personal biographical accounts and novels have provided a rich source of insight into the subjective experience of people with dementia, particularly during the early stages of the disease (Bernlef 1984; Davis 1989; Forster 1989; McGowin 1993).

In the case of a particular set of signs and symptoms it follows that two or more people may have different definitions of the situation. Thus someone could perceive themselves as ill, perhaps experiencing difficulty remembering people's names, while being defined as 'normal' by standard psychiatric assessment measures. Similarly an individual may meet diagnostic criteria for dementia but not perceive themselves as being ill. This contrast is problematic in the case of dementia for two reasons. First, a person with dementia not recognizing that they have an illness is exhibiting a symptom of the disease. Second, a formal diagnosis can only be confirmed at autopsy. The contrast remains important, however, because it highlights the potentially different definitions of the situation and that definitions of disease and illness are socially constructed.

Illness behaviour

A second key contribution from a structural functionalist perspective is the concept of illness behaviour. The term was first coined by Mechanic (1962) who defined illness behaviour as 'the way in which symptoms may be differentially perceived, evaluated and acted upon by different kinds of persons'. In other words, illness behaviour is about the social factors, which influence the way individuals view signs and symptoms, and the kinds of actions they engage in to deal with them. Individuals may recognize signs and symptoms as a medical problem, but they may choose to ignore them, or they may deal with the problem without seeking formal medical care. To date the use of medical services by people with dementia for their dementia has been reported in epidemiological studies (Philp *et al.* 1995; Boersma *et al.* 1997; Ely *et al.* 1997) but factors associated with reasons for seeking or not seeking medical help have not been the subject of systematic investigation. Studies of illness behaviour which are not necessarily associated with any specific diagnosis document the association between use of health services and social factors such as age, gender, marital status, social class, ethnic status, religion and education (Bond and Bond 1994).

Sick role

Perhaps one of the most celebrated concepts relevant to the study of health and illness to emerge from structural functionalism was the concept of the **sick role** which describes the expectations of people in society and defines the rights and duties of its members who are sick (Parsons 1951). Like all roles, the sick role has both rights and obligations associated with it. Parsons highlights two rights. First, the sick person, that is the one occupying the sick role, can claim exemption for normal activities and the responsibilities of other roles. Second, the sick person can expect assistance from, and be dependent on, others. The concept has been regularly criticized as being too simplistic. There is considerable variation in the way in which different individuals claim the rights of the sick role. Such variation will be associated with personality, gender, culture, material characteristics and particularly the varying cultural expectations of how one should behave when ill. How does one play the role of a person with dementia? The sick role will also be contingent on the social context of each individual. For example, if there is no one else to care for her husband who has severe dementia, a woman with flu will struggle to continue caring despite feeling extremely ill.

The first of the obligations associated with the sick role is that the incumbent should want to get better and to get out of the sick role as soon as possible. Yet for chronic conditions like dementia this is a problematic idea. When we

are ill we all, generally, want to get better. To this extent we should be conform-
ing to the expectations of the sick role. The experience of chronic illness, particularly a degenerative condition like dementia, is that there is no getting better.

The second obligation of the sick role identified by Parsons is that the sick
person should not only try to get better but do so by acting in an appropriate
manner: staying indoors as necessary or seeking medical care when required.
Leaving aside the problem of chronic illness, the major criticism of this obligation is that it does not allow for the different perspectives about what is
appropriate action. The sick person, other lay people and a doctor may well
hold different views about the relevance or appropriateness of specific treatments (Dingwall 1976). The carer of the person with dementia may well feel
that the cared-for person should take a course of antibiotics for his or her
chest infection whereas the general practitioner does not feel that this is necessary for the severity of the infection. Neither may have a clear idea of the
views of the person with dementia on this matter.

As an abstract idea the sick role is useful in providing an insight into the
way an individual is expected to behave in the face of acute illness. It is less
useful when considering chronic illness or disability. Many writers consider
that the concept has been over-used (Freidson 1975; Mechanic 1992) and to
some extent its importance is the way in which health professionals now use
the term to label certain categories of sick people. We return to the importance
of labelling theory below but for the present suffice to say that from the
perspective of labelling theory the term sick role becomes the label generally
used to describe people who are 'normally ill', in other words acutely ill.

Two critical challenges to the dominance of structural functionalism in the
study of health and illness emerged in the 1970s through the **political economy**
perspective and **symbolic interactionism** and it is to these which we now turn.

POLITICAL ECONOMY

Political economy, like structural functionalism, emphasizes the importance of
social structures rather than individual characteristics for the understanding
of human behaviour. This perspective encompasses two complementary approaches (Bond 1986) rooted in the writings of different schools of sociological
thought; Fabian sociology and Marxist critiques of capitalism. The common
threads which links these writings are: notions of class, ethnic and gender
inequality; and a focus on the relationship between the economic, political
and social structure of society and the impact of these relationships on the
distribution of material and social goods.

A key concept within the political economy perspective is that of **structured
dependency** (Townsend 1981; Walker 1981). This concept describes the development of a dependent status resulting from the restricted access to a wide
range of resources, particularly income. This is reflected in the large numbers
of older people who live in poverty (Townsend 1979; Townsend 1991; Johnson
and Stears 1997). It has long been recognized that older people are in the

lower levels of the income distribution because they are not in the labour market and pensions and other assets are generally inadequate to sustain a standard of living comparable to people in work. Older women are significantly poorer than their male counterparts (Arber and Ginn 1991) as are older people from ethnic minority groups (Blakemore and Boneham 1994), reflecting the triple jeopardy of older women from ethnic minority groups (Norman 1985). Retirement from the labour market contributes to the decline in older people's social networks and a reduction in social relations (Phillipson 1982). All older people are discriminated against by economic and social policies, which benefit the young employed and well off. Poverty in later life and the dependent status of people in later life continues to be related to low resources and restricted access to resources throughout the life cycle. Feminists and others have commented on the narrowness of this approach, which concentrates on inequalities resulting from poverty and economic disadvantage (Dant 1988) and ignores the increasing cultural diversity of the contemporary world. Yet structured dependency helps us understand **ageism** and aspects of **racism** in contemporary society.

Ageism

A key experience for older people is ageism and for people with dementia this is compounded by '**disablism**'. Ageism is endemic in UK society. Biological models of ageing have been used inappropriately to justify common perceptions of later life: disability, senility, powerlessness and loneliness (Bond 1997). Such negative attitudes have been not only a feature of this century but of earlier times in history (Featherstone and Hepworth 1993).

Ageism, the negative stereotyping of individuals on the basis of age, is institutionalized in the UK and other European societies. Older people are denied certain citizenship rights and have limited access to social, political and economic power. Ageist attitudes are expressed in the behaviour of personal social services and health service staff who treat patients and clients as dependent children through invoking use of the metaphor of childhood to describe older people (Hockey and James 1993). Practices such as infantilization at one level may be regarded as being an unfortunate but inevitable response to human dependency. On another level, however, the metaphor can be seen as one means of creating and maintaining the powerful social categories between 'them', the 'aged' and people with dementia, and 'us', the younger and 'abler' members of society.

One specific effect of institutionalized ageism is the implementation of age rationing for health services. Within the National Health Service (NHS) the definition of what medical services would be of benefit to individual patients has been that of the doctor, and different doctors clearly make different decisions, given the substantial variability in treatment rates throughout the country. As an age-stratified society both explicit and implicit discrimination is practised by health care professionals in response to the shortfall in health care resources (Bond 1997).

SYMBOLIC INTERACTIONISM

The other perspective, which challenged structural functionalism, was symbolic interactionism. This broad approach emphasizes understanding the individual by attempting to look at the world from the perspective of the other and appreciating how the world looks to them (Blumer 1969). To this is added learning the ideas, motives and goals which make people act (Mead 1934). Symbolic interactionists are also interested in the processes by which members of society define their own circumstances and respected identities. A particular application of this approach has come to be known as the labelling theory of **deviance**.

Labelling theory

The term 'labelling' refers to a social process by which individuals or groups classify the social behaviour of other individuals. In sociology, we are generally interested in understanding the processes by which labelling of particular individuals or groups evolves and the characteristics of the groups which fall within a given label. We include social groups regularly in our everyday conversations – feminists, the elderly, patients, and we label individuals – old, demented, frail – in order to classify them. The important thing to note about these examples is that the nouns refer to deviant groups, and the adjectives describe deviant attributes. They imply a shift in some respect or attribute which is away from the normal and valued attributes of the social group. In this way a state of health is the norm, as is being cognitively intact, while illness, and cognitive impairment, is deviance from the **norm**. There is general agreement that 'deviance always refers to conduct that is a violation of the rules constructed by a given society or group' (Berger and Berger 1976: 305). Deviance is therefore a matter of social definition. Two types of deviance have been identified: primary and secondary deviance (Lemert 1964).

Primary deviance

Whether a given label will have meaning within a social group will depend on whether that label is permanent and this, in turn, will depend a great deal on whether the person applying the label has the authority to do so. For example, if a man is labelled as mentally impaired by his wife or his lawyer this may not be accepted by others until a psychiatrist has legitimized this label by diagnosing the behaviour of this individual as dementia.

Secondary deviance

One of the important features of labelling is the effect it has on both the person being labelled and other people around them. This is called secondary deviance, to distinguish it from the attributes which initially triggered the label.

Being given a label is likely to affect the way individuals behave with others. In time, they are likely to act the role which the new label implies, because of the way others have behaved towards them, the possessors of the label. For example, if residents of old people's homes are called 'senile' or similar adjectives and, perhaps more importantly, if they are treated as if they are cognitively impaired then a frequent response is for residents to take on the behaviour of people who are cognitively impaired.

Stigma

Goffman (1968) has shown how secondary deviance has negative effects. Certain disease labels have stigmatizing effects on the holder of the label. Thus **stigma** refers to a relationship of devaluation in which one individual is disqualified from full social acceptance. Stigma is a social attribute, which is discrediting for an individual or group. It seems likely that people with dementia would be stigmatized because of the 'out of the ordinary' (Dingwall 1976) or problematic behaviours of those with dementia. The bizarre behaviours characteristic of people with the disease clearly challenge social norms regarding appropriate conduct. There is an absence of research-based evidence of the presence of stigma in dementia (Macrae 1999) but this may reflect the nature of the disease in which people with dementia may not be aware of others' negative response to their behaviour. However, biographical accounts written by people who were in the early stages of dementia indicate that some individuals experienced embarrassment and shame (McGowin 1993).

Goffman also coined the term courtesy stigma to describe the situation in which an individual 'is related through the social structure to a stigmatised individual' and the wider society then 'treat both individuals in some respect as one' (Goffman 1968: 30). There is stronger evidence of the presence of courtesy stigma among caregivers of people with dementia (Blum 1991), with both caregivers and other family members experiencing courtesy stigma.

Much of the research on courtesy stigma resulting from other conditions focuses on the management of stigma. Blum (1991) found that the management of stigma by the caregivers of people with dementia has two phases. In the early stages of the dementia caregivers collude with the cared-for while cooperating over the management of information and problematic social situations. Two strategies identified by Goffman (1961) are used: passing and covering. Passing involves concealment of damaging information or the management of undisclosed discrediting information. Caregivers and cared-for suppress evidence of symptoms of dementia from others outside the immediate close family. Passing should not be confused with denial whereby during early stages of a chronic illness people with the illness deny to themselves and others the presence of symptoms. Covering occurs once the stigma becomes visible in interactions. This strategy involves keeping visibility of the problem to a minimum. The second phase identified by Blum (1991) begins during later stages of dementia when the person with dementia can no longer maintain the collusion.

Information control is no longer the primary concern. Avoiding situations where inappropriate behaviours of the person with dementia are visible now becomes the main strategy. The caregiver now 'realigns and sides against' the person with dementia 'in order to maintain social order as well as preserve his or her own face' (Blum 1991: 281–2).

Macrae (1999) argues that 'since definitions of the situation are negotiated rather than given, affiliation with a stigmatised individual does not automatically result in courtesy stigma' (p. 60). Family members were found to manipulate or control others' definition of the situation so that their reactions would not be negative. Information control through concealment of the diagnosis or the behaviour of the person with dementia was used to make the situation invisible. Others openly referred to the diagnosis and medicalized the associated behaviour problems. Those family members who were able to manipulate others' definition of the situation by ignoring or challenging the others' perspective managed the stigma more successfully. But stigma management was easiest where others, although aware of the discreditable condition, were sympathetic or non-judgemental. But it will be at the societal level where most change must occur. The publicity generated by advocates of people with dementia and the coming out of celebrities with dementia will have greatest impact on making dementia a less discreditable condition.

PHENOMENOLOGY AND ETHNOMETHODOLOGY

Phenomenology is about perceiving the world as objects or events, which are in essential respects common – the same for others as they are for us. Its basic assumptions derive largely from the phenomenological philosophy of Edmund Husserl (1859–1938) who described the meaning of everyday life through human experiences and the 'essences' which underpin them. Only by grasping such essences do we have a foundation for all experiences, which enables us to recognize and classify it in an intelligible form. In order to grasp these essences it is necessary for the philosopher to disengage from our usual ideas about the world. The experience of dementia is one that is very much described through the eyes of the cognitively normal individual. To understand what dementia means to the person with dementia it is necessary, phenomenologists would argue, to suspend everyday assumptions and try to understand the experience from the perspective of the person with dementia. Thus dementia must be studied as experienced in everyday life and not the phenomenon observed and interpreted by scientists with their own particular view of the world.

Alfred Schutz (1899–1959) developed the phenomenological approach into the sociological study of everyday life known as **ethnomethodology**. Two key ideas of ethnomethodology are useful in our understanding of the everyday life of people with dementia and their informal caregivers. First is the idea that social order is achieved through what Schutz (1972) has termed our taken-for-granted assumptions, in other words, our expectations about what should happen in a normal day and how we expect others to act. For example, when driving to work in the morning we make numerous assumptions about the actions of other motorists and pedestrians in order to arrive safely. If we did not make these assumptions we would never leave home. One taken-for-granted assumption is that others, by and large, see the world as we do, something which is clearly not always borne out. Challenges to one's taken-for-granted assumptions occur more often when interacting with people with dementia although we can change our assumptions about the actions of a person with dementia in light of our experiences.

One way that the social fabric is maintained is through the use of 'typifications' (Schutz 1972). These are common ways of classifying particular objects, events or experiences but in ways which can be redesigned or adapted. The act of categorizing things, events and people into types functions to reduce the complexity of our social world by narrowing the focus of interaction to a small number of recognized types. Available typifications are a major determinant of how subsequent relationships are managed. They take account of the characteristics of the type, more so than those individuals who constitute the type. An important feature of typifications is that they are 'plan determined' (Schutz and Luckmann 1974). That is, the practical purposes underlying typification, and the circumstances in which it occurs, will influence the particular person types constructed. A general case of this arises, for example, when care staff typify 'good' or 'bad' patients or residents. In nursing homes, residents with dementia who wander may constitute particular problems while those who are 'too able' may be equally problematic, especially if they are also assertive. What constitutes wandering or assertiveness is, of course, context-specific.

The creation of meaning for people with dementia

'A phenomenological perspective requires that our understanding of dementing illness be empirically grounded in the "lived experience" of those who have the condition' (Lyman 1998: 49). The meaning and quality of life is only meaningful through the subjective definitions of individuals. This perspective is problematic within the biomedical or psychological model of dementia because of the expectation of profound loss of self. The phenomenological perspective challenges the deterministic biomedical model of disease progression in which dementia is characterized as an inevitable decline in cognitive function and development of associated behaviour problems. Accepting that dementia can be characterized by functional impairment, the phenomenological perspective argues that many of the problems of dementia are socio-environmental and not biomedical. It focuses on the experience of illness rather than disease progression. In contrast to the deterministic perspective of the biomedical model, which attributes an individual's functioning and behaviour problems to the neuropathology of dementia, phenomenology offers a perspective that modifies the social and environmental conditions affecting the illness experience. Living with dementia involves the active creation and recreation of meaning and identity, and the negotiation of empowerment, as part of the daily work of living with the condition. Sociological studies of the meaning of dementia from the perspective of the person with dementia and their carers have highlighted its complexity and variability (Gubrium and Lynott 1985; Gubrium 1986, 1987; Askham 1995).

Biographical accounts

Personal accounts of the experience of illness have a strong tradition in sociology particularly within the symbolic interactionist perspective. Sociological accounts of the subjective experience of people with dementia are limited (see for example Gubrium 1986), most accounts, particularly biographical accounts, being provided by **significant others** (Bayley 1998). The **life history** perspective (Johnson 1976) is built on concepts of career, a progression of events which relate to each other (Goffman 1961), and trajectory, the course and timescale of events associated with phenomena like dying and pain (Glaser and Strauss 1965). The use of these specific concepts and the generic life history approach relegates the individual to a passive subject shaped by outside forces and interpreted within the researchers' categories. In phenomenology the emphasis is on biographical work rather than life history. The distinction here is that **biography** is not so much the presentation of the facts of an individual's life that are ordered in relation to their life history but is the descriptive product of retrospective and prospective reflection, the representation of individual experience. 'To inspect biography is to display the work that enters into its production and subsequent reproduction' (Gubrium and Lynott 1985: 350).

The phenomenological approach uses dementia as a 'code' for rendering meaningful the general age-related troubles of late life (Gubrium 1986). By itself the code, dementia, provides us with little understanding of these troubles of later life; rather it provides a description of the end point of these troubles. Observing the cultural experience of dementia through the accounts of individuals goes beyond the experience of individuals and the meaning that the diagnosis might have for the individual. Treating dementia as biographical work reveals the condition's pervasively social character. It shows how dementia is dependent on the particular experience of those with dementia and how significant others in particular and society in general respond to the ageing of society's members.

Biographical work on the experience of dementia proceeds on two fronts. First, biographical accounts of the disease experience from the person with dementia and their caregivers provide insights into the personal nature of the disease. Second, biographical work involves examining the cultural context of the disease: public accounts, explanations, cultural images of dementia and shared knowledge and understandings. The interdependence of the individual experience and the broader cultural experience of the disease again highlights the social nature of dementia.

POSTMODERNISM

Postmodernism challenges the existence of a stable coherent self and the idea of human rationality. It doubts the notion that science and reason can provide an 'objective' foundation for knowledge and the idea that this knowledge will be 'truth'. Postmodernism rejects the existence of absolute truth which is independent of the interpretation of individuals and the belief that language accurately reflects 'reality'. Indeed, for postmodernists language does not reflect reality; it creates it. A key criticism of modernism is the use of binary logic in describing and explaining the world such as men and women, and rich and poor. The aim of postmodernism is to unravel modernist thought in such a way as to reveal them as artefacts of a particular way of knowing and looking at the world. Postmodernism achieves this through the process of deconstruction (Derrida 1982) which involves looking at an imputed opposition such as cognitively intact/cognitively impaired. By showing that the dominant privileged position (cognitively intact) is created out of contrast with the oppressed position (cognitively impaired) postmodernists argue that dualisms are not really opposites but are interdependent because they derive their meaning from an established contrast.

The loss of self in dementia has been examined from a postmodernist social constructionist view of the nature of **self** (Sabat and Harre 1992). From this perspective two kinds of 'self' have been identified. The first is the self of personal identity in which one's sense of personal agency supports continuity of purpose and meaning in life. The second sense of self is the one which persists 'behind' what Goffman called 'personae'; this is the self which is publicly displayed in everyday interaction (Goffman 1971). In their analysis of the construction and deconstruction of self in dementia, Sabat and Harre (1992) refer to the first as 'self' and the second as 'selves'. Linguistically we display the 'self' through indexical expressions such as 'I' and 'you'. Indexical expressions and the way we describe our own 'self' depend for their meaning on the context in which they occur. Understanding the personal identity, the 'self', of another is only possible when one has a knowledge of the individual and the context in which 'self' is described. In contrast, 'selves' reflects the variety of ways in which people behave in everyday interactions – interactions which will be dependent on the context in which they take place.

Social constructionist theory has provided new insights into our understanding of dementia. 'Self' remains intact during the course of dementia despite the loss of cognitive and motor functions (Sabat and Harre 1992) and perhaps the loss of the indexical creation of self. The threatened loss of self does not appear to be linked to the 'progress' of the disease. Rather it is linked to the related behaviour of significant others. They interpret the loss of the indexical creation of self as a loss of self and they interpret the presentation of 'selves' as indicative of loss of self. In so doing they create their own reality and language to describe the presentation of self by the person with dementia. In practice the resultant loss of 'selves' leads to loss of autonomy and loss of personhood.

FEMINISM

Gender is a key organizing principle of the social order across cultures. Oakley (1972) demonstrates the way different societies allocate roles and responsibilities differentially between men and women. But gender order is not just about the sexual division of labour. It is also about authority relations and social stratification on the basis of gender. Although feminist theory is not a homogeneous set of ideas (Evans 1995), it has a unifying theme in the critique of the gender order and the concept of patriarchy – an autonomous system of social relations between men and women in which men are dominant and women oppressed by men. Rather than being biologically or naturally determined, patriarchy is socially determined, designating social relationships between men and women. Yet feminism and the feminine viewpoint provide only one way of gaining insights. Women are never just women – they are also young or old, from diverse ethnic origins, partnered or not partnered, mothers or daughters, employed in the labour market, in public life or at home – and so a feminist viewpoint is contextualized among others (Gelsthorpe 1992).

Feminist theory has challenged the way we look at the world. It has also provided a key critique of the health care system and the role of women in health and illness, as well as highlighting the state's dependence on informal care for the support of people with dementia.

Formal and informal care

Formal care is undertaken in the context of **bureaucratically** structured organizations. Caregiving tasks are more often than not instrumental and are undertaken by specified individuals within a framework of professional or occupational hierarchical **accountability**. Informal care (provided by carers) contrasts with formal care (provided by care staff) by the attachment of caregivers to recipients of care rather than by a commitment to tasks (Bond 1992b).

This contrast is illuminated by Ungerson's distinction between caring for and caring about (Ungerson 1983). In the former instrumental activities necessarily predominate, while the latter highlights feelings of concern. A comparable distinction here is Blau's analysis of intrinsic and extrinsic aspects of social exchange (Blau 1964). Both aspects are the function of formal and informal care but only informal care is based on both affection and service (Graham 1983). Abrams (Bulmer 1986) concluded that the personally directed nature of informal care gives it a special quality, endowing social significance to the relationship between the caregiver and the recipient of care, which formal care organized within a hierarchical bureaucratic framework could never hope to achieve.

The gendered nature of care

Health care work is predominantly women's work, but it is controlled by men (Doyal 1985). Within feminism the relative importance of equality between men and women and difference between men and women is an ongoing debate (Evans 1995). To avoid this debate, C. Davies (1995) suggests that we turn the spotlight from women to gender. In doing this we make a clear distinction between men and women on the one hand, and masculinity and femininity on the other. The organizational context in which formal care operates is one which has been forged by historical processes where men were the key actors and cultural notions of masculinity dominate. The professional career, the bureaucratic structures in which we are employed and the very nature of professions are all gendered and gendered male.

In this male gendered world women typically have two kinds of labour, that in the domestic sphere, which is unpaid, and paid work (Yeandle 1984). But women's work is generally devalued and paid at low rates. We can trace the low pay of qualified and unqualified nursing staff to their position as women who did not have to earn the family wage but only support themselves. Nurses have always been regarded as a 'disposable' workforce (Mackay 1989) and so not worth investing in to maximize their potential.

The impact for people with dementia, the majority of whom are women, and for their informal carers, the majority of whom are also women, is the lowering of status within the modern health system where masculine values dominate and curing rather than caring has top priority. Being 'less important' from a male world-view, caring activities are left to women, particularly informal care.

Historically women have always been the carers. And even nowadays with the emergence of the male carer (Fisher 1994), women provide the bulk of caregiving to older people with dementia (RIS MRC CFAS 1999). Despite the male-oriented rhetoric of public policy on community care it remains the case that 'in practice community care equals care by the family, and in practice care by the family equals care by women' (Finch and Groves 1983: 494). Even where community care is outside the family, such as neighbourhood care, it is women again who provide the majority of support (Abrams *et al.* 1989). With the emphasis on gender in caregiving research, there has been little examination of ethnic or class issues.

A SOCIOLOGY OF DEMENTIA

In this chapter we have surveyed a range of sociological perspectives and examined concepts and ideas from these perspectives for their relevance to dementia. It is useful to consider here the often quoted distinction between the sociology of medicine and sociology in medicine (Strauss 1957). We can make a similar distinction here between sociology of dementia and dementia care and sociology in dementia and dementia care.

The sociology of dementia and dementia care has confirmed that dementia is very much a social state of affairs. We have seen from a range of perspectives how dementia exists within a social context; how it is perceived differently by the person with dementia, informal caregivers, health professionals and society;

and how the experience of dementia impacts in a variety of ways on the social world of people with dementia and their informal caregivers.

The chapter also provides insights into a sociology in dementia and dementia care through the examination of specific sociological concepts. By understanding concepts like primary and secondary deviance, typification, taken-for-granted assumptions, ageism and the social construction of 'self' and 'selves', formal and informal caregivers can begin to see how they could change their behaviour to improve the dignity, autonomy and personhood of people for whom they care. For policy makers the feminist critique of health and social care has the potential not only to increase the quality of life of people with dementia and their informal caregivers but the quality of working life of the predominantly female workforce providing formal care. Taken together, the sociological perspectives reviewed provide substantial insights into dementia and dementia care.

FURTHER READING

Bond, J. and Bond, S. (1994) *Sociology and Health Care: An Introduction for Nurses and Other Health Care Professionals*, 2nd edn. Edinburgh: Churchill Livingstone. An introduction to the mainstream concepts of the sociology of health and illness.

Bond, J., Coleman, P. and Peace, S. (1993) *Ageing in Society: An Introduction to Social Gerontology*, 2nd edn. London: Sage. Introduces the reader to sociological concepts within the broader context of ageing.

Gubrium, J.F. (1986) *Oldtimers and Alzheimer's: The Descriptive Organization of Senility*. London: Jai Press Inc. This classic text introduces the reader to the social construction of dementia.

Hill, T.M. (1999) Western medicine and dementia: a deconstruction, in T. Adams and C.L. Clarke (eds) *Dementia Care: Developing Partnerships in Practice*. London: Bailliere Tindall. A useful critique of the biomedical model of dementia from a postmodernist perspective.

4

PETER G. COLEMAN AND MARIE A. MILLS

Philosophical and spiritual perspectives

KEY POINTS

- Contemporary societies need to develop new cultures of dementia care drawing on insights from the world's faiths and traditions.
- Relationship is the key to maintaining identity in dementia, and is central to the Christian concept of the person.
- The term spirituality is used to encompass issues of value, meaning and relationship, and may or may not imply a transcendent reality.
- Spiritual well-being is increasingly recognized as an important component of quality of life.
- Caring for those who are sick in mind or body is itself a spiritual act.

INTRODUCTION: DEVELOPING A CULTURE OF DEMENTIA CARE

Dementia poses a challenge to many of our established ways of thinking about human life, the importance we give to memory, to rationality, to personal identity, what it is to be a person, and what is ultimately valuable about our existence. It is a condition of life most of us fear. But it is short-sighted to see dementia only as a problem for which we have to find practical solutions, eliminating it if possible. For dementia, in shaking our assumptions, provides opportunities to deepen our perspectives on life in general, to learn, for example, to accept and to value our own vulnerability, neediness and interdependence.

Within the European and North American perspectives on ageing, the history of dementia care appears as a story of neglect until very recently. As a result there is little or no tradition on which to build in formulating a more adequate conceptual framework, one that goes beyond the practical and emotional issues raised by the demands of caring for people with dementia, and which addresses questions of meaning and purpose. With rising numbers of the population now growing to an age where dementia becomes a likely condition of life, the need for **philosophical** and **spiritual** answers as well as practical ones has become urgent. We have to start, if only tentatively, formulating some very basic principles about living in a state of dementia, to try to build on them, and see how far they take us in moving dementia from the dark periphery to the mainstream of life.

In this chapter we will provide a brief exploration of current thought and practice which address existential issues arising from the experience of dementia. By the term 'existential' we refer to questions and answers touching on the meaning of existence. These questions can be **secular** and philosophical in character, or spiritual and/or **religious**. It is necessary to acknowledge the plurality of perspectives on the meaning of life that exist in contemporary society. Ideally, in a chapter such as this, we should address a wide selection of perspectives held by the general population. However, many of these views are not well articulated; they are also poorly studied and documented. We prefer to keep our focus on perspectives that are familiar to us. Our presentation therefore reflects our own particular backgrounds and chosen commitments in life. It is therefore on Christian thought that we shall draw most in discussing both philosophical and spiritual perspectives on dementia and their consequences for practice. However, the resulting limitations have to be acknowledged.

The history and culture of European society have been shaped in large part by Christianity, but in regard to dementia care its influence has been mixed. In fact the particularly aversive attitude to dementia in our society may be due in large part, as we shall see, to the emphasis on the human capacity for reason rather than relationship found among western, including Christian, philosophers. Nor is it only dementia that is marginalized within Christian thought. Ageing in all its aspects is given less attention than in other world religions (Achenbaum 1985). As a result it is often not in Christian culture that one finds the best examples of dignified care of the old and frail. Other cultural and spiritual thought patterns appear more intrinsically favourable to the old, and more systematic investigation is needed into the patterns of caring for people with dementia observable in such cultures.

Kitwood has stressed how the human need to be cared for and to care develops within a culture. Caring, he argues, 'is facilitated in some cultural settings and is marred and distorted in others' (Kitwood 1997b: 3). But we are not only passive recipients of culture; we are also responsible for its continuation and development. We not only maintain traditions; we reform and renew them, and on occasions dare to innovate and change. For the study of ageing this is a very important point. Culture has usually developed as the friend of ageing, in contrast to biology, which appears as its enemy (Baltes 1997). In the course of human evolution it is the development of culture that has compensated for the failings and weaknesses of age, and provided older people with valued roles and purposes. But although in the course of human civilization we have developed a variety of cultural environments suitable for older people, human innovation in this field has not managed to keep pace with the recent rapid growth in numbers of the very old and frail. We have much more culture building to do if we are to create a society fit for all ages.

Kitwood envisaged the creation of environments in which caring for dementia 'feels natural'. The traditions we have inherited from the past contain many false beliefs and inept practices relating to dementia care, which we would be better off jettisoning. Although it is said we do not possess instinct-like drives to help us when it comes to looking after those who are old and frail in the same way as we care for children, this may not matter if we can develop strong cultural norms of caring for the old. In fact we can perceive that such norms exist in stronger forms in some other cultures and we can imitate and learn from their practices.

One of the defining features of ageing is loss. Dementia is loss writ large, since it deprives people often of what they value most in terms of sense of security, a continuous identity, memories of person and place, and powers of reasoning. The degree of loss can go beyond what is normal and acceptable, appearing an affront to human dignity and self-respect. At the same time it may attract unworthy behaviour on the part of family and professional carers that corrupts and lowers standards. Kitwood referred to this phenomenon with the term 'malignant social psychology'. Such poor standards of care feed on ignorance and uninformed prejudice about the dementing person's behaviour, that develop in the absence of proper training and emotional support. But they also reflect a real cultural poverty. Our own interviews with residential staff suggest that negative attitudes to care work and disappointment with lack of felt **reciprocity** in interactions with older people mirror the (lack of) earlier positive relationships with older generations in the personal background of the care staff themselves (Coleman 1992).

Although there are many older people present within modern western societies, the meanings related to being old are less clear than before. At the same time we appear to have lost from our culture the folk stories about midlife and ageing whereby people in the past acquired insight into the developmental issues of the second half of life (Chinen 1989). In the folk stories we do retain which address, mainly for children's benefit, the challenges of growing to adulthood, older people appear predominantly as figures of guidance. Hence perhaps the disappointment young people feel with older people who no longer appear to retain that role. But it is unrealistic to expect older people always to be there for us in this capacity of wise guide. We need to become mature adults ourselves who can let older people follow a different path at the end of life and simply be themselves.

PERSONALITY, PERSONHOOD AND DEMENTIA

We shall begin by considering the changes that occur in the human person as a result of dementia and how we should best conceptualize them. Complex issues arise. Does personality change? If so, what is the implication for personhood? In what sense is the person with dementia still the same person, in what sense a different one?

Psychology distinguishes the study of cognition from that of emotion and motivation, and in line with western biases has always given more attention to the former. Dementia likewise has been conceptualized primarily as a disorder of cognitive and especially memory processes. Although assessment of dementia focuses on cognition, this is largely an artefact of the relatively more developed technology which is available for measuring cognitive than personality processes. In recent years there has been some increased attention given to personality and dementia with the recognition that incipient personality change is one of the markers of early dementia and also that it is the aspect of the condition that carers find hardest to deal with.

What is personality? Successful definitions need to be broad: for example, the motivations, attitudes and behaviour that characterize an individual (McAdams 1995). McAdams conceptualizes three different levels of personality enquiry. The first level consists in the broad 'traits' on which individuals can be distinguished from one another (for example, extraverted, neurotic). The second level, which McAdams refers to as 'personal concerns', denotes the specific motivations and interests, values and coping styles that mark a person out in time, place or role. The third level, which he refers to with the term '**identity**', is an aspect of personality particularly well developed in the modern western world. It encapsulates the unity and purpose shown in the individual's life, and is best represented in narrative form as the story of a person's life seen from the inside.

The destruction of personality in dementia appears to occur at all three levels. People lose contact with the course of their lives, as memories become more difficult to retrieve. Their particular skills and interests become harder to express, and even characteristic personality traits may disappear, as people lose inhibitions and cease to be restrained by conventions of social behaviour.

Dementia can be frightening to behold. It seems to threaten or actually to overwhelm the essence of what makes us who we are. Something fundamental appears to be changing as in a horror film. The reality of this fear is indicated in the efforts of those practitioners who emphasize that stability is to be found beneath the change.

Recent academic discussion has focused a lot on the third level of personality, that of identity and self. In what sense can it be said that dementing people retain a self? For example, linguistic research has examined the use of both first person (i.e. the internally defined self) and second and third person (i.e. the externally defined self or 'persona') references in conversation by, with, and about dementing people (Sabat and Harre 1992; Small *et al.* 1998). The findings reported are both positive and negative. Self and personae are susceptible to decline in dementia, but even in severe dementia they are referred to in a variety of ways. We do not cease to refer to ourselves and to others as individual selves.

Nevertheless, disquieting questions remain about the nature of the change brought about by dementia, as Goldsmith (1999a) explains:

> ...although the (physical) illness may conquer their body, it does not conquer their spirit. But this is not the case with dementia. People cope with loss in different ways; it may affect their personality, but it does not necessarily do so. But with dementia the very person seems to change. This raises basic questions, which have a spiritual dimension, such as 'Who am I?' and 'Which is the real me?'
>
> (Goldsmith 1999a: 128)

In these and other passages dealing with personality change in dementia we can note the frequent and often interchangeable use of words as 'individual', 'person', 'self' and 'real me'. It is insufficiently acknowledged, however, that these are words with complex meanings and the way we choose to use them reflects our philosophical and spiritual understandings of life.

The Christian concept of the person

> The very essence of the person is the image of God, and this remains despite every disfigurement.
>
> (St John of Kronstadt)

It is important to stress that the concepts of person and personhood as we know them arose in the course of **theological** developments within the Christian Church. The classical and ancient world had our notion of individual but quite a different conception of person. The Latin word 'persona' referred to the theatrical mask that classical actors put on and took off. It referred to the role – often transient – which the individual played in society. In contemporary postmodern thought this has become again a familiar way of thinking about human intercourse. All we really perceive are shifting appearances. We construct solid realities out of this flux, including our own selves and lives. But the interpretation always remains problematic. We only have the 'text'; we cannot penetrate beneath it (Bruner 1986; Freeman 1993).

In the first centuries of the Christian era the concept of 'person' took on quite a different meaning. In pondering the nature of the Christian revelation, theologians moved from seeing God in terms of different modes of being or operation – God as one but manifesting Himself in different ways, as Creator of the World, as Son of God, and as Spirit working through all things – to appreciating God, as a 'community' of 'persons'. This affirmed both the distinct individual realities of the three persons of the Trinity, but also their essential interrelationship. This remains an aspiration for all human beings. In Orthodox Christian thought we are individuals who are called to be persons in that deeper sense of wholeness in relationship (Zizoulias 1985). These are fundamental theological ideas but their practical consequences have still to be unfolded.

For, although the Trinity is central to the Christian conception of God, its significance for human relationships has been neglected until recently. In the west we have been more influenced by medieval scholastic interpretations of how humankind is made in the image of God. Rather than emphasizing our capacity for relationship and **community**, these stressed humankind's rational faculty, just as in contemporary processes of law, people with dementia were excluded for consideration because they did not meet the necessary standards for capacity for autonomous action (Dworkin 1986). The result of this emphasis on autonomy, reason and competence has been the tragic neglect of those beyond typical **pastoral** discussion involving reason and argument.

In a pioneering study, Petzsch (1984) has examined the problems for the Christian churches in providing effective pastoral care for dementing people because of this theology of man as a rational being. It has also led to the exclusion of dementia from recent theological reflections on ageing.

The importance of memory for personal identity is also strongly emphasized in the western tradition. How, it is asked, can one be the same person if one cannot remember who one was? This has severe consequences for someone suffering from dementia. Indeed it has to be admitted that memory is a very important aspect of the Judaeo-Christian tradition which builds upon faith in historical events and in particular the recollection of God's saving acts in history. In their central act of worship, the Eucharist, Christians are urged to 'do this in remembrance of Me'. Yet as Goldsmith (1999a) points out, the ability to remember, to be able to record what they believe, becomes increasingly difficult for people with dementia. However, perhaps more important to stress, he argues, is our faith that we are remembered by God, and that God is not bound by our limitations however great they become. The temptation of relying on human logic, rather than Divine purpose, in interpreting our destiny is very great indeed, and one to which western Christianity has been particularly prone. To avoid such a fate, we have to listen with our heart as well as our mind.

The distinction we have referred to between individual and person is a very important one to future developments in Christian thinking on dementia. 'Individuality' refers to our fragmentation, in that we are separated from one another and broken up within ourselves. 'Personhood' refers to our deepest essence, that is distinct from that of others, but through which we are called into relationship with humankind and God. When St Paul writes that we carry things holy in broken vessels, he captures both notions. Our brokenness and our need for relationship go together. The conception of a person, which we inherit from our Christian culture, therefore, is a spiritual one and cannot be equated with the sum of our present personality characteristics, even including the highest level of identity. Rather personhood is the spiritual identity given to us by God and to which we aspire.

Dementing persons present their brokenness clearly to us but, as Kitwood has so eloquently written in theorizing about dementia care, we are all damaged, frail and vulnerable (Kitwood and Bredin 1992c). The only difference between 'us' and 'them' is that whereas 'they' are more likely to admit their problems we hide and defend ours. Kitwood, although not writing as a Christian, has recognized, like some others in this field, that the key to improving dementia care is the concept of 'person':

> ... the core of our position is that personhood should be viewed as essentially social: it refers to the human being in relation to others. But also, it carries essentially ethical connotations: to be a person is to have a certain status, to be worthy of respect.
>
> (Kitwood and Bredin 1992c: 275)

Relationship is central to this conception of personhood. Of particular importance in twentieth-century theological discussion of relationship is Buber's ([1923] 1937) 'I and Thou' which contrasts two ways of being in the world, two ways of forming a relationship, the first being purely instrumental, the second involving commitment. To be a person is to be related to in the second sense, to be addressed as 'Thou'. At the other extreme is the 'I–It' mode of relating. It is significant that it is for this very reason that eastern Christian Churches insist on the use of 'Thou' in addressing God. In so doing they want to emphasize both the total otherness but also the infinite closeness of the person of God to every human being.

It is no coincidence that the particular significance of Buber's 'I–Thou' mode of relationship for understanding dementia was recognized and promoted by Kitwood. He saw that modernity, as a product of western reason and logic, had brought with it a distancing and objectification in human relationships (Kitwood 1997a; Wilson 1999). The consequences for treatment of madness, the institutions that were built to confine those who offended against rationality and good order, have been recorded by Foucault (1967). Dementing people have suffered especially from this approach of isolating and analysing people as separate individuals rather than as persons in relationship. However, we will turn later to recent attempts to correct this imbalance in research and practice which draws on Bowlby's **attachment theory** for understanding the behaviour and needs of dementing people as well as the responses of those caring for them (Miesen 1992).

SPIRITUALITY, SPIRITUAL BELIEFS AND DEMENTIA

Spirituality is a term increasingly used in health care (Sloan *et al.* 1999). It is recognized that most if not all people have spiritual needs and that the way these are responded to in a health context may materially affect physical outcomes as well as well-being (King *et al.* 1995). Such attention to spiritual needs has now been extended to people with dementia. In the UK a recent report on the spiritual needs of older people in residential care (Regan and Smith 1997) and a reader on spirituality and ageing (Jewell 1999a) have both given ample attention to dementia. However, at the same time they also illustrate a common problem: the lack of a shared definition of 'spirituality'. As Regan and Smith note, many people who are religiously non-aligned reject the concept of spirituality because they see it as the language of religion. This applies both to those cared for and to those doing the caring.

Nevertheless, there is a growing consensus that the language of spirituality raises important questions about well-being, in later life in particular, which are not answered within a purely psychological, sociological, economic or political frame of reference (Howse 1999). For example, there is a suggestion in the psychological literature of ageing that issues of self-esteem become less important, and issues of meaning more so (Coleman *et al.* 1999). Jewell (1999a) also points out that spiritual questions, although common to all humanity, appear to find a special focus in old age.

Bruce (1998) describes the following as distinct qualities of spiritual well-being: moments of transcendence (that is feeling one's perspective to belong outside the natural world); having a sense of connection with something beyond the individual; experiencing feelings that are deep and mysterious; experiencing moments of awe and wonder; being concerned with deeper values; finding some meaning in life; feeling that the universe will endure; and having a point of reference from the individual to the universal. Although such experiences can be described in a religious framework, they need not be. The definition provided by the Office for Standards in Education, referred to by Regan and Smith (1997), includes four dimensions of spirituality: reflectiveness, attribution of meaning to experience, valuing the non-material parts of life, and intimations of enduring reality. They adopted this definition for their own research, although, significantly, they added a fifth dimension of 'connectedness'.

We doubt that a common definition of spirituality can be constructed. The concept of spirituality will necessarily be used differently by those who ground their experiences in a non-material reality, whether defined as transcendent or immanent (that is sensing God's presence within His creation), and by those who wish to accept them simply as psychological experiences to which humans are inclined. Whereas religious people, and many non-religious people, believe in a supernatural power or force, many non-religious people wish to avoid any such assumption. The important point to note is not the distinction between religious and non-religious, but between those who believe in a spiritual reality and those who do not. Although religious affiliation has declined in the UK, the evidence suggests that most people still ascribe to spiritual beliefs of some sort (King *et al.* 1995). It is better to acknowledge the differences between religious, spiritual and non-spiritual beliefs than to pretend that they all mean the same thing.

Where perhaps a greater degree of agreement can be reached is around some of the constituent parts that have been identified in the search for a concept of spiritual well-being. This applies especially to questions of values, relationships and the discovery of meaning in life. Older people can have spiritual concerns sometimes related to the past, sometimes to the present and sometimes to the future. All have to be addressed (Metropolitan Anthony of Sourozh 1999). Older people with dementia may have concerns in the same areas, and we must not underestimate the potential for helping them. For example, even as regards the past it is possible to sustain and sometimes to recover a person's narrative identity for a while by patient detective work and counselling, and even to achieve a measure of reconciliation with past disturbing experiences (Mills 1998).

Even when certain avenues close for the dementing person, others will likely open. A person, for example, may cease to be able to connect present and past identities. This may appear sad but it is important to realize that it is not a negative state to live in the present moment alone. In fact, many spiritual traditions emphasize the importance of aspiring to such a state. Feelings, desires, imagination, will and moral being still exist in dementing persons, and can be appreciated sometimes better by stepping into their world. Indeed, to be more rooted in the present is perhaps one of their greatest lessons to those of us who are not yet dementing.

Spiritual well-being also finds its anchor in optimism, in future hope, for oneself, for one's family, for one's community, for humankind, for all creation. In Christian terms the concept of the person made in the image of God provides a promised unique identity which the label of dementia cannot expunge. Present activities and goals are given meaning by reference to these distant horizons of meaning (Marcoen 1994). In Christian and other spiritual traditions these promises of eventual salvation and reconciliation at the end of time are very important indeed (Gerkin 1989). But we need to be reminded that redemption and eternity also exist in the present and now, and not only in the future.

Perhaps the most tangible aspect of spiritual well-being, certainly for those with dementia, is relationship. As we have seen relationship is central to the concept of the person, and it is personhood that has appeared to be most at risk in dementia. Both Christian theology and **humanistic** discussion would suggest that fear of loss of personhood with dementia becomes less a problem when we accept frailty and brokenness in relationships as our common condition. Dementing people help us to confront a reality that they no longer can hide. All of us feel the need to reach out, whether in appealing for understanding from another person, or through the lighting of a candle. For many this is the archetypal expression of prayer, of contact with ultimate reality, mysterious, unknowable and unspeakable, but calling us into relationship.

We now turn to how practice and research in the field of dementia care has changed in recent years as a result of the acknowledgement of the importance of spiritual well-being. Again our emphasis is on developments within Christian ministries, but we do refer to other spiritual faiths, and in the final sections we return again to relationships as the key to promoting spiritual well-being in dementia.

DEVELOPING THE PRACTICAL EXPRESSION OF SPIRITUALITY IN DEMENTIA CARE

King *et al.* (1994) found in their study of 300 patients in a London hospital that 232 participants had religious and/or spiritual beliefs. Certainly spiritual awareness and experiences have been reported as existing widely in the adult population of Britain (Gallop 1986). However, spiritual awareness is not the sole province of any belief system but encompasses the many different faiths contained in our increasingly secularized society. Although these many voices have tentatively begun an active dialogue, especially at community level, there is little unified discussion of the spiritual needs of people with dementia. Nonetheless, debate is forthcoming and has emerged out of a growing public realization that people with dementia may have unmet spiritual needs.

Traditionally, within the United Kingdom, the Christian Church has supported endeavours to help the dependent 'needy', including those people who are old and frail. This practice has continued in relation to dementia. It is expected other faith communities will increasingly offer their own unique insights into dementia and spirituality (Jewell 1999b), including the sacred importance of relationship and commitment to the other (Abdalati 1975; Sears 1998; Gyatso 1999).

Various Christian initiatives are now beginning to reach out to embrace other faiths and beliefs. The previous lack of dialogue can partly be explained by the strong emphasis that many spiritual traditions place on care as being the responsibility of the family and/or the faith community. For instance, Islamic beliefs include the fundamental principle of caring for frail older people within their families (Abdul-Rauf 1982). This is borne out by the very few Muslim homes for older people, and the tendency for existing homes to be for Muslims without relatives. Equally, Judaism believes that Jewish communities should care for their dependent members. This includes retaining an active responsibility for their physical and spiritual well-being when they are cared for in non-Jewish environments (van den Bergh 1997).

The Christian Council on Ageing (CCOA) began the debate with the publication of 'Dementia: a Christian Perspective' (Froggatt and Shamy 1992). Froggatt found a need for theological reflection and spiritual understanding in the paradigm of dementia care. She identified carers of people with dementia who felt isolated and abandoned by the Church and who desperately wanted guidance and support. Further, her respondents suggested that pastoral visitors and clergy had little knowledge of how to treat the person with dementia. Shamy highlighted the need to nourish spiritual well-being in dementia. She argues that the Church has a unique opportunity to offer constant commitment to meeting spiritual needs 'with at least as much informed concern as is given to providing physical care'. Shamy (1997) also emphasizes the importance of focused, simple and well-prepared rituals based on previous experiences of worship. From this work a significant literature has developed, committed to the practicalities of effective work in this field (see for example Treetops 1992, 1996). Other examples of good practice from the group include the 'memory box project' (Treetops 1999).

THE STUDY OF SPIRITUALITY AND DEMENTIA

Bruce (1998), reporting on a longitudinal study of quality of life and death of people with dementia, argues for a broad description of spiritual well-being which can be encouraged by a range of interventions. Although Kung (1980) argues that there is an ultimate reality which lies in the heart of all world religions, Kitwood *et al.* 1995 suggests that 'the fragile web of well-being in dementia' does not allow the strength to pursue this goal. However, Barrance (1999) issues a word of caution, arguing that we should not assume that we can determine the spiritual needs of all people with dementia. She questions 'Who owns the spirituality?', pointing out that it is often others who determine the needs of people with dementia. Nonetheless, the trend towards early diagnosis of dementia, together with possible pharmacological interventions, suggests that there will be an increasing number of people with mild dementia more able to verbalize their differing and diverse spiritual needs.

Barrance (1999) points out that seeking spiritual expression may be aligned to the more moneyed leisured classes. This criticism has also been levied at the humanistic approaches. Nonetheless, one of the strengths of humanistic psychology is its commitment to individual fulfilment and personal well-being. Csikszentmihalyi (1992: 53) found that a strong sense of well-being was generated by the 'flow' of peak experiences, 'when all a person's relevant skills are needed to cope with the challenges of a situation . . . and that person's attention is completely absorbed by the activity'. Similar types of experiences appear to be generated by the use of multisensory enhancements in dementia care. Barker and Pinkney's (1992) study exposed patients to varying levels of pleasurable sensory stimulation for three hours a week over a four-week period. Comparing baseline to post-session measures, they found a significant increase in levels of 'happiness' and 'level of interest', together with some lessening of 'sadness' and 'fear'. Further, Baker *et al.* (1997) suggest facilitation of verbal expression and memory recall through the use of multisensory enhancements.

Pool (1999) argues that **occupation** maintains a maximal sense of identity for people with dementia in which the sense of self is fully engaged with the activity. These findings suggest that occupation and activities can give meaning in dementia and support McColman's (1997: 211) view that the expression of spirituality 'begins with trusting life's wonder rather than fearing life's risk'. Perhaps one of the most typical forms of spiritual expression in dementia, and frequently observed by carers, is that of wonder in the face of small examples of beauty (Mills 1997). However, for people with dementia this sense of wonder requires careful nurturing. It will disappear if the experience is too great or overwhelming, probably because the task of processing extensive information is no longer possible.

ENABLING SPIRITUAL EXPRESSION THROUGH CARING RELATIONSHIPS

There are some arguments to suggest that the **altruistic** nature of caring is both biologically and culturally determined (Brown 1986; Toates 1996). Hardy (1966) goes further and boldly contends that spirituality also has a biological basis, with spiritual awareness having a survival value for our species. Certainly Bradburn (1969) found a significant association between reports of spiritual well-being and personal happiness (see Bowling 1991).

Cassidy (1988) suggests that caring for those who are sick in mind or body is a spiritual act. Especially so when the acknowledgement of the precious nature of being underpins an instinctive response to meeting unmet needs. Barrance (1999) points to the spirituality inherent in dementia care tasks where the 'utterly mundane' is undertaken with genuine respect. Further, Moffat (1996) perceives the individualization of dementia care leading to the meeting of spiritual needs. She argues that in order for spirituality to relate to everyone it must have human feelings and relationships as its focus.

Kitwood (1997a) maintains that people with dementia may continue to express spiritual well-being through relationships and in caring for others in simple ways. This implies that people with dementia need the provision of a facilitating environment where one is allowed simply 'to be' together with carer awareness of spiritual needs. However, Moffatt (1996) warns against the over-intellectualization of this task, suggesting that this may lead some carers to assume it is beyond their capabilities.

A recent survey suggests that many young dementia care workers may have few, if any, strong religious or spiritual beliefs (Williams and Norton 1999). Certainly, Tobin (1991) gives evidence that the lack of belief of service providers negatively influenced clients' and respondents' willingness to disclose their religious beliefs, whereas student researchers who believed in an afterlife found respondents to be very open and cooperative.

In addition, many carer staff may be reluctant to engage in a discussion of the 'Sacred' with clients, or to encourage spirituality-seeking behaviours, perhaps seeing this as an intensively private matter or one in which they have little to contribute. Of further concern is the realization that the spiritual needs of older people with and without dementia do not tend to be readily identified in care plans or, perhaps, to form part of keyworker/client activities. Moreover, an assessment of spiritual needs may never have been undertaken by a social worker in a needs assessment interview (Parsloe 1999). This lack of awareness amongst those who deliver care is troubling. Parsloe (1999) notes that many university social work courses largely omit spirituality and religious matters in the syllabus. In addition, most NVQ courses in direct care also overlook this topic, although directing students to allow clients freedom of religious and spiritual expression. It can be argued, therefore, that many training and academic courses pertaining to the delivery of care are negligent in this regard. Parsloe speculates that this omission may contribute to older people's inability to discuss these topics with others. Those involved in the delivery of care may have little awareness of their own spiritual needs, or indeed fail to differentiate them from religious beliefs. We would suggest that all care education should openly and positively address the wide variety of spiritual and religious expression, and to acknowledge that to be human is, as McColman (1997) states, 'to have the quality of being related to spirit'.

A COMMUNION OF COMMUNITIES

The notion of being related to spirit runs through all faiths and beliefs, whether these faiths and beliefs identify with the creator, the created or the process itself. Moreover, we find they contain common themes of peace, **justice** and a desire for positive change, even in such seemingly disparate beliefs as African traditional religion, Sikhism, Druidry and the Islamic principles of Sufism. At the heart of all spiritual belief systems is a gentleness of holding and supporting the other, a desire to reach out to help and assist. The Hindu Gospel of Sri Ramakrishna describes Ramakrishna telling Narendra, 'The roof is clearly visible, but extremely hard to reach. But if someone who has already reached it drops down a rope, he can pull another person up.'

Gyatso (1999) states that a healthy community contains a ready and mutual acceptance of the other, including their weaknesses. Perhaps better known as the Dalai Lama, this author also points out that 'compassion and love for the other is the source of all spiritual qualities'. Indeed, McColman (1997) argues, 'We are not excused from relating to the other, even when there are significant differences.' In the paradigm of dementia, Goldsmith (1999a) asks, 'Who is the real me?' We propose that the answer is the 'me' who needs you, the 'other', with your powerful mind to support the vulnerability of my mind and my fragmented sense of identity. However, the onerous nature of dementia care suggests that even the strongest of us require support. Kitwood (1997a) argues that humans are best designed to carry burdens as a communal group, which in turn is shaped by the culture of the wider community. We are community, writ both large and small.

Community, in essence, is about relationships. In Christian thinking the highest and most mysterious community of relationships is the Trinity. Inherent in this concept is a willingness of followers to relate, believe and trust in this mystical unknown. This trusting relationship with the unknown Sacred is, of course, shared by all other faiths. Moreover, it can be argued that the nature of all close human relationships share in this intrinsic 'unknowingness' and uncertainty, no matter how well explored. How well do we truly understand the other? Perhaps we might ask how well do we truly understand ourselves? James ([1892] 1960) has succinctly described 'that pit of insecurity beneath the surface of life, where, at times, the awareness of one's personal vulnerability is made sharply manifest'. To be human, therefore, is to exist in a certain introspective state of anxiousness, to have a desire for certainty while contending with uncertainty.

THE IMPORTANCE OF RELATIONSHIPS IN DEMENTIA

Mikhail Bakhtin ([1929] 1984: 287), the Russian philosopher, states that 'I cannot manage without another, I cannot become myself without another; I must find myself in another by finding another in myself (in mutual reflection and acceptance).' Heard and Lake (1997) argue that our ability to form relationships with others is given to us through evolutionary and social influences. Building on the need of the other for survival purposes, humans have developed non-verbal and symbolic patterns of relating (Trevarthen 1979; Stern 1985). This is most clearly demonstrated in the attachment between mother and child, where Bowlby (1969) argues that caregiving and care-seeking attachment behaviours in the caregiver/child dyad are adaptive and instinctive. Moreover, attachment behaviours are thought to often operate outside conscious awareness (Bretherton 1985). Attachment theory contends that the need for safety and reduction of anxiety triggers infant attachment behaviours that are activated in times of stress. Moreover, a psychodynamic perspective, which argues that the irrational unconscious influences many of our behaviours, suggests that these experiences will be represented in a variety of ways throughout vulnerable periods in the lifespan.

Miesen (1992, 1993) hypothesizes that the vulnerability associated with feelings of permanent loss and fearfulness in dementia will also reawaken such attachment experiences (Munnichs and Miesen 1986). These feelings may generate behaviours, such as parental seeking or, as is so frequently and distressingly observed in the later stages, the calling out, crying and need to be close to another. Thus it is within the uncertainty of dementia that the need for the 'certainty' of the other is made most manifest. It is only the positive nature of the relationships in dementia which make the condition bearable (Kitwood 1997b; Mills 1998).

Kitwood (1997b: 11) argues that the maintenance of personhood in dementia 'requires a living relationship with at least one other, where there is a felt bond or tie'. The older person with dementia, viewed as a 'broken vessel carrying the holy', is held and carried by the 'Thou' of the other. It is paradoxical, perhaps, that this type of relationship is less problematic in dementia which effectively destroys psychological defences but can permit the person with dementia to relate more 'authentically' to another (Kitwood and Bredin 1992c). This vulnerability of being can allow the discarding of defences by those of us without dementia, making it possible to glance over the barricades of years, if only for a brief moment. In this brief meeting of 'person to person' it becomes possible for both to experience a true reality of being and unconditional acceptance from another (Mills 1997). Although often unrecognized, we argue that this form of spiritual encounter is frequently observed in good dementia care. We have argued elsewhere that it is, perhaps, this type of mutually empowering relationship, based on attachment experiences, which attracts people to the work (Mills *et al.* 1999). We suggest that it is within this work that the practical expression of spirituality in dementia is made most manifest.

Throughout this chapter we have continually returned to the topic of relationships in their many secular and spiritual guises. We have examined them against the present culture of dementia care and their influence on personality and personhood. We consider that they have a profound influence on our own spirituality and spiritual beliefs whatever our faith, creed or path to enlightenment. Moreover, the impenetrable nature of spirituality has close associations with the inherent 'unknowingness' which is part of many relationships. Dementia is also about not knowing and not being known. This state of being should be no bar to spiritual expression. What is merely required is another to help us to find our own particular spiritual light.

FURTHER READING

Jewell, A (ed.) (1999) *Spirituality and Ageing*. London: Jessica Kingsley.

Kimble, M.A., McFadden, S.H., Ellor, J.W. and Seeber, J.J. (eds) (1995) *Aging, Spirituality and Religion: A Handbook*. Minneapolis, MN: Fortress Press.

ACKNOWLEDGEMENT

We would like to thank Dementia Voice Bristol for their assistance in the preparation of this chapter and our colleagues Revd Prebendary Peter Speck and Dr Fionnuala McKiernan for their helpful suggestions.

5

JANE GILLIARD

The perspectives of people with dementia, their families and their carers

KEY POINTS

- It is only recently that attention has been paid to understanding the perceptions and views of people with dementia.
- We need to understand the different perspectives of people with dementia, their carers and their wider families.
- Our understanding of the perspectives of people with dementia is still limited.
- There is evidence that given the right opportunities, people with dementia are able to express views and preferences about a wide range of matters affecting their lives.

INTRODUCTION

When we consider the numbers of people affected by dementia, any statistics are almost certainly an underestimate. They take no account of any of the other players who are involved – the spouses, children, grandchildren, siblings, friends and neighbours. The diagnosis of dementia has been likened to throwing a stone into a pond (Tibbs 1995). The ripples spread out across the pond (Gilliard 1996). If the point where the stone lands represents the person with dementia, the ripples spread out to encompass the main or **primary caregiver**, often a spouse. They then move on to cover the **secondary carers**, who might typically be adult children who support one parent who is caring for the other parent. Finally the ripples continue outwards becoming ever more gentle, but still

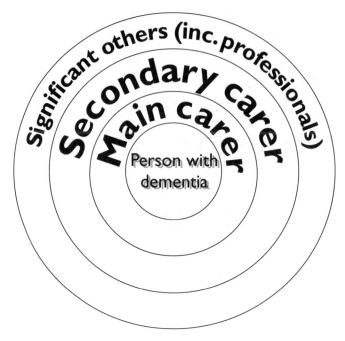

Figure 5.1 The ripples in the dementia pond

affecting a third group, whom we might call significant others. Significant others are often the children of the secondary carers, or sometimes the brothers and/or sisters of the person with dementia and/or the main carer, and often the friends and neighbours of the main players.

It can be helpful to change the analogy from a stone thrown into a pond, and consider the effect of the diagnosis of dementia as the lighting on a stage. Traditionally the main spotlight has focused on the carer of the person with dementia. Service provision attempted to address their needs but scant regard was paid to the needs of the person with dementia him/herself. **Respite care**, for example, was seen as an opportunity to give the carer a break, but little attention was paid to what happened to the person with dementia while he or she was in respite care. The development of the 'new culture' of dementia care (Kitwood and Benson 1995) moved the spotlight. Now it began to focus on the person with dementia. But as this person's condition deteriorated, he or she slipped further into the shadows at the edge of the stage. Already in the shadows were the secondary carers and significant others. They had never been in the spotlight. What is needed is a stage that is fully lit; where the person with dementia is centre-stage; and where the other actors also receive their share of the limelight.

The organization of most service provision only allows the spotlight to focus on one or possibly two players in the drama. The way family life is often arranged means that people are not so easily isolated. Those who **commission** and plan services, as well as those who provide them, should take a more holistic view of the impact of dementia. This chapter will address the experience from the perspectives of all players. It will first consider what we understand of the subjective experience of dementia, that is from the point of view of the person with dementia. It will then move to consider the family's experience. Finally, it will address the needs of others involved in the care of someone with dementia, including the role of, and the impact on, paid carers.

THE SUBJECTIVE EXPERIENCE OF PEOPLE WITH DEMENTIA

Carers are often left bewildered by the changes that they observe as their relative struggles to cope with the onset of cognitive impairment. Practitioners report that carers sometimes say that they wish they could get inside the head of their relative to really experience what the person with dementia feels. If only the person experiencing dementia could say what it feels like. In this, dementia is no different from illnesses causing physical pain. We cannot experience the pain of others, but we can begin to understand it from their descriptions. In dementia care we lack such descriptions, although there are a few examples:

> It's one thing I've been getting for quite a time now and that is a distant feeling that things are misting over and that I'm trying to remember. There's things coming through faintly that I'm trying to remember what they are. There was a patch of that and it's in a shroud of mist and I can't remember what it was I was trying to remember.

> It's as if my head was full of little bubbles, like a glass of lemonade and sometimes the bubbles all rise to the surface and my head clears. Then it slowly fills with bubbles again.
>
> (Keady and Gilliard 1999: 248–9)

Kitwood (1997b) has suggested seven 'access routes' by which we might be able to further our understanding of the subjective experience of dementia:

- the accounts that have been written by people who have dementia during a period when their cognitive powers are relatively intact (for example, McGowin 1993);
- careful listening to what people say in some kind of interview or group work (for example, Cheston 1996; Goldsmith 1996);
- attending carefully and imaginatively to what people say in the ordinary course of life;
- learning from the actions or behaviour of people who have dementia;
- the possibility of consulting people who have undergone an illness with dementia-like features and who are able to experience something of what they have experienced;
- the use of our own poetic imagination (for example, Killick 1997);
- the possibility of using role play, or acting the part of a person with dementia.

Maybe one of the reasons why we have so little information about the subjective experience of dementia is because we simply have not asked. Dementia carries with it a stigma that feeds our fears, and a concern that we will open a Pandora's box if we ask too many, or even any, questions. For many there remains a conviction that people with dementia are unable to communicate with us at all, so to ask them what they are feeling is a waste of time. Experience in practice and in research studies is that people with dementia have plenty to say to us if only we take the time and trouble to listen (for example Keady *et al.* 1995). The challenge is to open up the channels of communication so that we can hear what people with dementia want to tell us.

The traditional staging of dementia is based on a medical model:

- healthy;
- questionable dementia;
- mild dementia;
- moderate dementia;
- severe dementia.

But this model tells us little, if anything, about the personal experience of having dementia. A nine-stage process, defined by Keady and Nolan (1994b, 1995) and informed by the experiences of people with dementia, is a more useful framework for considering the process. The stages they identify are:

- slipping – the person gradually becomes aware of lapses in his or her memory but discounts them;
- suspecting – the lapses become more frequent, cannot be so easily discounted and the person suspects that something is not right;
- covering up – the person makes a conscious effort to hide his or her difficulties;
- revealing – the person shares his or her concerns with someone close;
- confirming – outside help is sought and a diagnosis obtained;
- maximizing – the person adapts by using coping strategies;
- disorganization – there is a diminishing ability and awareness;
- decline – the demands of care become more prominent;
- death.

Further exploration of this model, in a study involving people who were aware that they had Alzheimer's disease and willing to talk about its impact, shows that it gives us greater insight into the complex process of adaptation and adjustment to dementia (Keady and Gilliard 1999). This study demonstrates that the transition into Alzheimer's disease is often a very secretive process. People often recognized their difficulties but kept their fears to themselves:

> At the beginning it was so dark, I couldn't believe I was doing these things. I felt so stupid and didn't want to share it with anyone else. I had trouble getting the right word out and forgetting people's names. It was awful.
>
> (Keady and Gilliard 1999: 241)

The participants in the study demonstrated strategies for keeping their feelings and concerns secret. They also went further and used strategies for 'covering their tracks', for example:

• keeping my fears and feelings secret;
• keeping any further memory loss to myself;
• making up stories to fill in the gaps.

Fairbairn (1997) has commented on how insight and lack of insight can create tensions for people with dementia and for carers. He quotes lack of insight as probably the commonest cause of lack of cooperation within care. Conversely, insight may be a crucial factor in asserting the right to remain independent.

Some of the people with dementia in the Keady and Gilliard (1999) study were able to sustain a prolonged period of subterfuge in an attempt to keep from others the reality of their difficulties. Sometimes, those around them tacitly colluded with the strategy. For example, one wife described how she was becoming concerned about her husband's driving abilities, but was reluctant to confront him. And at the same time he was becoming concerned about his ability to manage in other areas of his life. Neither told the other of their concerns, but eventually both decided to confide in a third party. By coincidence they chose the same person and their friend was able to act as broker in encouraging them to share their concerns with each other.

Eventually, though, a point is reached where the subterfuge can be maintained no longer. There follows a period which Keady and Gilliard (1999) call 'sharing the load'. That is, the key players are forced to confront the fact that something is amiss, that one of them is experiencing difficulties in maintaining everyday life. Sharing the load involves telling another about one's concerns. In the example above, the husband and wife partnership made separate and independent decisions to share their thoughts with a close friend. Among the participants in the study this was an unusual decision. Much more common was the move to share one's worries with the person to whom one is closest, and that was usually one's spouse. Interestingly, the expression of concern led no further. It was often the case that those involved in the drama still found excuses for why this was happening – adapting to retirement, bereavement, general ageing. Only as the difficulties persisted, worsened, and reached a stage where they were interfering with everyday life and activities, did those in the study make a conscious decision to seek outside help. This is the stage that Keady and Nolan (1994b and 1995) call confirming, and it marks the start of the process by which people with dementia are assessed, possibly receive a diagnosis, certainly take on board the label of 'dementia' and begin their journey through the system of services.

In practice what generally happens at this stage is that people who are concerned about their cognitive functioning visit their own doctor who will form an opinion about what is going on. As a result of geographical accident in some cases, and of the interest or otherwise of the general practitioner in other cases, some people will be referred for a more thorough assessment. Even if this happens, the likely result is that the individuals and their families will be left to deal with the situation on a day-by-day basis until, as things deteriorate, they eventually reach a point at which they can no longer cope without support. Those who work in health and social services often comment that they only become involved with people with dementia at a time of crisis and, they say, 'If only we could have known about the situation earlier . . .'

SUPPORT AND INFORMATION NEEDS OF PEOPLE WITH DEMENTIA

We know relatively little about the information and support needs of people with dementia in the early days when they are adjusting to their new situation. McGowin (1993), in her first-hand account, *Living in the Labyrinth*, shares some of her thoughts about what would have been helpful to her. In particular, she would have liked a peer support group – a group of fellows travelling through the same maze with whom she could have shared her feelings and learned from the experience of others. As a result of the publication of her book and the emergence of the person with dementia as someone with a voice, there has been a growth of such **support groups** for people with dementia in the USA. This has not been a trend that the UK has followed. While there are small pockets of work being carried out by inspired individuals (Cheston 1996; Bender 1999b), there has been no consistent widespread development of support groups. There is an ongoing project evaluating psychotherapeutic support groups for people with dementia. The groups are small, approximately six to eight people, and time-limited. They are facilitated by at least two staff members and seek to support people with dementia as they come to terms with their condition (Cheston and Jones 2000).

Although the main focus of the Keady and Gilliard (1999) study was the process by which people adjust to their dementia, they also uncovered some views on the support people in the early stages of dementia would appreciate. These included having someone to talk to and an opportunity to learn how to improve their memory. Support groups may meet both these goals. Individual counselling may also create an opportunity to explore issues such as loss, changing relationships and adjustment (Whitsted-Lipinska 1999). The evidence to support the need for qualified counselling compared with, for example, volunteer befriending is still thin. It seems that there is still plenty of work to be done in identifying what support would be most beneficial in the earliest days. Many of the respondents in the Keady and Gilliard (1999) study expressed their apprehension about the assessment process. For example:

> I could manage most of the questions but not all of them. I got scared as the time went on as I wanted to do well and had trouble working out what was happening.
>
> (Keady and Gilliard, in press)

Perhaps a system of pre- and post-assessment counselling, as established in the HIV and AIDS services, would be helpful.

Keady and Gilliard (1999) asked the participants in their study about their need for information about dementia. The authors identified five areas of information most frequently requested. They were:

- technical information about what was happening to the brain;
- information about the causes of Alzheimer's disease;
- practical information about services and benefits;
- advice about the changing relationships with family members;
- information to be provided in accessible forms – for example, large print or on audio cassette.

Kitwood's book, *Dementia Reconsidered*, is subtitled '*The Person Comes First*' (Kitwood 1997b). Often when people are working to adjust to the losses associated with dementia and finding it difficult to maintain their former social façade, other people around them are finding it even harder to adjust. Fear and ignorance may lead them to distance themselves from the person experiencing dementia. The dementia becomes the all-important aspect, and fear of doing or saying the wrong thing leads to a situation where it is difficult to focus on the person, even in situations where people have known each other well for a long time. Kitwood exhorts us to take a view of 'the PERSON with dementia', rather than 'the person with DEMENTIA'. Some people may take the easy way out and avoid social contact with the person with dementia as much as possible. This leads to a vicious circle where the person with dementia becomes increasingly isolated. It may also serve to reinforce a negative self-image.

We still have a paucity of information about the views of people with dementia as service users. Goldsmith (1996) first highlighted this gap in our knowledge. His work opened the debate and created awareness that we should take account of the views of people with dementia in assessments for services and in the review procedures. The care in the community legislation (NHS and Community Care Act 1990) requires **care managers** to seek users' views when making assessments, but people with dementia have often been marginalized in this process. The carer is treated as their advocate and yet there is anecdotal evidence to suggest that the needs of people with dementia and the needs of those who care for them are often quite different.

Ongoing work at the Dementia Services Development Centre at the University of Stirling is seeking practical ways in which we can hear the views of people with dementia as service users (Allan 2000). Allan is considering ways to hear the views of people in the later stages of dementia when verbal communication is limited. The project includes the imaginative use of creative arts, the interpretion of behaviour, the use of pictures in offering choice and in eliciting views, and the use of third party approaches (for example, asking people with dementia how they would describe a service to others who may want to attend). This work has served to highlight how little we know about the subjective experiences of people in the later stages of dementia. Perhaps the best known example to date of work that seeks to understand this is the writing of John Killick (Killick 1997; Killick and Cordonnier 2000) who uses the words of people with dementia to create poetry.

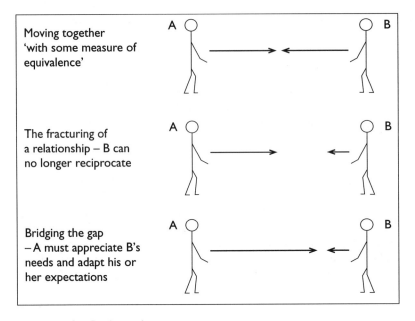

Figure 5.2 Bridging the communication gap

Dementia almost inevitably leads to a difficulty with language. This makes it hard for people with dementia to describe their experience to others. Reaching out to understand these experiences requires an extra effort on the part of those of us who do not have dementia. Crimmens (1996) has eloquently and graphically shown how those who do not have dementia need to go the extra distance to facilitate communication with people with dementia. Figure 5.2 shows how she demonstrates the breakdown in normal patterns of communication when someone develops dementia, and how the onus is on those who do not have dementia to bridge the gap when dementia fractures the relationship. This may require all our imagination, skill, patience and a good deal of time. The reward will be the empowerment of people with dementia in a way that challenges traditional thinking. For further discussion of communication see Chapter 9.

THE SPOTLIGHT MOVES TO THE CARER

There comes a point in the career of a person with dementia where it is difficult to separate the needs of that person from those of the family. To use the earlier dramatic analogy, it is as if there has been a spotlight on the person with dementia and a spotlight on his or her nearest relative (by now identified by others, even if not by him or herself, as the carer). Now the play has reached a stage where the interdependency of the two main actors is such that their spotlights are moving towards each other to become one. In actual fact, what tends to happen at this stage is that the carer's spotlight eclipses that of the person with dementia, and there is a move towards a requirement for outside services, which have been designed to rescue the carer and contain the person with dementia. Fortunately the growing acceptance of the 'new culture' means that there is a growing movement towards meeting the needs of people with dementia as well.

THE CARERS' EXPERIENCE

Our ignorance about what it feels like to have dementia from the point of view of the person with dementia seems especially unbalanced when compared with the wealth of studies that consider the experience of being a carer. There are studies on spouse carers (for example, Fitting *et al.* 1986; Cahill 2000), adult children who are carers (for example, Cahill and Shapiro 1998), male carers (Harris 1993; Fisher 1994), female carers (Parker and Lawton 1990a, b), black carers (for example, Patel *et al.* 1998), and gay carers (Alzheimer's Society 2000).

From these we learn, for example, that men often manage caring by framing it in an occupational role – seeing it as a job of work (Fisher 1994). This fits with the way they have been used to living their lives. In this respect they may manage caring better than women because they are not afraid to ask for time off – after all, that is what you expect when you work. In addition, women are socialized to care so it is expected that they will slip more easily into the caring role. Men are therefore often more successful in their requests for support from statutory services than women in similar positions. Other research has demonstrated that wives cared for their husbands because they wanted to, whereas daughters generally felt that they had to care (Cahill and Shapiro 1998; Cahill 1999).

The emergence of silent or hidden groups, for example black or gay carers, is a relatively new phenomenon. The literature is scarce but there is an emerging awareness of their needs being distinct and separate.

The difficulties faced by those who care for someone who has dementia were highlighted in an early but still standard text, *The 36-hour Day* (Mace and Rabins 1985). As its title suggests, the 'job' of being a carer can be all-consuming, but often unrecognized. In the same way as dementia develops insidiously and almost imperceptibly, the changing roles of a partner who becomes a carer slide gently from one phase to the next. Keady and Gilliard (1999) found that some of the coping strategies adopted by people with dementia were mirrored by their nearest family member. There was, for example, often a tacit collusion between carers and the people with dementia. When the people with dementia 'covered their tracks', the primary carers also often covered their tracks for them.

Family members and others who provide care often do not recognize themselves as fulfilling the role of 'carer'. They may need to be introduced by professionals to the idea that they have become carers. At what stage does a wife, for example, cease this role and become instead 'a carer'? Some would argue that they never lose the original role, while others would point to the changes brought about by dementia and accept a change in status. Sometimes this makes it easier to take on the mantle of 'carer'. The process has been described as a 'living bereavement' (Taylor 1987). The phrase caught on and many carers identify with its sentiments. But I have argued elsewhere (Gilliard 1992) that there are aspects of the traditional model of bereavement as described by Kübler-Ross (1970) that are not helpful in the caring situation. The final adaptive and moving-on stages are particularly irrelevant for those who grieve for someone whom they perceive they have lost to dementia but who remains a live and present reality.

One of the legacies of Taylor's (1987) ideas about 'a living bereavement' has been the negativity associated with caring for someone with dementia. Many studies share a negative language, using emotion-laden terms like 'burden', 'stress', 'victim'. While it would be naive to suggest that it is not difficult to care for someone with dementia, carers can feel ground down even further by this negative stereotyping. It was as long ago as 1987 that it was first suggested that we should take a more widely critical view of caring (Motenko 1987) but we still frequently hear reference to 'sufferers' and 'victims'. Nolan *et al.* (1996) suggest a more balanced approach, looking at carers' satisfactions as well as their difficulties (for discussion see Chapter 11). Their work provides a British context for earlier work undertaken in Canada, which sought to raise the profile of positive aspects of caring (Cohen *et al.* 1994). To reframe the caring role, and to enable carers to see some of the more positive experiences they have had and the new skills they have learnt, can be an empowering process for them.

We can also empower carers by providing them with the information and support they say they need. Gilliard and Rabins (1999) identify six main areas in which carers want information:

- *The diagnosis* – they need to know what is wrong with their relative, even if this confirms their fears. Although many people have heard of Alzheimer's disease, many are still uncertain of exactly what it means for the person with dementia. In addition, many will not be familiar with other forms of dementia.
- *The prognosis* – carers often want to know how long their relative will live, and the course of the condition. This information helps them plan for the future. Many carers will want their relative to live as long as possible, perhaps on the premise that while there is life there is hope. Others will say that they find it difficult to witness the effects of dementia and argue that they do not want their family member to suffer.
- *The practical implications for the person with dementia and for the family* – information about what to expect in the future enables carers to develop strategies for coping. The challenge is to know how much or how little information to give. Training for carers has been shown to be an effective tool for enabling them to care well and to feel good about their ability to care (Brodaty and Gresham 1989; Magni *et al.* 1995).

- The health and social services which may be able to help.
- Financial entitlements.
- Legal aspects.

These last three aspects of information enable those who have to impart the information to balance the difficult news about the diagnosis with more positive elements. Carers can build a library of material that they can dip into at various points of their caring career. Allowing carers to hold this information leaves them with some control over the way they deal with the situation. Sadly, many carers are not given this basic information. Or those giving the information think they have done their job, but the information has not been accessible to the listener. Carers need the information to be presented to them clearly, without the use of jargon, in a format that is accessible to them, and they may need to hear the same information repeatedly (Gilliard and Rabins 1999). The result of misheard information, or simply a lack of information, may be a downward spiral of helplessness, lack of self-worth and feelings of an increasing inability to continue caring (Seligman *et al.* 1968).

While working to empower people with dementia and to empower their carers, practitioners are often faced with a dilemma. There is often a tension between what people with dementia feel they need and what their carers want. A typical example is when a carer reaches the stage of needing a break, but the person they care for cannot understand the need to go to day or respite care. Many practitioners are faced at this point with the dilemma of deciding whose needs are paramount, and which person is their 'real client'.

Those who provide services have to work with the tensions between service users and carers and recognize that carers are often very protective of the person they care for, for example, Maguire *et al.* (1996) who report on a study conducted in Dublin. This study found that, while 71 per cent of carers would want to be told their diagnosis if they thought they had dementia, only 17 per cent of those attending a memory clinic with a relative wanted their relative to be informed. Other studies have found it difficult to gain access to talk to people with dementia without a carer being present (Gillies 1995; Keady and Gilliard 1999). This protectiveness, and a feeling that caring is a duty and an act of love, may lead to low take-up of formal services (Canadian Study of Health and Aging 1994).

In addition, there are sometimes tensions between carers' needs and what service providers can offer. Despite the exhortations of the NHS and Community Care Act 1990 that services should be 'needs led', provision in the UK is still often dominated by traditional models and the need to make the client fit the service. This may lead to added frustration and stress for carers, as well as exacerbating their feelings of guilt. It is time to break the mould of traditional service provision for people with dementia and to begin to give some lateral thought to alternative models, perhaps borrowing in examples from other fields (like learning disability) or from other countries. It may be, for example, that there would be less tension between people with dementia, their carers and professionals if the services provided had more to offer all those involved.

THE WIDER FAMILY AND OTHER PEOPLE

This chapter has considered how dementia affects the various parties involved (see Figure 5.1 above). The circles start with the person with dementia
and spread out to include the primary carer. The ripples continue outwards
to encompass those whom I called secondary carers, and finally significant
others. Little attention has been paid to the impact of dementia on these
other key players. Studies focusing on carers have considered the impact of
dementia on the primary carer, whatever the relationship may be, but have
tended to overlook the importance of secondary carers. These may be adult
children supporting a parent who is the main carer. The fact that they too
have a relative who is developing dementia will inevitably impact on their
lives. If primary carers experience aspects of a 'living bereavement', secondary carers too will experience a variety of emotions associated not only with
the dementia in one relative, but also with watching the emotional impact on
another.

Secondary carers are often women, usually daughters, and they may well
be in the now-recognized situation that the British call the 'care trap' and
that Americans call the 'sandwich generation' (Brody 1981). That is, they are
in a position of balancing a dependent family and ageing parents, possibly
with a career as well. More and more women will find themselves in this
situation, as they delay having children until later in life, as they place more
importance on developing their careers and as the older generation continues
to live longer.

Other secondary carers will be, for example, siblings or good friends of
those who have dementia. There is often a tension for them in balancing their
own feelings with a need to support the primary carer. Grief takes many
different forms and a friend will grieve differently from a spouse. There is
anecdotal evidence that secondary carers work to conceal their own feelings
from the primary carer so that they can appear to give wholehearted and
unconditional support.

There are also those whom I have called significant others; people who
know the person with dementia. They may, for example, be grandchildren,
work colleagues, friends, neighbours and acquaintances. Our knowledge about
these groups varies. We have little information about how grandchildren relate to grandparents with dementia. Work in the Netherlands is demonstrating how caring for people with dementia and for toddlers in the same facility
can have a positive outcome for both parties (Mercken 1998). There may be
more we can learn about the interactions between children or young people
and their relatives with dementia.

Carers often complain about the isolation that they find in caring for someone with dementia. Friends and neighbours begin to drift away until they
cease to visit altogether, their fears fed by uncertainty about what to say, how
to respond and what to expect from dementia.

Another important group of people affected by dementia includes those
who come into contact with people with dementia through their work. This

chapter has already considered the role of the care manager in listening to the views of people with dementia, and the challenges that this raises. Others find themselves working with people with dementia almost by accident. Many care assistants are unqualified and untrained. They may be very caring, but they do not have the knowledge or experience that allows them to provide best quality person-focused care. The work is unglamorous and it may even be difficult to own publicly that this is how you spend your days (Packer 1999). Those who work in dementia care have a duty to work to raise its profile as worthwhile and fulfilling. Training and empowering all those who work with people with dementia, in much the same way as we have argued we should do for unpaid carers, may go some way to redressing the balance.

Finally there is the general public. Those of us who are passionate about our work in dementia care become frustrated by the fear and lack of understanding in the general public that leads to comments about how depressing this work must be (Downs 2000). There is a need to address this fear at source and to continue the work of raising public awareness and education.

PERSONAL AND FICTIONAL ACCOUNTS

Finally, it may be helpful to widen our reading about dementia beyond the academic literature and to consider first-hand and fictional accounts. Two remarkable books by McGowin (1993) and Davis (1989) give very different accounts of the experience of dementia and serve to reinforce the notion of the individuality of each person with dementia (Kitwood 1997b). Similarly, accounts written by carers not only serve to highlight the frustrations and occasional joys of being a carer, but also act as reminders of the reality of dementia in everyday life. The most notable recent examples are the books of John Bayley (1998) and Linda Grant (1998). Works of fiction, too, can communicate a view of dementia in a powerful way. The novels of Forster (1989) and Ignatieff (1993), for example, have a telling and dramatic effect. Dementia has even reached our television screens, in documentaries, in dramas and even in 'soap operas'. Few who watched the programme *Malcolm and Barbara – A Love Story* (Granada Television) will forget seeing Malcolm and Barbara as they struggled to manage his dementia on a day-to-day basis. A recent story line in *ER* (Channel 4) about a doctor who tried to continue working while he slipped into the early stages of dementia had a similarly powerful effect.

CONCLUSION

Perhaps the fundamental question we should ask ourselves is not how we treat people with dementia, but rather why should we treat people with dementia differently from anyone else.

FURTHER READING

Goldsmith, M. (1996) *Hearing the Voice of People with Dementia: Opportunities and Obstacles*. London: Jessica Kingsley.

Mace, N. and Rabins, P. (1985) *The 36-hour Day*. London: Age Concern.

McGowin, D. (1993) *Living in the Labyrinth*. Cambridge: Mainsail Press.

SECTION 2

Practice knowledge and development

6

CHARLOTTE L. CLARKE

Understanding practice development

KEY POINTS

- There is a current drive to promote 'evidence-based practice', but there are many ways of understanding evidence with different implications for practice.
- Health and social care practitioners need to be able to both use and create knowledge for their own practice.
- Research can be used to advance the care of people with dementia, not least through practitioner research, but there is a need to consider some of the methodological difficulties in this area.
- Practice development research is about: being part of good practice, collaboration and mutual learning, change in a local environment, challenging and examining key concepts and values, being led by clients.
- Interpersonal, inter-professional and organizational processes, such as ownership, can make or break developments in practice.

INTRODUCTION

Health and social care practice is now under intense pressure to be accountable for its actions, and consequently able to articulate a therapeutic and economic rationale for interventions with clients. In seeking to respond to such public and professional demands, practitioners have turned to the **knowledge base** which informs their particular profession's practice, and at times found not just that knowledge base wanting but, moreover, the practitioners' awareness of that knowledge base sadly lacking. As the knowledge base has come under scrutiny, a strong critique of the nature of knowledge has been apparent, with the National Health Service even ranking knowledge on the basis of the **methodology** used to create it (DoH 1996). In parallel, investment has been made in engaging practitioners in that knowledge through mechanisms such as clinical guidelines, to ensure that wherever possible the most highly rated knowledge is central to care decision making. However, this approach to accountability – demonstrating 'best practice', '**evidence-based practice**' and 'clinical effectiveness' – becomes rather problematic in some areas of care and for some client groups, not least people with dementia, grounded as dementia care is in multiple understandings of philosophy and practice.

KNOWLEDGE AND PRACTICE

The concept of practice development is poorly defined in literature, although one way of understanding it is as a concern about how we use and create knowledge to inform our understanding and practice of client care (Clarke 1998). However, knowledge is not neutral or objective. Rather, the knowledge that is created and valued is subject to political vagaries, societal norms and professional interpretations of care. There can be few areas where this is more apparent than in dementia care. The history of dementia care can be used to illustrate this, with the nature of intervention emanating from the dominant moral framework of the time. The early twentieth century heralded a movement to exclude people with mental illness from the rest of society, and to contain them within large institutions. Now this has been replaced by the 'new culture' of dementia care (Kitwood 1997b) which emphasizes the personhood of people with dementia and their right to a lifestyle in which they are valued members. The criteria used to determine good practice have shifted in line with societal shifts in defining that which is 'good'.

Evidence about 'good' practice cannot be separated from beliefs about that which is valued and correct in any society. Enquiry which is inconsistent with societies' beliefs will probably never be sought, funded, articulated or disseminated because it is not near the top of the agenda of research or practice development activity. Further, in utilizing evidence, we become increasingly aware of not only what we know, but also that which we do not know. We do not know the effectiveness and efficacy of a great many health and social care interventions – this is not to say that they are not effective and efficient, but simply that the evidence for their effectiveness is beyond current knowledge.

These societal beliefs and values about dementia care impact on the perspectives of knowledge for different professional groups; the knowledge held by family carers and by people with dementia themselves. These differential knowledges result in many understandings of an individual's care. The variety of issues that arise from the application of different knowledge bases are explored in Example 6.1.

Example 6.1   Continence management

The management of care for people with dementia is dominated by risk assessment and management, which emphasizes the maintenance of personal physical safety and that of others (Baragwanath 1997; Clarke and Heyman 1998). Further, services are largely reactive in their care, intervening at the points of crisis. The points at which services 'can't cope' act as triggers for changes in service provision. This may even result in a change in care environment for individuals as they are moved on to the next level of service provision, one which supposedly provides the resources to cope with their needs. This may involve, for example, moving from family care to residential home, to nursing home and to NHS continuing care (Davison and Reed 1995). However, although continence care for older people with a mental illness presents a number of challenges to services, it does not play a major part in these primary determinants of service provision: the physical risk of incontinence is perceived to be restricted to potential spillage and skin damage. Also, continence management rarely acts as a 'can't cope' point for services because it is a problem that can, quite literally, be contained. Similarly, although troublesome, the management of incontinence does not appear to be as much of a source of burden for family carers as is disruption to their relationship (Keady 1996).

However, the instrumental management of incontinence obscures the impact of events of incontinence on the individual, with associated disturbances in behaviour and consequently their relationship with those who care for them. Continence care for older people with a mental illness becomes of great importance when their sense of well-being is considered (Gold 1992). For example, Dowd (1991) found that for women with urinary incontinence, the central issue was its threat to their self-esteem and self-respect. These are recognized as key features of **well-being** for people with dementia (Kitwood and Bredin 1992c). Most people are able to demonstrate periods of insight, despite the apparent severity of their dementia (Fairbairn 1997) and will recognize times when their dignity is being compromised, such as happens when they are incontinent or when the pads associated with a containment form of management require to be changed.

Thus continence care for people with dementia may be regarded as troublesome but manageable, and consequently it rarely acts as a trigger for preventative intervention or as a major issue when carers are faced with other more demanding needs which require to be met. However, continence care may also be regarded as a central aspect to the well-being and self-esteem of the person with dementia. It has such a major impact on the relationship between people with dementia and their carers that Gold (1992) describes continence care as more than a quality of care issue, but rather a quality of life issue.

Practice development is not concerned solely with the *use* of evidence by practitioners in effective care, but also with the role of practitioners in *creating* knowledge. The capacity to create knowledge is a concern within both health services and social services (Fuller and Petch 1995; MacDonald 1997) and is central to the ability of a profession to define its own knowledge base (Fish 1998). However, the role of practitioners in knowledge creation is considerably less clear than their role in knowledge use, and while the responsibility to deliver care is unquestioned, the responsibility to develop that care and contribute to a professional knowledge base attracts considerably more ambivalence (Kitchen 1997).

The ways in which practitioners create knowledge is quite distinctive. It is very explicitly located in the context of the particular client group characteristics, and in the environment of care. This knowledge may result in a development in the cognitive understanding of the care of people with dementia (which may or may not translate into altered practices) rather than visible and overt practice change. This is what Brown (1995) describes as the contemplative growth process that typifies knowledge development. Indeed, Bell and Procter (1998: 68) call for 'a recognition that the association between "doing" research and "using" research is not linear . . . Practice development thrives on an association between "thinking" and "working" which is articulated by "meaning" as depicted in the developmental model of change'. It is this reconceptualization of care need and care delivery that is arguably most important for health and social care practitioners in working with people with dementia and their families.

Dementia care knowledges

Knowledge, research and practice are very interrelated. These are cyclical in relationship to each other, with practice being determined by the value placed on knowledge and the sources of knowledge by professional groups and by society. Research is an activity that generates knowledge and so it is a conduit between practice, knowledge and society. At various points it describes, challenges, critiques and explains social and health policy and practice, as illustrated in Example 6.2.

The relationship between knowledge and practice is particularly apparent in the area of risk knowledge and management for and by people with dementia. The particular and individualistic knowledge of family carers is very different

---

Example 6.2   Carer experience

Throughout the 1980s, research into the quality of life of carers was defined by stress and burden such that caring was seen to be an overwhelmingly negative experience with a potentially deleterious effect on carer health. Eventually, the validity of such a restricted conceptualization of caring and indeed of burden itself was questioned (Vitaliano et al. 1991), and carers' stress was even challenged as a creation of the stress researchers (Kahana and Kinney 1991; Opie 1992). It is only recently that more qualitative and interaction research such as that by Wuest et al. (1994) has highlighted how central the caring relationship is to the caring experience. Thus there has been a transition from developing services as external buffers to stress (for example, respite care) to recognizing the internal complexities of the caring relationship (for example, lifespan reciprocity).

---

to the collective and technical knowledge of health and social care practitioners, yet it is from these knowledge bases that each frames its ideas of risk and need (Clarke and Heyman 1998). Tied up in family caring are risks associated with the biography of the individual and the family, and interpersonal aspects of their relationship. These perceived risks colour the nature of care and the location of that care such that, for example, care outside the domestic environment may be seen as a substantial threat. This is a perspective that may identify different needs than those identified by practitioners. However, until different knowledge bases and their impact on the construction of care are recognized, professional practice will fail to engage with individuals in a way that respects, and works in partnership with, individual understandings of their own care needs.

We can explain this further by examining the knowledges of dementia care and their impact on professional practice. Just as different types of evidence are appropriate for different circumstances, so different knowledges of dementia and dementia care all have a valuable role to play. Indeed, Berg *et al.* (1998), based on interviews with 13 nurses caring for people with dementia, discuss the close interrelationship of different sources of knowledge that inform care. They note 'the delicate interpretation process required, to adapt care to the individual patient, was based on knowledge about the patient's personality, life history and disease progression in combination with the nurses' interpretation of the current situation' (p. 271). The diversity and complexity of knowledge bases is demonstrated in Section 1 of this book.

The different knowledges of dementia and dementia care have important ramifications for the way in which we understand professional practice. Health and social care is largely orientated to the identification of need and the management or resolution of problems identified. However, identification of need is as diverse as the knowledge bases upon which it rests (McWalter *et al.* 1994). For example, in a study which compared a new residential facility for people with dementia with a traditional care home, McAllister and Silverman (1999) found that the new home used a social and family-orientated model of care working which emphasized a balance between safety and autonomy. This was quite different to the traditional care home that emphasized safety through a medicalization of physical care, rigid work routines and a task orientation. In another **qualitative** study, of a special care unit for people with dementia, Morgan and Stewart (1999) identify the relationship of need to physical environment, and propose a model of dementia care environments which are based on the tripartite relationship between physical and social environments and the organizational context. However, such diverse understanding of need is usually subsumed beneath the dominance of physical safety as the primary driver of care management, Caldock (1996) arguing that even in social care, medical needs and assessment dominate. For example, in early onset dementia, Tindall and Manthorpe (1997) argue that the perceived needs of people are currently located in beliefs about norms of society, justice and equality, rather than in a knowledge base informed by research. Thus there remains a need to develop further theoretical frameworks to inform professional practice in early onset

---

Example 6.3   Negotiating compliance

Take, for example, the potential (and frequent) dilemma faced when a minibus arrives to take a person with dementia to the local day centre, to find that the person firmly refuses to go; the family carer is fraught, has had little sleep and despairs at the possible lack of a break that day. To what extent is it acceptable to cajole, not to say coerce or bribe, the person with dementia into the minibus? Accept the biomedical model and the answer becomes relatively easy. Even working within a psychosocial model, it can be argued that day care provides necessary stimulation and social contact for the person with dementia and relieves the stress of the family. However, working within an interactional model creates unresolvable dilemmas, as cajoling is seen to destroy just a little more of the individual's self-determination and rights.

(Clarke 1999: 14)

---

dementia. Example 6.3 illustrates the impact of these differential knowledges of dementia on professional practice.

Gaps in knowledge

It is important to remember that any knowledge base is incomplete. Indeed, a knowledge base tells us as much about what we do not know as what we do know. This is essential since it helps us to determine priorities for future research. However, 'not knowing' is obviously problematic in practice and results in a patchwork of knowledge about care which has holes in it. The fragmentation of knowledge perpetuates a task-orientated interpretation of health and social care practice (Kendall 1997). For example, interpersonal communication models have been promoted through pre-qualifying education programmes, yet this reductionist approach (such as maintain eye contact, sit at the same level) obscures the context of that communication as being within a practitioner–client relationship, to the detriment of its therapeutic potential (see Chapter 9 for further discussion of communication).

It is also vital to consider the context in which the evidence is being applied. For example, can you act on the evidence that indicates effectiveness of patient self-medication if your patients all have limited visibility or indeed dementia? What else must you do to ensure the safe implementation of the evidence in these situations? As Ross and Meerabeau (1997) argue, service delivery is dependent on the context and process of change:

robust evidence on current management of leg ulcer treatment will not produce real health gains if the factors associated with patient compli-ance and the organizational issues implicit in the process of care are not understood.

(Ross and Meerabeau 1997: 5)

There is a lack of knowledge about some quite fundamental issues concerning dementia care. One issue is that of the relationship between practitioners and family carers and the person with dementia (Lyons and Zarit 1999), and this lack of knowledge has resulted in care interventions which have been unknowingly abusive of the relationship between the person with dementia and their carer (Carter 1999). Most often this abuse has resulted from assumptions of involvement based on gender and kin relationships (e.g. Ungerson 1987). Carers who are spouses have been exploited by policies and practices that have failed to recognize the tensions in a relationship that is both caregiving and marital (Parker 1993; Carter 1999).

PROMOTING PRACTICE DEVELOPMENT

The increasing requirement to be accountable to a technical rational knowledge base creates several problems for health and social care since this knowledge concerns only one part of the knowledge which practitioners must use in working with people with dementia and in developing care practices. However, contemporary health and social care emphasizes the role of practitioners in using evidence generated by the research of others, rather than the role of practitioners in creating knowledge for their clients and their profession. Undoubtedly, promulgating the latter model is not without difficulty. Street (1995) and Brown (1995) both identify the inconsistency of knowledge-generating work with practice or care delivery work, although others would argue that practice and research are inextricable (Ritchie 1995; Waterman et al. 1995). Further, the dominant definitions of good quality research, which emphasize **objectivity** and **generalizability**, may not be appropriate criteria for research which is inherently located in and relevant to practice (Reed and Procter 1995; Rolfe 1998).

Using and creating knowledge as a practitioner

The complexities of applying research-based evidence to practice are increasingly recognized. The emphasis on the individual care environment is strong, with Sackett et al. (1996) stating that evidence must be contextualized, that is put into the context of specific practice settings and to individual patients, and that national guidelines must be customized to local settings (Eccles et al. 1996). There is an enormous effort nationally to make sure that evidence is available to practitioners as close as possible to the point of clinical decision making.

Some of the more common ways of communicating evidence to practitioners is through **systematic reviews** of research and the development and dissemination of guidelines. A systematic review uses a research strategy to evaluate all research on a specified topic area and produces recommendations based on the collective message of all this research. Kendall (1997) argues that evidence-based practice implies this thorough evaluation of the evidence and is therefore more than research-based practice. The recommendations from a systematic review are then published in journals, for example *Evidence-based Nursing* or *Evidence-based Medicine*, and as guidelines. Guidelines are produced at both national and local levels and so you may find more than one for a specific topic.

However, the impact of these strategies on practice has been limited by being targeted at individual practitioners rather than systems of care delivery, or in being isolated bits of knowledge, which require application to particular services and clients. For practitioners, very often the technical knowledge is not available or does not fit the unique client care situation they are faced with. Practitioners are left to rely on their tacit, that is unstated knowledge (Meyer and Batehup 1997) and their creativity in evidence use (Fish 1998). It is important to acknowledge and explore the impact which educational experience can have on an individual's capacity for thinking and challenging practice.

Mechanisms that foster such thought in practitioners include professional development programmes, and individual and group **reflective practice** which encourage people to learn from their experiences (for example through **supervision**). In this way, supervision is not seen as a mechanism for checking and monitoring individuals or case management but rather is seen as a support and review framework to promote change processes and the development of ideas. There is consequently no need to see supervision as simply a manager–employee relationship. Indeed, breaking down this hierarchy may be very productive. While managers may be able to act as gatekeepers to some resources, the hierarchical position may also inhibit an open critique of current practice. More fruitful patterns of supervision may emerge from peer supervision (with a respected colleague, preferably self-selected), group supervision (with colleagues from a single area), professional supervision (with a colleague of a similar professional background), and even specialized forums such as critical incident groups (which allow people to learn through shared exploration and examination of incidents). In these non-hierarchical situations the supervisor's role becomes one of facilitation and sharing.

These other forms of supervision are perhaps suitable for the development of practice. In particular they can allow an agenda of concerns to emerge (capturing the 'grumbles') and an action plan to be formulated. In a group supervision situation, this agenda is immediately negotiated with all those present so the complexities of 'selling' an idea to colleagues are minimized. The cycle of reflective practice, that is critical appraisal of current practice, action planning and evaluation, is maintained.

The strategies of communicating evidence also fail to accommodate more experiential forms of knowledge creation, such as that by practitioners themselves, carers or people with dementia. It is these latter forms of knowledge which result in practitioners and services critically challenging definitions of user need and so reconceptualizing care. A development culture locates people with dementia as a central focus of care and addresses the sustainability and plurality of knowledge and practice.

There are some key areas of practice development work which need to involve research activity, including evaluating changes, identifying the perspectives of the users of the service, challenging the professional assumptions of practice, surveying and predicting the outcome of particular forms of intervention. The development of practice is often very fluid and responsive to the developing awareness of the needs of that practice environment. As such some of the traditional research models may be of limited use since they emphasize a static, 'outsider' view of services. Some of the **action research** and participatory action research frameworks may be useful to consider because they allow the simultaneous gathering of data, changing of practice, and questioning of professional roles (for example, Hart and Bond 1995; Meyer and Batehup 1997).

A model of evidence use, rather than knowledge creation, also places health and social care practitioners in a passive role. This is not a problem if professional practice is accepted as serving society, furthering its established values and beliefs. However, it is problematic if practitioners and professions are understood to have a role in shaping society and therefore in shaping its values. This is not an abstract debate, unconnected to all but the most politically active practitioners. Just one example is of the policy and research drive for early diagnosis of dementia, although user perspective research indicates how private the early stages of dementia are (Keady 1997). Another example is that of the tension between assessing carer need and pathologizing family care through the creation of a category of pseudo-client or patient in which carers are seen to be dependent on services (Clarke 1997). Yet another is the conflict between the sanctity of human life and the right of the individual to practise euthanasia (Goldsmith 1999b). These are all debates in which practitioners and their professional bodies may wish to be very active. However, if practitioners and professions wish to play a part in shaping society and in articulating the nature of care for people with dementia in order to validate and develop that care, then some methodological challenges lie ahead.

THE CHALLENGE TO PRACTICE DEVELOPMENT RESEARCH METHODOLOGY

The holistic nature of practice with people with dementia

The holistic nature of health and social care practice with people with dementia and their families is not well served by research methods that fragment knowledge. More inclusive methodologies include qualitative or reflexive enquiry that searches for, as Meyer and Batehup (1997) describe, 'a different type of knowledge more appropriate for practice disciplines'. These approaches to developing knowledge do not try to strip away the context of the situation that is being studied, as approaches such as **controlled trials** do, but rather they are entirely context-specific. The challenge is to understand the impact of that practice context on the care of people with dementia. These results are not generalizable in a conventional sense, but they are transferable to other situations so long as the details of the context in which they are located are described in detail.

The visibility of people with dementia

The visibility of people with dementia in research needs to be enhanced. Notions of personhood and biography are hard to reconcile with the enumeration found in **quantitative research**. McKee (1999) graphically describes walking into the home of a family and walking out with a number that purported to represent that family but which said nothing about them. The vast majority of dementia care research to date rests on the proxy voice of the family carer and it is only very recently that research has attempted to access the views of people with dementia themselves, for example Keady (1997) who interviewed people in the early stages of dementia.

The organization of care

As society engages, as it has done, in a process of redefining some areas of care as a social rather than health concern, so research must pursue questions which challenge the boundaries of care interfaces and the responsibility of different professional and family groups. Researchers, and this is where practitioner researchers have the advantage, must therefore be present with people in care homes and in the domains of health, social, **independent sector** care.

The role of service users in creating knowledge

Not only must practitioners be seen as creators of knowledge, but so too must service users themselves. How to engage people with dementia in this process is complex and challenging. In working towards this we perhaps need to recognize the advice of Eraut (1994) who calls for practitioners to replace their drive for a technical–rational knowledge base with expertise in context-specific knowledge. Similarly Fish (1998) suggests the artistry of professional practice is developed through enquiry and experimentation within and as part of practice.

There are, then, some fundamental principles about practitioner research, and indeed practice development, which we need to recognize in seeking to develop practice for people with dementia (Reed and Biott 1995; Clarke 1998). Thus practitioner research and practice development should be:

- *Part of good practice* – they are not activities that should be added onto a role, undertaken after the 'work' has finished or be regarded as 'not normal' practice by managers or colleagues. Similarly, they are not activities that can be undertaken by someone from outside the environment of care delivery, although they may usefully act as a facilitator in examining concepts of care.

- *About collaboration and mutual learning* – practice developments are not sustainable if they are thought to be possible only by 'special' people who are particularly clever, obsessed or employed to do it. Developing practice must involve everyone and is an activity in which everyone can learn. Furthermore, it is an activity that has no end point – as more is learned so more is seen that needs to be learned.
- *About changing practice in a local environment* – the development must therefore take place in a location, or with an aspect of care, over which people have some control. Practitioner research and practice development is not primarily concerned with applicability to other settings or traditional research criteria such as 'generalizability' but rather emphasizes an evolving nature, relevance to practice and transferability to other settings through articulation of the local contexts of care policy, delivery and receipt.
- *About challenging and examining key concepts and values* – not about perpetuating inherited aspects of professional practice. Thus it will involve reorienting ourselves to a view of health and social care which is led by clients rather than services and organizations. It includes a theoretical aspect of the work of practice development which, for example, allows exploration about what is truly meant by 'better' practice – for whom are we improving practice and what criteria do we use to evaluate a better practice?

Earlier in the chapter, we discussed the particular issue of continence care for people with dementia, and following on from this Example 6.4 describes one study that was undertaken and that illustrates the four principles of practice development research (Clarke and Gardner 1999).

THE CONTEXT OF DEVELOPING PRACTICE

In addition to understanding the nature of knowledge and its impact on practice, practice development activity has to take place in a service context. This context includes the client groups themselves; the structure and resourcing of the service; and the skills of the people involved in the development. Perhaps more important, though, is an appreciation of the processes that are going on in an organization and between groups of practitioners. This section highlights just a few of the key areas. Without addressing these, practice development activity is likely to fail to reach its full potential. Certainly in the example above of developing continence care, the full potential of the study was not realized. Multiple staff changes meant that those most interested in continence care were not able to sustain involvement (and those remaining has less of a sense of ownership of the study), and the profile of the patients changed, resulting in continence care becoming less of an issue for staff.

Example 6.4   Developing continence management

This study was undertaken in one clinical area, a ward that provided acute assessment care for older people with mental health problems, with a clinical issue that was identified by the ward manager: continence care. The research team was modest, involving project management from the local university, data collection from a practitioner in the Trust who was seconded to work on the project for one day a week for six months, and participation from a core group of four staff on the ward. The intention was not that 'someone else' did the research, but that it belonged to the ward staff – an ambition that was not always realized because of the movement of staff onto other wards during the project.

The study used a participatory action research approach that holds the central values of exploring practice concepts, involving practitioners and being specific to the local context of care and client characteristics. The study had three concurrent strands of activity. First, 'evidence' was identified from three sources: existing research, policy and practice guidelines; interviews with a few family carers; and focus groups with staff on the ward. Second, a monthly Collaborative Learning Group/Project Management meeting was held and attended by both the research team and ward staff. The function of these meetings was twofold: to plan the subsequent stages of the study, and to appraise the evidence from strand 1 in relation to ward practice, identifying potential changes in practice where appropriate. The meetings were tape recorded, acting as both the focus groups of strand 1 and as data about the decision making of practitioners. The third concurrent strand provided a description of continence care on the ward over the time of the study. At the start, mid and end points of the study, data was collected by participant observation and by abstracting information from case notes.

The proportion of incontinent patients on the ward did reduce dramatically over the period of the study. However, it is not possible to attribute this change to the study – among the many changes in the organization at that time, the ward had new consultants who introduced different admission criteria. As a result the patients admitted were substantially less likely to have continence problems.

However, the study did demonstrate the very complex issues faced by practitioners. For example, they had to balance accountability to the evidence base of good continence care with accountability to the expressed autonomy of the patient. For instance, a patient at any one time may wish to do nothing about his or her incontinence, and the tolerance of the staff of episodes of incontinence were situated in the specific context of that time. In this way, an episode of incontinence was not tolerated in a public area because of the perceived impact on other patients, but in a private area staff were more tolerant of any expressed wish to do nothing about the situation. Furthermore, the study highlighted the complex relationship between continence management and developing a therapeutic relationship with a patient. At times dealing with incontinence was postponed so that the trust between the staff and the patient was not threatened. However, incontinence was also a factor that limited access to some therapeutic activity such as day trips.

Support

Support for developing health and social care practice comes from a number of sources (Waterman *et al.* 1995). Internal to an organization managers, care staff, domestic staff and indeed all other staff may be in a position to 'make or break' a development. There may be several sources of support available within an organization including personnel (for example, research and development staff) and material (for example, financial and time support for undertaking professional development courses). Outside an organization, support may be financial (from a funding charity for example) or may include families and friends who can act as a 'sounding board' but who may also need to be tolerant of the effects of change upon the individual (and these should not be underestimated). Waterman *et al.* (1995: 60) write that 'Support for change ... can at the same time, on different levels, have a positive and negative influence, thus giving rise to tensions some of which need to be confronted to allow change to take place'.

Power and ideology

Developing practice in situations involving more than one professional group often confounds developments and, certainly in nursing, this has been recognized for some time. Hunt (1987) wrote of professional autonomy only existing when other people 'fail, or decide not to exert, power' – she refers specifically to managers and medical staff, as do Waterman *et al.* (1995). Similarly, Lacey (1994: 987) writes that 'the biggest deterrent to research utilisation appears to be the lack of perceived autonomy – some nurses feel unable to challenge medical colleagues and organisational managers and so fail to make use of research findings available to them'.

Ownership

Not only do organizations change but the people within them change roles, for example Waterman *et al.* (1995) found that staff members left so the initial educational input had to be covered again. Baron *et al.* (1995) found that as organizations change the future of service provision is questioned. Also any one person will have a fluctuating level of involvement with practice developments over time. There are obvious implications for 'bottom-up' approaches to development if ownership of the ideas and support needs to be frequently negotiated and is difficult to sustain. Nor is it clear at what level in an organization it is appropriate for a development to be 'owned', although it is recognized that for clinical guidelines to be implemented there must be local ownership of the guidelines. Without managerial ownership a development is likely to be starved of resources and may not be seen to be a legitimate activity. However, without ownership of all practitioners and colleagues, the development is unlikely to be sustainable.

Facilitation

Because so little health and social care can be changed without impacting on other groups and their activities, the facilitator of practice developments becomes a negotiator, a manager, a collaborator, an inspirer of others (perhaps even conspirator), a planner, a problem solver and so on. A framework of characteristics that may be needed by a facilitator can be drawn up, in part from the work of Waterman *et al.* (1995):

- *Ability to cope with uncertainty.* To develop practice on the basis of evidence is to also work at the edge of what is known and what is not known – sometimes known as the 'cutting edge'; that is potentially painful and always involves a fine line between safety and problems. Not only is the limit of knowledge unknown but people's reaction to it and practice change is unknown. Consequently, a practice development facilitator needs to be able to live with the uncertainty of practice change within an ever-evolving culture and structure of service delivery.
- *Experience of managing learning.* Depending on the specific role of the facilitator, there may be no need to manage 'formal' teaching sessions. However, there is a need for facilitators to take people with them through the development of practice, and also to create opportunities for them themselves to challenge, to be challenged and to learn from their experience. In this way a facilitator does indeed need to be an educationalist.
- *Intellectual curiosity.* Having a reputation as someone who wants to know the ins and outs of everything, and to know what is going on, is probably a good indicator of someone who has intellectual curiosity. Unless someone wants to challenge existing practices and unpick professional assumptions about care, then they will see no need to change practice. Moreover, it is necessary to have the facility to respond to others in a way that engages with their ideas.
- *Openness to change and clarity of purpose.* Similarly, someone who has an idea and doggedly attempts to see it through by steamrolling all opposition and problems is most likely to fail. Being open to change requires **reflexivity** in problem solving and a willingness to amend plans in the light of new information. This must be balanced, however, with the need for facilitators to have clarity about their purpose, to be able to make decisions and manage the consequences of them.
- *Commitment to the project.* All projects go through cycles of optimism and despondency. At times, it will feel as though there is no way forward, that the obstruction to change is immovable, perhaps even that the purpose of the change is questionable. These are the times which are hardest to manage, and when support from others will start to waver. Practice development

facilitators need not only to have commitment themselves, but also need to be able to facilitate commitment in others. That said, though, there may be times when deciding not to pursue a development is the correct decision, and the facilitator has a role in helping all the team members to realize what they have learned from the work and so redirect commitment into another area.

- *Respect for others involved.* This is perhaps one of the most important characteristics of a facilitator. Collaborative developments in care, which have the commitment and involvement of others, can only be nurtured by acknowledging the expertise that others bring with them to a project. One key stage of collaborative working is to identify these differing knowledges and to capitalize on them for the benefit of the development.

- *Access to authority.* Sustainable practice developments need to fit into organizational frameworks. This may be structural: for example, developing a service which demands altered patterns of resourcing, staffing and work patterns needs to be negotiated from the outset with managers. Alternatively, it may be strategic for example, a development may be inconsistent with the strategic direction of the organization in which case it will fail to be recognized and supported. It is important that a facilitator identifies the gatekeepers in the organization (and indeed in other organizations if need be) and works with them to create developments which marry practice need with organizational direction.

- *Credibility in the eyes of others.* Just as the facilitator needs to respect others, so they themselves need to be respected. It is important to consider the criteria of credibility which others will value; for example, academic experience, research skills, management position, practice skills and experience, and ability to 'graft'.

CONCLUSION

If there is one thing that we need to know about practice it is how to ensure its responsiveness to client need in all its diversity. If practice development is about better understanding that need and positioning care interventions and services to respond to that need, then we will be advancing care and the professions. Achieving this, though, requires us to know what knowledge base is informing our current care practices. It also requires us to be able and prepared to engage in the application and even the creation of that knowledge. To do otherwise will compromise the responsiveness of our care and result in a failure to meet the needs of clients. We do need to be accountable to a technical–rational knowledge base, but equally we must know the limitations of that knowledge and create ways in which people with dementia can inform the artistry of our practices.

FURTHER READING

Eraut, M. (1994) *Developing Professional Knowledge and Competence*. London: Falmer Books.

Fish, D. (1998) *Appreciating Practice and the Caring Professions – Refocusing Professional Development and Practitioner Research*. Oxford: Butterworth Heinemann.

Reed, J. and Procter, S. (eds) *Practitioner Research in Health Care: The Inside Story*. London: Chapman and Hall.

7

DAVID STANLEY AND CAROLINE CANTLEY

Assessment, care planning and care management

KEY POINTS

- Assessment, care planning and care management are three distinct processes within a continuum of practice.
- The values base of relationships between service providers and service users is crucial.
- Different stakeholders in different service settings adopt different approaches.
- Multidisciplinary and multi-agency working are central.
- The needs of people with dementia and their carers should prevail.

INTRODUCTION

This chapter discusses concepts of assessment, **care planning** and **care management** from a range of practitioner-oriented perspectives. For the purposes of reviewing the material, three distinctive processes of assessment, care planning and care management are identified. However, each of these processes is part of a continuum which begins with referral and results in an **outcome** for action which is subject to ongoing review. This continuum in turn needs to be understood in the broader context of the experiences and 'life-space' of the person with dementia – ranging from diagnosis on the one hand to the physical care environment on the other.

Each of the processes of assessment, care planning and care management occurs in a wide variety of settings: hospitals, GP practices, domestic homes, residential and nursing homes, uni- and multidisciplinary teams. Each of the processes can also mean different things to different people in different contexts. For example, assessment as a process has often been seen as a problem-oriented activity (Nocon and Qureshi 1996) and the distinction between needs-led and service-led assessments has been long recognized (for example in the NHS and Community Care Act 1990). Care planning can be seen as the specific domain of different professions and conversely has been experienced by service users and professionals alike as an activity for which no one takes overall responsibility (Øvretveit et al. 1997; Stanley et al. 1999). Care management has been associated with a very specific definition since the introduction of the NHS and Community Care Act in 1990. However, the term is commonly used in two different ways: first, to refer to a combined process of care planning and implementing a care package; and second, to refer to ongoing management of day-to-day service delivery.

In addition the field is further complicated by the fact that within and across professions there are different theoretical underpinnings to assessment, care planning and care management. So for example: health care practitioners' perspectives are largely informed by biomedical considerations; social care practitioners' perspectives are informed by broad psycho-social considerations; and the perspectives of people with dementia and their carers are founded equally in whole-life canvas issues as well as the minute detail of their day-to-day experience. We need to take full account of this range of perspectives and we need to ensure that we do not make unwarranted assumptions about their relative importance. It is equally important to be aware of our own orientation and how this affects our conceptions of, and assumptions about, assessment, care planning and care management.

In order to explore the complexities of assessment, care planning and care management, this chapter deals with each process in turn. However it is, first of all, important to consider the value basis of these activities.

VALUES

Kitwood (1997b), in the first chapter of *Dementia Reconsidered* entitled 'On being a person', wrote:

> There is, however, a very sombre point to consider about contemporary practice. It is that a man or a woman could be given the most accurate diagnosis, subjected to the most thorough assessment, provided with a highly detailed care plan and given a place in the most pleasant surroundings – without any meeting of the I–Thou kind ever having taken place.
>
> (Kitwood 1997b: 12)

Kitwood, drawing on the work of Buber ([1923] 1937), was making a distinction between the 'I–It' form of relationship and the 'I–Thou' form of relationship (also discussed in Chapter 4). In the 'I–It' relationship the individual is not valued or responded to as a unique, whole being and this type of relationship is characterized by coolness and detachment. The 'I–Thou' relationship on the other hand is about valuing and responding to the whole being and is characterized by warmth, acceptance and involvement. It was from this basis that Kitwood developed his notion of personhood. If processes of assessment, care planning and care management are to achieve individualized, person-centred care, they must be founded on 'I–Thou' relationships between service providers and service users.

The appropriate values of professional activity are at one level incontrovertible. We see this in the array of existing codes of conduct, standards of practice and protocols of professional ethics. These values systems are rooted in common in: the **Rogerian** principles of genuineness, empathy and respect for the service user; the provision of high standards of service; and notions of accountable practice within a framework that accords the service user dignity, choice and **self-determination**. Most professions have regulatory bodies in place to ensure compliance, and those that do not are in the processes of regulatory development. However, it is not necessary to look very far to find cases where these principles are openly flouted.

Within the context of acceptable standards of practice there are many contested areas, with sophisticated arguments as to why particular canons should not be applicable in particular circumstances (ethical issues more generally are dealt with in Chapter 13). One of the most significant overarching principles in dementia care, as in much community care, is that of supporting independence over dependency. We see this, for example, in O'Donovan's (1994) framework for assessment and care management for the person with dementia within NHS continuing care wards. This framework aims to take account of individual needs and abilities and to foster independence. It emphasizes the importance of shifting nursing care away from a task orientation that tends to increase the patient's passivity and dependence.

Kramer (1995) sees the philosophy of care as a fundamental part of a 'jigsaw' in which the picture includes the care environment and staff, residents and education alongside assessment, care planning and case management. The value framework of Cox et al. (1998) includes reference to the importance of knowing the person; maintaining and reinforcing family and community networks; the need to protect individual **rights** and the centrality of person-centred planning.

Diagnosis is often an important precursor to, or part of, the assessment process. It can be a key event for people with dementia and their carers and for those involved professionally. The processes of reaching and sharing a diagnosis can confront professionals with a variety of ethical challenges when the intent of ethical values interacts with the pragmatics of practice (see also Chapter 13). In noting the complementarity of philosophies of person-centred care and care management, Mackie (1997) defines person-centred as being where the 'diagnosis is not ignored but it ceases to become *the* determinant of care practice' (our italics).

Overall, then, a values-driven approach is at the heart of person-centred care, in the sense that it should demand that the best and most comprehensive services be available.

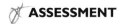 ASSESSMENT

Diagnosis

Within a biomedical framework diagnosis is a first and essential stage in assessment. It is also often a requirement for access to other services, including more broadly based assessments.

One survey of carers by the Alzheimer's Disease Society (now the Alzheimer's Society) (1995a) found that 60 per cent of GPs, when consulted about memory problems, did not administer a memory test, that 40 per cent did not offer a diagnosis and that 36 per cent of those who made a diagnosis did not make a specialist referral. In recommending that GPs pay greater attention to the value of early diagnosis, the report reflected the critical importance attached by service users to being able to have confidence that professional services are providing informed and consistent responses. Evidence-based guidelines for primary care (Eccles *et al.* 1998) review the available assessment scales and include recommendations about the initial diagnostic tests for general practitioners to use with patients with suspected dementia.

Diagnosis is not a matter for the GP alone. The Alzheimer's Disease Society (1995b) explores the role of the GP in linking with secondary services and social services. Highlighted here is the need to assess the physical, mental, behavioural and social conditions and to ensure that the administration of a functional assessment by doctors is linked with assessment by other members of the primary health care team.

Models of assessment

One of the central themes of dementia care practice is to focus on the person and the associated dilemma of actively maintaining personhood while ensuring that it is not undermined (Kitwood 1997b). Following from this, the prime imperative must be to approach assessment from a positive perspective. Garratt and Hamilton-Smith (1995) point to the proactive stance that must be adopted in order to ensure a positive approach. They argue that 'assessment needs to focus upon strengths, competencies and personal resources; care planning and management must provide an environment where these can be realized for as long as possible rather than suppressed' (p. 12).

The diversity of existing assessment processes means that we need to differentiate between those tools and functions which are designed to track the level or progress of the disease and those which are designed to inform matters of service provision. There are substantial qualitative differences between, for example, assessing the individual's mental state (Robertsson *et al.* 1997), assessing levels of well-being (Kitwood and Bredin 1992a; Perrin 1997b), and assessing for needs related to enabling the individual to continue living in the community (DoH 1991). Yet we would also argue that these different levels of assessment should be interdependent and inform each other. The reality of practice is sometimes that different types of assessment are conducted in isolation one from the other (Reed *et al.* 1998). In a related sense Nocon and Qureshi (1996) refer to notions of an 'hierarchy of complexity', where there is basic screening, followed by core assessment, followed by detailed assessment procedures.

Notwithstanding the interrelationships between the various approaches to assessment, we can understand them as falling within a number of general categories. Social, psychological, health and mental health are the four main broad categories, though each of these in turn has sub-categories. It can also be argued that some of the sub-categories assume greater significance in the context of individual circumstances. For example, a **Maslovian** approach to human needs (Maslow 1970) might well identify that financial assessment in association with the provision of basic physical needs is initially the most important issue to be addressed.

Each of the above categories and sub-categories of assessment have to be understood in the broader context of agency and legal requirements. So, for example, there are clear statutory responsibilities for local authorities in respect of assessment for service provision. This has been extended by the duty to assess the rights of carers under the Carers (Recognition and Services) Act 1995. Service delivery itself raises legal rights and responsibilities, indeed the norms of casework have been and continue to be defined at least in part through litigation and individual or group challenge to agency interpretation of statutory duties (Dimond 1997).

The nature of assessment is determined by the location as well as the purpose of the activity. For example Carr *et al.* (1998) describes specialist occupational therapy (OT) assessment as relating to the person with dementia, the carer and the environment. It comments that a more useful picture will be obtained if the assessment is undertaken in the person's own environment rather than in the hospital setting. This position does, of course, leave open questions about whether it is always possible to be clear about the 'own environment' in a situation where the person is in transition from his or her own home, through hospitalization to residential or nursing care. However, it is evident that the assessment should occur in the most appropriate environment.

The Department of Health Social Services Inspectorate (DoHSSI 1996) uses the results of an exploratory study to produce a checklist for agencies reviewing their assessment processes. This includes the following key questions:

- Do assessors understand how dementia affects people and their ability to communicate and make judgements?
- Is information available to help people access the judgement of people with dementia?

- Do procedures exist for early identification of people with dementia?
- Do community care assessments include trigger questions to help assessors recognize dementia?
- Do assessors seek appropriate advice to distinguish between dementia and other conditions?

While the community orientation of many of these items is clear, there are many which are equally applicable in other settings.

Based on discussions with four local authorities, a report by the Social Services Inspectorate (Barnes 1997) highlights the importance of early referral, the need for constant review and clear trigger mechanisms known to all involved. It proposes a similar checklist to the bullet points above, highlighting how good services for a particular user group are predicated upon good practice per se, followed by the application of specialist knowledge.

CarenapD (McWalter et al. 1996) has been developed as an assessment tool for people in community or day care settings. The tool assesses need for different types of help rather than dependency or the need for specific services. It is designed to be used by trained staff, of any profession, as part of the assessment process and in conjunction with care planning. CarenapD uses a range of 'subscales' (health and mobility, self-care and toileting, social interaction, thinking and memory, behaviour and mental state, housecare and community living together with checklists for housing and nutrition) to assess whether there is 'no need', 'met need' or 'unmet need'. For unmet needs it goes on to identify the type of help required. CarenapD assesses the person with dementia and carer separately. For further discussion of assessing carers of people with dementia see Chapter 11.

There is wide variation between authorities and services in both the content and the quality of their assessment approaches. For example, Challis et al. (1996) found little attention given to assessment after admission to the continuing care home environment.

Multidisciplinary approaches to assessment

Effective multidisciplinary assessment can have a profound impact on service delivery. For example, multidisciplinary assessment, in conjunction with individual care programmes which are regularly reviewed and updated, is identified as being among the key components for achieving effective individualized care (Alzheimer Scotland – Action on Dementia 1996). Equally, multidisciplinary assessment is presented as being crucial to the determination of the most appropriate placement. This report also points to evidence of a substantial level of inappropriate placement and suggests that this may be explained by the insufficient health expertise of local authority care managers and to resource-led, rather than needs-led, allocation of placements.

Sturges (1997) identifies some particularly apposite lessons about multidisciplinary working in dementia care. Based on a study of a community mental health team for older people with a single management model across health and social services, Sturges concludes that:

- there is a risk that dementia can be lost in wider mental health teams;
- the assessor/provider split is meaningless to people with dementia and can lead to too much emphasis on assessment at the expense of long-term support;
- some staff like the blurring of roles as generic mental health worker while others prefer their specific professional identity;
- if teams are based in secondary services their links with general practice are unlikely to be as successful.

This final bullet point reinforces the view that general practitioners and primary care teams are well placed to play a central role in the care of people with dementia (cf. Downs 1996). For further consideration of the broader professional and organizational factors that affect multidisciplinary working see Chapter 15.

The views of people with dementia and their carers

Davis *et al.* (1997) studied the assessment of people with disabilities and reported that teams tended to treat users and carers as separate 'units' of assessment rather than as interrelated entities. This ran counter to the way that disabled people experienced caring in their lives and could lead to a tendency to create or exaggerate conflict of interests. This issue of potential conflicts of interest has been increasingly recognized in dementia care as more attention is being paid to listening to the views of people with dementia rather than simply using their carers as proxy (for further consideration of this issue see Chapters 5 and 18).

From the perspective of people with dementia and their carers the processes of assessment are often unclear. Moriarty and Webb (1997, 2000) explored the experiences of assessment (and care planning) of older people with dementia in 14 social work teams. Interviews were undertaken with the assessor, the person with dementia and a carer or proxy. This study identified that 20 per cent of referrals to area teams concerned people with dementia, rising to 70 per cent in specialist teams. Almost 50 per cent had received a joint user/carer assessment. The carers and proxies were generally unaware that there had been any multidisciplinary assessment, neither were they clear about who had actually been involved. Two-thirds of the carers had been told of the dementia diagnosis by either a GP or an old age psychiatrist. While some people with dementia understood the underlying purpose of assessment, others did not. However, Moriarty and Webb are clear that many people with dementia are able to express views about what they want and that this should be incorporated in assessments.

For broader discussion of these issues see for example Phillips and Penhale (1996), which among other issues explores needs-led assessment in the context of user **empowerment** and interprofessional working.

The outcome of community care assessments

Moriarty and Webb (1997, 2000) report that over 25 per cent of the referrals in their study resulted in residential or nursing home placements and almost 60 per cent of the referrals led to an increased provision of community-based services. This study also found that few community packages broke down in the near future, with most assessors being qualified social workers or others with relevant experience, suggesting that this is an area where skill and knowledge do make a difference. Over an 18-month period there was considerable movement between community, hospital and residential or nursing home care. The probability of long-term care related to several factors: severity of dementia was the strongest predictor and, with the provision of day care, admission was delayed.

CARE PLANNING AND CARE PLANS

As with assessment, care planning is as much an integral part of the wider process of providing dementia care as it is a feature in its own right. In the context of community care it has been defined as that part of the cycle which lies on the continuum between assessment of need and service delivery (DoHSSI and Scottish Office 1991). It is therefore critical to the effective delivery of services. In common with assessment it is essential that planning is conducted in a positive way that builds on the retained abilities of the person with dementia. One definition of care planning then is that it uses the data of a person-centred assessment to construct an appropriate package of care for the individual person with dementia as well as ensuring support for their carers.

There is a certain amount of ambiguity in the literature concerning the use of the term care planning, especially in the context of care management. Burton *et al.* (1997: 21) define care management as 'the stage where you identify the action to be taken, based on assessment of need, and begin to plan what services can be utilised'. However, another useful definition is to think in terms of a care plan, sometimes referred to as a care package, that is a product rather than a process.

The value of care planning in community care and residential settings for older people has been well established. The King's Fund (1986) sets out principles for care planning for people with dementia which emphasize the importance of enabling the person with dementia to retain skills, strengths, preferences and relationships and of enabling them to use these capacities. In the context of residential care, *A Better Home Life* (Centre for Policy on Ageing 1996) reinforces that care plans are essential for individual care, record keeping and facilitating good communication. The application of these principles in dementia care again focuses on maintaining a positive approach. Elgar and Marshall (1998) highlight the challenges:

> The label of 'dementia' tends to prompt very negative stereotyped responses and as a result care plans tend to be couched in terms of risk, dependency or disability. This can lead to self-fulfilling dependency spiral

and decline. The low expectations of staff, and the assumption that the people with dementia cannot do much, lead to an enforced reliance and dependence on support.

(Elgar and Marshall 1998: 25)

The principles described above are supported by the Department of Health Social Services Inspectorate (DoHSSI 1993) which identifies that:

- agencies should have clear policies and procedures on how users are involved in individual programme planning;
- individual programme plans should reflect users' wishes;
- individual programme plans should be implemented;
- the review of individual programme plans should involve users and provide an opportunity for changes to earlier decisions;
- individual programme plans should address what risk taking is appropriate for that individual;
- individual programme plans should address equal opportunities.

Different care planning systems proliferate in care homes and other settings. Examples specific to dementia care include Simon's nursing assessment manual (O'Donovan 1994) and the system of Oyebode *et al.* (1996), both developed in NHS continuing care settings, and Model Care Plans developed in care home settings (Fleming *et al.* 1996).

Care plan content

A Better Home Life (Centre for Policy on Ageing 1996) provides detailed advice on the ideal content of a care plan. It recommends that care plans include: personal details; social information; preferences about food and daily life; the role of relatives and friends; health record; risk assessment for safety, manual handling and pressure sores; extent of confusion or challenging behaviour; medication and medical treatment; any nursing care; self-care ability; help required and preferences about how; preferences about future care; religious, spiritual and cultural background; and wishes concerning death and dying. Garratt and Hamilton-Smith (1995), more specifically in dementia care, advocate that the following key elements should exist in the document:

- each care goal;
- how and when the goal is to be attained;
- what strategies are to be tried;
- who is responsible for implementing each strategy;
- when it needs to be evaluated.

Their approach adds an operational dimension onto the descriptive component of the care plan. They also make the point that the care plan is a formal, official document and therefore must be accorded the respect of its status, requiring signature and legible changes where applicable. While legislation is silent on care plans, Mandelstam (1999:148) makes clear that 'inadequate care plans can amount in some circumstances to unlawfulness'.

Overall these various models provide a considerable variation of perspective and philosophy, as well as implications for human and financial resources.

User involvement

Throughout the literature on care planning the involvement of the person with dementia and of carers is reinforced time and time again. Myers and MacDonald (1990) in their study of social work departments in four regions of Scotland look at this issue in some detail. They refer to the tension between user participation and resource allocation, and to the structural and practice barriers to its implementation. Some discrepancy was reported in the comments of workers who suggested that although they recognized that people with dementia were able to express views, they were not thought to be able to make an informed judgement. In relation to people with dementia it seemed that the voice of the carer was deemed to be more legitimate. This highlights the gap that frequently exists between the rhetoric of 'hearing the voice' of the person with dementia and the meaning of subscribing to a person-centred approach in practice.

In care homes and other long-term care settings a variety of approaches have been developed to try to ensure that the interests, likes and dislikes, values, personality and biography of the person with dementia are fully reflected in care plans. A frequently used method is the compilation of life histories. Oyebode *et al.* (1996) describe the introduction of personal care planning in four NHS continuing care units. This approach used a personal profile to give a picture of the individual's life experience. As the profiles were written from the point of view of the person with dementia they helped staff to 'walk in their shoes'.

Overall the aim must be to ensure that plans are drawn up in partnership with the person with dementia and his or her family. This is one way in which agencies can try to ensure that service providers' needs do not override plans for maintaining or improving the quality of life of the person with dementia.

CARE MANAGEMENT

If care management is the final dimension of the continuum with which we began it is clearly dependent upon the assessment and care planning processes. Care management is about effective service delivery in the sense of implementation and ongoing review of a care plan. It is beset by the potential for conflict between user and professional perspectives similar to those discussed above. We have already seen that people with dementia and their carers do not themselves differentiate the processes of assessment, care planning and care management. They can be at a loss to make sense of what might seem to them to be an array of language that masks rather than illuminates their needs. Studies have demonstrated that neither older people, nor their carers, moving through the transitions from community to care homes, whether via hospital placement or not, identify with the term 'care manager' (Stanley *et al.* 1999). If the people representing the care management function are not identifiable then the process itself is even more elusive to the service user. It is therefore important that the various professionals involved are able to be confident that this process makes a positive contribution to service delivery and does not become merely an arcane professional construction.

Care management for people with dementia is not without its attendant difficulties. A Social Services Inspectorate report (Barnes 1997) identified these as including:

- working with people with dementia who cannot articulate their needs;
- building in flexibility and response to change;
- the negotiation of higher cost care packages;
- managing a strategy for people who are reluctant to accept services;
- acting as **advocate**;
- balancing confidentiality with sharing information to ensure that a person is living alone with an acceptable and agreed level of risk.

Tools for practice delivery

The Department of Health Social Services Inspectorate (DoHSSI) and Scottish Office (1991) advocates a single integrated process for identifying and responding to individual needs. It describes care management as a seven-stage process which includes publishing information, determining the level of assessment, assessing need, care planning, implementing, monitoring and reviewing. The ten key benefits of this approach are identified as:

- tailoring services to individual requirements;
- individual care planning specifying desired outcomes;
- division of responsibility of assessment/care management from service provision;
- more responsive services as a result of linking assessment and commissioning;
- wider choice across statutory and independent sectors;
- partnership with users and carers;
- improved opportunities for representation and advocacy;
- more effective meeting of needs;
- greater continuity of care and greater accountability to users and carers;
- better integration between and within agencies.

This definition represents the major professional perspective in which management refers to a process for ensuring effective service delivery, rather than a more specific focus on the delivery itself. A rather different approach, combining these two aspects of care management, is advocated by McWalter *et al.* (1996). Their multidisciplinary needs assessment tool, CarenapD collates data on met and unmet needs and makes a contribution to the care management function by monitoring dependency. One practical application of CarenapD is its identification of a 24-hour/seven-day planner which identifies support and gaps in support. CarenapD aims to achieve the delicate task of sustaining a positive approach through building on strengths and avoiding the fostering of dependency. It also aims to: avoid change as much as possible; use knowledge of the past as a foundation; address the needs of ethnic minority groups; and incorporate regular, systematic review. Thus it is a tool which builds upon a theoretical approach to deliver a tangible service.

Care management approaches

The Department of Health Social Services Inspectorate (DoHSSI 1998) found that authorities have different approaches ranging from differences in professional representation in the care management system to differences in the way budgets are managed. This study emphasized the importance of developing links and reciprocity between local authorities and the NHS, particularly primary care services, whose staff contribute to assessment and care planning and also provide an important access point to services (see also Chapter 15). Significantly, this report also identified that links between care management and strategic commissioning of services were not equally developed in different areas, an important issue since care managers can only purchase the services that are available.

A second issue is the extent to which care management for people with dementia is linked with the **Care Programme Appproach**. The Care Programme Approach provides a health service-led framework for managing the care of people with mental health problems in the community. Different areas vary in how they apply the Care Programme Approach to people with dementia. Although *Building Bridges* (DoH 1995a) stresses that the Care Programme Approach and care management (a social services-led system) are based on the same principles and should be capable of being integrated, there is variability between areas in the extent to which this is achieved (DoHSSI 1999).

A third issue of concern in dementia care is the approach that authorities take to financial assessment and to ensuring proper management of the resources of the person with dementia. Means (1997) reports that staff often have little knowledge of the legal safeguards available including **enduring power of attorney, receivership** and **appointeeship**. More particularly there was often a lack of recognition of the vulnerability of people with dementia and little attention to ensuring that appropriate procedures were in place to protect them.

SPECIFIC USER GROUP ISSUES

Throughout this chapter we have emphasized the importance of a person-centred approach to assessment, care planning and care management. It is important to end, then, by recognizing that in all three processes we need to be able to work with the diversity of people who have dementia. This means taking account of the different abilities of people with dementia and developing the skills to enable them to participate as fully as possible in determining the care that they receive.

Recently we have seen an increased awareness of the service needs of people with early onset dementia (for an overview see Cox and Keady 1999). Cantley *et al.* (2000) summarize the findings of a study of one community team for people with early onset dementia. This concludes that team members develop specialist knowledge and skills in a number of areas of assessment, care planning and care management. However, it is also clear that many of the issues involved in working with people with early onset dementia are common to dementia care for older people and indeed to community care more generally.

Kerr (1997) points out that the assessment of people with learning disabilities who develop dementia is likely to involve a wider range of practitioners since service users will already be in touch with services. Stalker *et al.* (1999a) outline some of the key issues in working with this group of service users. Kerr suggests that one difference is that in working with people with dementia practitioners generally would try to adopt a '**substituted judgement**' approach to decision making. However, in working with some people with dementia and learning disability there will have been existing doubts about competence and a '**best interest**' approach may therefore be more appropriate (see Chapter 13 for further discussion of ethical issues).

The assessment of people from minority ethnic communities raises a range of issues (cf. DoHSSI 1998). Jenkins (1998) focuses on the importance of communications with people with dementia and their carers, particularly in exploring the divides of culture and language, and examines ways of developing more effective communications skills when working in a multicultural context. Patel *et al.* (1998) caution against using a 'checklist' approach in identifying and responding to the needs of minority ethnic communities. They argue that this can lead to narrow stereotypical pictures of needs and preferences. If services are to avoid this they must be open and receptive to understanding the individual in a much broader social context.

The assessment and care management of people with challenging behaviour presents particular challenges for a wide range of service providers (see also Chapter 10). Moniz-Cook (1998) reviews research which focused on a psychosocial intervention approach to challenging behaviour in care homes, providing an overview and identifying practice implications. Crump (1992) similarly describes wandering behaviour and explores its assessment and causes, and good practice for its management.

Finally there are the issues of assessment and care management for people with dementia who may be subject to abuse or who are considered 'at risk' in other ways. Seaton (1995) presents practice guidelines for staff in identifying and responding to potential or actual situations of the abuse of vulnerable older people, and the article covers a range of perspectives from staff training to developing procedures. Guidance on multi-agency working is provided in

No Secrets (DoH 1999c). Penhale (1999) reviews the research evidence relating to people with dementia and argues that they are more likely to experience abuse, particularly if their behaviour is disturbed and disruptive. Discussing risk management for people with dementia living at home, Baragwanath (1997:103) argues that 'duty of care concerns are too frequently raised by professional staff as an excuse for inadequate *individual* assessment and inflexible and restrictive care plans'. She advocates more imaginative approaches and open discussion of how best to balance concerns about safety against the rights and quality of life of the person with dementia. Counsel and Care (undated) similarly provides guidance on balancing risk and empowerment for vulnerable older people in residential settings.

CONCLUSION

Perhaps the ultimate message of this chapter is the need for awareness that different professions have different approaches to assessment and care planning which underpin their specific professional tasks and aims.

An integrated approach to assessment, care planning and care management – with the provision of as 'seamless' a service as possible – is dependent upon effective multidisciplinary working with the professionals involved. It also requires effective partnership with people with dementia and their carers (cf. DoHSSI 1997), using advocacy as a medium where appropriate. The key principles which emerge are concerned with ensuring that practice is undertaken within a person-centred, values-based approach which sustains a focus on positive action and which actively works to ensure that dependency and negativity is always minimized. These principles are equally applicable across all stages in the process, across all professions and across all service settings.

FURTHER READING

Archibald, C., Chapman, A. and Weaks, D. (1995) *Dementia: A Practice Guide for Community Nursing*. Stirling: Dementia Services Development Centre.

Burton, A., Chapman, A. and Myers, K. (1997) *Dementia: A Practice Guide for Social Work Staff*. Stirling: Dementia Services Development Centre.

Carr, J., Garton, C. and Munroe, H. (1998) *Dementia: A Practice Guide for Occupational Therapy Staff*. Stirling: Dementia Services Development Centre.

Mandelstam, M. (1999) *Community Care Practice and the Law*, 2nd edn. London: Jessica Kingsley. Judgments, case examples and an authoritative interpretation of the law in relation to community care practice.

8

MARIA PARSONS

Living at home

KEY POINTS

- Most people with dementia live in their own homes for a substantial part of their lives.
- Informal carers, whether co-resident or providing daily support from outside, are a key element in enabling people with dementia to remain at home.
- In meeting the needs of people with dementia attention needs to be paid to social, psychological and spiritual needs as well as physical requirements such nutrition, mobility, and continence.
- The daily living needs of people with dementia from black and minority ethnic groups are less likely to be met by formal services.
- Housing, adaptations, aids, equipment and assistive technology are important components of community care for people with dementia.
- Effective services should be needs-led, coordinated, consistent, and flexible.

INTRODUCTION

Most people with dementia are able to live at home in the community for a substantial part of their lives. The quality of their lives and their capacity to preserve independence depends, to a large extent, on personal and social characteristics and on the availability and quality of informal and formal care. Hence, each individual has a different experience of and response to dementia shaped by personal biography, physical health and personality and structured by social class, gender, age and ethnicity. However, critical elements in enabling people with dementia to remain at home are the extent and level of care and support offered by informal carers and, when it is required, that of health, social care and housing.

PEOPLE WITH DEMENTIA LIVING IN THE COMMUNITY

Measuring the prevalence of community-dwelling people with dementia is problematic and some underestimation is likely to occur. Although most people with moderate to severe dementia usually become known to statutory agencies (Spicker *et al.* 1997), intervention is often prompted by the ill health of carers (Levin *et al.* 1989). Between 36 per cent and 53 per cent of people with mild or moderate dementia live in the community, and another 35 per cent of those with high dependency needs also live at home supported by carers (Melzer *et al.* 1997).

GPs, usually the first professionals to be contacted by concerned individuals and families, are generally reluctant to look actively for dementia or make a diagnosis (Audit Commission 2000). People with mild dementia often dismiss, deny, or mask early memory difficulties, making detection and diagnosis more difficult. The transience of this group also makes planning and commissioning for community services an inexact science. One study of older people with dementia showed that each year a third died, while another third were admitted to institutional care (Spicker *et al.* 1997). Early onset dementia shows a different progression, and higher care demands which, coupled with a paucity of appropriate community-based services, triggers earlier institutionalization (Harvey 1998). Overall more women are affected by dementia than men (reflecting comparative longevity) but this does not hold for people aged less than 65 years (Harvey 1998). It is estimated that in the UK there are some 5000 people with dementia from black minority ethnic groups (Patel *et al.* 1998).

In addition to age and gender, socio-economic status, education, and ethnicity are also associated with known risk factors for dementia. Problems relating to healthy lifestyle, hypertension, diabetes and alcohol abuse are highest in lower socio-economic classes and among some black minority ethnic groups. Psychiatric morbidity, which appears to increase risk of Alzheimer's disease, is highest in social classes 1V and V, and among women. By contrast, longer life expectancy with fewer years of disability (including dementia) is associated with more privileged socio-economic status, especially among men. Education appears to have a protective effect during neuro-degeneration and may also boost neural networking, enabling active neurons to continue functional tasks as others die (Orell and Sahakian 1995).

Informal care: living with others

Daily support from informal carers is a crucial factor in enabling people with dementia to continue dwelling in the community (Melzer *et al.* 1996). Up to

60 per cent of those caring for older people are likely to be co-located (Levin *et al.* 1992) and most younger people with dementia live with spouses or partners (Harvey 1998). Female kin continue to be the bedrock of much informal support for disabled relatives across all communities. Carers of people with dementia experience very high levels of stress and burden, especially women who carry out personal care over longer periods of time. Men are less likely to be involved in personal care, and spend less time caring, adopting a more structured and task-focused approach (Burns and Rabins 2000).

Living alone

Demographic change, social trends, and individual preferences have given rise to growing numbers of people living alone, especially among 30- to 50-year-olds and those over 85 years. An estimated 154,000 people with dementia live alone in the UK, a figure expected to grow to 245,000 by 2011 (Alzheimer's Disease Society 1994). Women over pension age without close family support make up most of this group (Wenger 1994).

The social, cultural and economic context

The way in which people respond to dementia and manage their lives is influenced by social, economic and cultural factors. Dementia is conceptualized in different ways among different UK communities and these differences often reinforce existing patterns of social inequality and exclusion. While cultural support, adequate and adaptable housing, material and financial security enables some of those with dementia and their families to mitigate, to a certain extent, the impact of dementia, social disadvantage and discrimination can exacerbate the marginalized position of people with cognitive disability.

MATERIAL RESOURCES

Home and housing

The majority of people with dementia want to remain at home, a place which usually provides psychological and physical safety and in which people are in control of their lives. People with dementia, however, often encounter difficulties in trying to adapt to their physical environment or in adapting the built environment to their needs. This can result in their functioning at a less than optimal level. Memory loss, disorientation, sensory deficits, hallucinations, anxiety, depression, rigidity and slowness can all impact on the ability to move safely around at home and to carry out self-care and other practical daily activities. Some 18 per cent of older people with dementia live in houses that do not have central heating, that need major repair, or that lack satisfactory sanitation (Spicker *et al.* 1997).

Various design features can compensate for such problems and address excess disability. 'Dementia friendly' design ideas have been applied in the planning and building of specialist residential or nursing homes to enhance the 'legibility' of built environments, that is the ease with which they are understood, through the provision of cues and prompts. Very little new domestic housing, however, is adapted specifically to meet the needs of people with disabilities, and where this exists, it tends to address the needs of those with physical disabilities.

Modification of existing housing is the responsibility of local authority housing departments and Housing Improvement Agencies (HIAs) which have statutory duties and powers relating not only to adaptations but also to repairs, or general improvements. Instead, people with dementia whose homes may need adapting rely on social services and housing agencies working together to assess and meet disability needs. Work may be major, such as adding a downstairs toilet, or minor in the fitting of grab rails. Much of this activity is carried out in conjunction with health and social services.

Independent living can also be enhanced by the use of aids and equipment available from health, social services and housing agencies, or from independent providers. The huge range, from wheelchairs to adapted tin openers, is set to increase with the introduction of devices using technology, which can enhance safety and communication, provide entertainment, prompt memory, and monitor health and movement. Some items use low technology, which is readily available, for example, mobile phone messages to remind someone to take medication, while surveillance systems installed as part of sophisticated 'smart houses' are more complex.

Practitioners carrying out assessments to identify needs which might be met through the use of technology need to act ethically in making decisions to introduce such assistance (Marshall 2000). Careful assessment is also required in order to ensure that environmental and technological recommendations meet specific needs. For many people with dementia, especially in the early stages, physical capacity to carry out activities remains intact but memory loss coupled with depression and agitation reduces confidence. Hence, removing or minimizing physical barriers such as taking off cupboard doors to make contents visible, or changing door handles, may help reduce anxiety, prompt memory, and encourage orientation. Later, community alarms and gas cut-off devices may enable daily activities to be continued but provide additional safety for those who are vulnerable.

A more coherent support strategy for people with dementia in their own homes needs to be developed to address the problems experienced by formal and informal carers in accessing information and equipment from health and social care purchasers, providers and the private market (Mandelstam 1997). Statutory sources of funding for aids equipment and adaptations are often constrained. However, the obstacles to seamless provision of housing, care and technical support for people with dementia are largely organizational, with few housing agencies fully involved in joint planning for community care (see Chapter 14 for further discussion of community care policy and planning).

Finances

Dementia usually results in individuals and their families incurring extra costs such as paying for services. Overall, it is likely that informal care costs are underestimated (Stewart 1998). The material implications of dementia for younger people are profound. They are more likely to be home owners, have dependants and be in employment which usually ceases not only for the person with dementia but more often than not for the spouse who becomes the primary carer. Families often become dependent on benefits (Harvey 1998) as carers forego earnings.

Occupational pensions skew income inequalities among elderly people and many older women are among the estimated two million people of pension age who live below the poverty threshold. One study showed that 24 per cent of older people with dementia relied solely on state pension, 39 per cent were in receipt of additional disability or carer benefits, and 37 per cent had a private income of whom 15 per cent also received disability or carer benefits (Spicker *et al.* 1997).

The need to safeguard and manage finances may be overlooked as families struggle to come to terms with dementia and access services. Guidance about a range of financial and legal options for both younger and older people with dementia is available from a number of national and local organizations and some solicitors specialize in the law regarding people with dementia. Social services are often best placed to help families, but coherent local authority policy and practice in respect of money management has been found lacking, 'even though a failure to handle money in terms of paying bills, buying food etc. can soon undermine even the most sophisticated care package' (Langan and Means 1995: 49). The development of comprehensive policy, **protocols** and training for community professionals would lead to more consistent and informed approaches to helping people with dementia manage their financial affairs. The development of direct payments and independent care advisors and/or advocates may offer people with dementia more opportunity to control and tailor public or private funding for their care.

PRACTICAL ASPECTS OF DAILY LIVING

Activities of daily living

People with dementia often need assistance in meeting basic needs (such as eating, washing, dressing, grooming and toileting), instrumental activities (such as managing medication, preparing food and cooking, housework, laundry, gardening and managing money) and more complex psychosocial needs (such as self-esteem, love, spirituality, and sexuality).

Co-morbidity is very common in dementia, and poor physical health or worsening of chronic conditions can trigger admission to hospital or institutional care. Minor but untreated sensory, oral, dental and podiatry problems, frequently experienced by older people with dementia, can exacerbate non-cognitive symptoms of dementia (Burtholt *et al.* 1997).

Occupation and activity

The maintenance of meaningful and culturally relevant occupation and activity is important for self-esteem and personal independence. Activities and skills most successfully maintained at home are those which do not rely on episodic and semantic memory, but which relate to individual motivation and habits. Sensory cues appear to provide additional routes to memory retrieval for everyday activities such as making tea or baking. Often, tasks such as dressing or grooming can be simplified or shared with a carer who can prompt where necessary. As people with dementia become less responsive, the focus of engagement may take the form of providing stimulation through music, walks, or a gentle hand massage.

Continence

Not only does incontinence of the bowel and bladder result in loss of dignity, autonomy and discomfort, but people with dementia who are incontinent, particularly of faeces, are more at risk of institutionalization. Many people with dementia develop incontinence when they are severely disabled. Continence, however, does not necessarily accompany dementia although the coexistence of depression increases the likelihood of incontinence developing.

Initial assessment and clinical evaluation is usually undertaken by GPs, or other community health professionals, who can also offer advice and support in managing continence at home. Often, reversible or transient causes of incontinence such as mobility problems, pain or urinary tract infections (UTIs) deter people from making the journey to the toilet. Side effects of some medication can contribute to incontinence with certain neuroleptics causing lethargy, whilst cholinesterase inhibitors have been implicated in constipation. Changes of any sort, particularly in familiar routines and surroundings, can also trigger incontinence. Strategies and practical support may include medication and toileting regimes. Specialist continence advisers are available if problems become more intractable (Jenkins 1999).

Mobility

Dementia can affect mobility in different ways. Some people, especially those who have Parkinson's disease or dementia with Lewy bodies, develop specific gait difficulties. Cognitive disability affects the capacity to judge depth and distance between objects, and can lead, for example, to people attempting to sit down in the gap between chairs. It may also lead to the mis-processing of information, such as busy patterns on carpets, resulting in accidents when people are walking.

Falls at home are a major cause of accidents among older people (Carter *et al.* 1997) although risk of falling is not found to be associated with the severity of dementia but with the functional capacity of the person, the risk increasing in the more capable (CHSR 1998). Detailed assessment of risks for falls may help identify whether they result from cognitive disability, which hinders navigating obstacles, or from underlying physical problems such as arthritis, fatigue, or from the side effects of medication (Shaw and Kenny 1998). Assessment also aims to identify hazards in the environment such as ill-fitting clothing and shoes, furniture that is badly placed, chairs which are light and tip over, or rugs which slide.

Walking

The constant walking or 'wandering' behaviour of many people with dementia often causes concern to families and formal carers. Wandering indoors is often viewed as purposeless. Outside the risk of getting lost is substantial with some 40 per cent of people getting lost outside the home. Research into the mobility behaviour of 104 people with dementia living at home with carers over a five-year period (or until their death) found that:

- most people who got lost only did so on one or two occasions as carers took steps to limit the possibilities of their spouse exiting the home unaccompanied;
- poor mobility was found to be very strongly associated with subsequent institutionalization;
- neurophysiological tests of topographical memory (i.e. memory for interpreting pictorial information – a requisite for route finding and returning) suggest that this is more impaired in those people who got lost.

(McShane *et al.* 1998)

Careful and systematic assessment may reveal alternative explanations for walking and provide different options for intervention (Allan 1994).

Nutrition

Dementia impacts on eating and nutrition in different ways and can lead to nutritional deficiencies and weight loss. People with dementia may have difficulties in concentrating sufficiently to eat and in recognizing food and its significance. Physical difficulties with eating and the effects of medication may also contribute to nutritional problems. People from black and minority ethnic groups may be at particular risk as vegan and vegetarian diets, observed by some groups, can lead to iron deficiency. Offers of culturally inappropriate foods and non-compliance with customs can lead to food refusal. Towards the end of their illness, people with dementia often have difficulties in opening the mouth, chewing or swallowing food (VOICES 1998).

Ensuring the person with dementia has sufficient food and drink is one of the major concerns of carers. Good oral and dental care is important. Carers under stress are also at risk of weight gain or loss, therefore meeting their needs may result in better outcomes for those they care for. Guidance is available to both informal and formal carers (VOICES 1998) as is referral to dieticians and specialist services.

Transport

Older people are less likely to be car owners or use private transport to get about. Those in rural areas may be reliant on public transport, which becomes more difficult for people with dementia and their carers to use over time. Transport is a key item in community care provision. Statutory and voluntary agencies often make their own separate arrangements, involving the use of hospital or community transport, or private taxis. If those attending facilities such as day centres are collected on a circuit, delays can occur, especially if people are collected over a wide area. The Audit Commission (2000: 56) noted that 'In some areas, it was not uncommon for people to spend over two hours in an ambulance before reaching the day hospital'. In rural areas, transport is a major cost factor in service provision, especially for smaller voluntary agencies. The development of locality-based services, mobile units or services which use community facilities for some activities has been very useful especially for people in rural communities.

For many people, especially younger men with dementia, giving up driving is a blow to pride, independence and control (Parsons 1999). Following diagnosis of dementia, physicians are obliged to inform patients of their responsibility to notify the Driver and Vehicle Licensing Agency (DVLA) that they are no longer able to drive (O'Neill 1992). Where a person with dementia insists on driving when there is evidence that they are clearly no longer able to do so safely and responsibly, the doctor can breach confidentiality and inform the DVLA.

SOCIAL ASPECTS OF DAILY LIVING

Sexual needs and sexuality

People with dementia remain sexual beings with needs for emotional security, self-esteem, affection, and physical closeness. Most studies focus on heterosexual experience and it is only recently that attention has been drawn to the needs of the gay community. Symptoms of dementia, and associated stress, anxiety, depression, or medication can all impair the capacity to satisfy sexual needs. Inappropriate expression of emotional or sexual needs, preoccupation with sex and sexual disinhibition are often difficult areas for carers and professional helpers, especially when those with dementia are older (Sherman 1999).

Capacity to cope with stresses engendered by dementia in marriage is related to the quality of previous relationships, which can be protective. Equally stress may reactivate previous long-standing problems. As dementia progresses, the level of intimacy between carer and cared-for tends to diminish; however, wide variations have been reported in the amount of affection given, and sexual intimacy achieved, where one partner has Alzheimer's disease. Couples achieving high affection and more regular sexual intimacy tend to be men with Alzheimer's disease and their wives.

Beliefs and spirituality

On one level, understanding spirituality involves finding out about the way in which someone makes sense of his or her life and identity; on the other it is about practising faith, usually in a ritualized way, with other people (for further discussion see Chapter 4). In an increasingly secular society, it is nevertheless important to establish an individual's faith history (Frogatt and Moffitt 1997). If the person concerned has a place of worship, it is important to maintain this and many more churches are enabling members of their congregations with disabilities to participate in services. Those who have ceased to be active churchgoers may nevertheless experience satisfaction in singing religious songs or hymns, or chanting. However, Barnett (1995a) suggests that it would be remiss of those caring for people with dementia to focus solely on 'meeting spiritual needs' without acknowledging that 'we need love in order to be able to give to the person with dementia what they most deeply need' (p. 42). Similarly in providing practical services to help carers, their spiritual and emotional support needs should not be overlooked.

DYING WITH DIGNITY

In the final stage of their life, people with dementia are often more frail, spend more time resting and need more physical care. For people who have been living at home, admission to hospital or nursing home often takes place at this stage. Identifying when a person has entered the final stage of dying with dementia is difficult for formal and informal carers who may for some time have regarded their relative as 'already dead' or 'as good as dead'. Hence such 'social death' precedes clinical or biological death (Sweeting 1997). Working alongside informal carers to enable them to continue caring for as long as they want to, demands skill, creativity and cultural awareness. Community professionals and care staff need to ensure that a person's values are integrated into the process of dying.

One study contrasted the quality of support available for those dying of cancer and their carers and those with dementia. Patients with dementia were reported as experiencing more unrelieved psychological and physiological discomfort for longer periods, saw their GP less often than cancer patients, and rated GP services less highly (McArthy et al. 1997). The comparative use of

hospice facilities by the two groups indicated that while this care was appropriate for people with dementia often it was not available to them. Service
users, families and formal carers favour **palliative care** but appropriate
arrangements need further research.

THE DAILY LIVES OF BLACK AND ETHNIC MINORITY PEOPLE WITH DEMENTIA

Few studies shed light on the way in which dementia is constructed among black
and minority ethnic groups, although it would appear that dementia is often
construed as 'normal ageing' (Patel *et al.* 1998). High levels of risk and unmet
needs of those with dementia in minority ethnic communities are associated
with changing familial, social circumstances or compounded by social disadvantage and discrimination, and untreated physical problems such as diabetes
and hypertension (Lindesay and Jagger 1997). Use of GP services is high but
referrals to specialist psychogeriatric services are low and access to other statutory community based services appears to be problematic (Ellen *et al.* 1998).

Services need to acknowledge diversity in carer response to dementia and
actively challenge stereotypes that black minority ethnic groups look after their
own relatives and therefore help is not required from statutory services (Patel
et al. 1998). Carers need services which take account of their specific cultural
needs, and in the absence of culturally appropriate formal services, self-help
and separate development takes place (Haringey Housing and Social Services
and Alzheimer's Society 1998).

SERVICE SUPPORT

Effective services to meet the changing needs of people with dementia and their
carers should go beyond mere maintenance and safety, to promoting choice,
control and citizenship and positively reflecting socio-cultural diversity. Prevention marks the beginning of good care, with public and primary health
care programmes, and preventative work being carried out by social services
and voluntary organizations, needing to be 'joined up' to create a dementia-
specific strategy for those living in the community.

Identification of people with dementia living in the community and early intervention is not as yet a high priority. Eligibility for community care services
remains tightly drawn by prioritising the needs of people with more severe
disabilities, people who live alone, or whose behaviour is causing concern
(DoH 1996). The response of primary care to individuals and families seeking
help needs to be improved. Less than one-half of carers had been asked if
they needed any help or given information about mental health by GPs (Audit
Commission 2000).

Families themselves are increasingly making contact with social services
(Moriarty and Webb 2000). Effective care pathways begin with comprehensive

multidisciplinary assessment (DoH 1996) involving people with dementia and their carers in discussions about care choices (see Chapter 7). Such choices may well be extended by Direct Payments arrangements (see Chapter 14) and the development of advocacy for people with dementia. Assessment is often undertaken by community mental health teams for older people. The use of such teams to provide and manage multidisciplinary and interagency services in given localities has grown rapidly (see Chapter 15 for further discussion).

Home care continues to be the service most used by older people with dementia and relied on by carers (DoHSSI 1997). Specialist needs are often best met through the provision of intensive or augmented home care, which is rated most highly when there is continuity of formal carers (Riordan and Bennett 1998). There may come a point, however, when formal services merely shore up existence rather than providing quality of life. Kitwood (1997b) suggests that there is another side to the 'homely coin':

> The darker possibility is that many people with dementia will continue to stay at home – for economic reasons – long beyond the point when it is consistent with their well being or that of their carers. Those who live alone face an even more dreadful prospect – that of being imprisoned in terrifying loneliness and personal danger as they await their packages of care.
>
> (Kitwood 1997b: 77)

Referral to day and respite care has been shown to extend duration of community living (Levin *et al.* 1992; CHSR 1998). Carers may need relief but, as Moriarty and Webb (2000: 94) note, 'offers of short term breaks pose uncomfortable dilemmas', because the person cared for may be distressed by the experience. Since those with dementia and their carers are often also physically frail, there is a need for services which provide rapid responses particularly to emergencies when temporary intensive support is required, especially at weekends, night times, and for holiday breaks. Community-based provision should be matched with cost flexibility, as peaks and troughs in the needs of both individuals and carers require both planned and unplanned services to be made available, sometimes at very short notice (Svanberg *et al.* 1997).

Over time, the social world of people with dementia and their carer contracts and formal services are frequently the only social contacts remaining. Since social isolation and receipt of meals at home strongly correlate with risk of institutionalization and reduced survival, maintaining social networks is particularly important. Activities such as accompanied walks, visits to places of interest and meals out were the most highly rated aspect of a home-based support service for younger people with dementia operating in a largely rural county (Parsons 1999).

Professionals and care staff who support people with dementia in their own homes often experience dilemmas between respecting autonomy and self-determination and protecting service users and others. Insofar as people with dementia demonstrate a general slowing down of responsiveness to environmental stimulation and experience increasing difficulty in interpreting information, they are likely overall to be more at risk in certain situations. However, people with dementia and their circumstances vary considerably, and professionals undertaking assessment and care planning need to strike a careful balance between safety and over-emphasis on security. A systematic approach to assessment is required in which strengths and positive factors are identified as well as hazards which predispose people to risk in certain circumstances. Dangers need to be clearly assessed as to the likelihood of their occurring. Common hazards, especially those associated with the environment, are often underestimated (Carter *et al.* 1997) and other risks, for example of abuse, have only been rendered visible relatively recently.

Support offered by a carer is crucial, and often irreplaceable. Local authorities vary a great deal in the extent and level to which they fulfil statutory duties to assess carers' needs. Households with carers receive lower levels of formal help (Burtholt *et al.* 1997). Professional intervention needs to take account of relationships and family dynamics. Carers may well refuse a service if it appears to replace an activity which is important to them or which undermines attempts to normalize their lives (Clarke 1999).

The range of choices for carer support needs to reflect real life needs and concerns. For example, in offering more support for carers who wish to maintain employment through services such as respite care which comes into the home. Some carers may benefit from more structured psycho-educational carer training programmes, others from family intervention. Many carers value consistent and reliable support from community psychiatric nurses (Audit Commission 2000). In future services will have to take into account the social consequences that the increasing use of anti-dementia drugs (see Chapter 1) will have for individuals and for carers.

CONCLUSION

This century growing numbers of people with dementia will live in their own homes. They are a far from homogeneous group and their experiences and responses will differ. It is therefore important that those involved in providing support to meet needs listen carefully to what people with dementia want in order to be able to live their lives at home. The development of individualized coordinated, flexible, and reliable services to support daily living and enable people with dementia to achieve the best quality of life possible remains a major challenge.

FURTHER READING

Cox, S. and Keady, J. (eds) (1999) *Younger People With Dementia.* London: Jessica Kingsley.

Gillies, B. (1995) *The Subjective Experience of Dementia: A Qualitative Analysis of Interviews with Dementia Sufferers and their Carers, and the Implications for Service Provision.* Dundee: Joint Information and Research Group, Tayside Health Board.

9 | **ANTHEA INNES AND ANDREA**

Communication and personhood

KEY POINTS

- The personhood of people with dementia can be maintained by effective communication.
- Only recently have systematic attempts been made to understand the words of people with dementia.
- Life history knowledge provides new opportunities for communication with those who have dementia.
- Diagnostic categories and labels are not always helpful starting points for communication.
- Responding to the feeling expressed by a person with dementia may be more fruitful than focusing on the actual words.
- Reflexivity is required of caregivers when working with people with dementia if personhood is to be maintained.

INTRODUCTION

One of the most common difficulties caregivers report in working with those who have dementia is a feeling of inadequacy in understanding and responding to the person's attempts to communicate. Communication pervades every area of care practice, and its importance can hardly be overemphasized, as good practice in any area of care provision is crucially dependent upon its effectiveness.

Difficulties in communication often arise as a result of the reduced, disordered, or fragmented speech which tends to form a significant part of the mentia syndrome'. Kitwood (1997b) has pointed out that many of the so-called 'problem behaviours' exhibited by people who have dementia can also be understood as attempts to communicate non-verbally. For example, a person unable to make a verbal request to be taken to the toilet may engage in various kinds of behaviour suggesting frustration and discomfort, for example pacing or moaning, grabbing hold of people nearby or attempting to move them in a particular direction. If the message is not understood it may lead to 'problem behaviours' such as 'inappropriate urinating'. Such behaviour may then be interpreted as an inevitable result of dementia rather than as a failed attempt to communicate.

PERSONHOOD AND THE SELF

Central to Kitwood's (1997b) thesis on person-centred care for people with dementia is the notion of personhood. He defines personhood as 'a standing or status that is bestowed upon one human being by others, in the context of relationship and social being' (1997b: 8). According to Kitwood, maintaining the personhood of each person with dementia is a crucial aspect of well-being. If we deny people with dementia their personhood then their well-being will diminish and the person-centred care many care workers strive to achieve will not become a reality. Thus, personhood is a concept that can be used to explore many facets of the experience of dementia and working with people with dementia.

A complementary concept of use in discussions around communication and personhood is the 'self'. Sabat and Harre (1992) suggest the 'self' we enable a person with dementia to present influences the way in which they can be heard and understood. They divide the self into two parts, 'self' and 'selves'. 'Self' is how an individual perceives and constructs his or her own personal identity. 'Selves' is how others construct and perceive the person. It is very easy to construct identities for people with dementia. For example, care workers' interpretations of behaviour can lead to their constructing those with dementia as 'difficult' people (Innes 1998). It is perhaps harder to accept the 'self' the person with dementia is trying to portray.

Cohen (1994) argues that anthropologists concentrate on the 'basket of selves' which any individual can draw upon in a given situation. This is useful if we wish to explore the culture of care people with dementia live within and to understand the way in which carers perceive the person with dementia. If we wish to explore the personhood of a person with dementia we need to explore the self presented to us by the person with dementia. Sabat and Collins (1999) suggest that within the social constructionist (see Chapter 3) approach to the self there are three ways in which selfhood can be expressed. The first, Self 1, is similar to the 'self' of Sabat and Harre (1992) where individuals use pronouns such as I and me to present their self. Self 2, according to Sabat and Collins (1999), is the attributes one holds, and beliefs about these attributes; thus this adds another dimension to 'self' as discussed by Sabat and Harre (1992). Self 3 is the personal personae presented to and interpreted by others which is similar to the 'selves' of Sabat and Harre, and similar to Cohen's (1994) 'basket of selves'. If we wish to enhance and maintain the personhood of each person with dementia then it is vital that we explore not only the carer's interpretation of the 'self', but also the self as understood by the person with dementia. If we do not hear and strive to understand the attempts of people with dementia to communicate we are in effect denying them a channel to express their personhood and diminishing their sense of self. Hearing and understanding requires a capacity for 'active listening' on the part of caregivers (Stokes and Goudie 1990).

LOCATING THE PROBLEM

Standard medical texts on dementia tend to relate speech and language problems primarily to damage in specific areas of the brain, but it is worth bearing in mind that in any living person this could never be more than a 'best guess'. There are no diagnostic tests or technologies currently available that would enable deficits to be localized in this way. What is more, this approach offers little potential for creative problem solving in the context of care practice.

Unorthodox or disordered speech patterns and usage of words are characteristic of verbal expression in dementia. Often these are given labels that seem to carry some form of diagnostic power (for example, perseveration, confabulation, dysphasia, echolalia). In reality these labels merely re-describe the person's incapacity in pseudo-medical terms; all they really convey is that 'he repeats the same thing over and over again'; 'she makes things up'; 'he gets his words mixed up', 'she repeats what she has just heard' and so on. One of the greatest problems with this tendency to attach diagnostic labels is that it can encourage care workers to give up very easily on attempts to understand the underlying message, on the grounds that 'it's just part of the illness'. A person with dementia will only be able to communicate effectively when he or she is heard and responded to and Table 9.1 describes suggested ways of responding to some common problems. The suggestions do not offer a solution to every problem that will arise in care practice; they will not work in each and every situation. They do, however, provide a positive context for communication. The person will know that he or she is being listened to, that someone is interested, that his or her personhood is recognized.

ASSESSMENT AND COMMUNICATION

At present the forms of linguistic expression adopted by people who have dementia are widely viewed as being part of the 'disease process'. As Sabat and Collins (1999) note, much of the available information on linguistic competence in dementia is derived from scores on standardized tests of cognitive function carried out as an aid to diagnosis. Thus, from the outset, assessment of linguistic 'incompetence' is viewed as part of the diagnosis of dementia.

Table 9.1   Common communication problems and suggested responses

Communication problem	Diagnostic label	Suggestions for person-centred responses
The person repeats key words, phrases, questions, e.g. 'When's Joan coming?'	Perseveration	The person may be worried about something, need reassurance, or want something to change. The real underlying message may be 'I'm lonely; there's nothing going on here.' What can you do to help?
The person's speech may appear to be inconsequential, vague and 'go round in circles'	Paraphasia	Try to go with the flow. Pick up on any phrases or points at which the person seems to become particularly animated and respond to these; be on the lookout for possible word games, songs or rhymes that you can incorporate into conversation.
The person may call you by the name of someone else, frequently a member of his or her close family	Nominal dysphasia	Whether or not the person really believes you to be someone else, or merely can't remember names very well, they are actually paying you a great compliment by associating you with someone so close to them.
The person may repeat your own words back to you when you ask a question or offer information	Echolalia	This could be a request for clarification, or for you to slow down a little. On the other hand it might just be a game. If the person seems to enjoy this kind of interaction go along with it.
The person may appear to cover up memory problems by turning questions back on you or giving information you suspect is inaccurate or irrelevant	Confabulation	If you need information for record keeping or other 'official' purposes it will usually be easy to check accuracy with other sources. The person may enjoy storytelling, or may be feeling a need to make him/herself 'more interesting'. Give people the message that they *are* interesting.
The person may rarely or never speak	Aphasia	Make sure that you are waiting long enough for a response. Slow down your own tempo as far as possible. Be on the lookout for non-verbal indications of what the person may be feeling.
The person may have difficulty in selecting the 'right' words and become anxious or frustrated about this	Dysphasia	Try to respond to the 'sense' of what the person is saying and give positive, non-verbal signals; ask 'Would you like to show me?' Offer cues, rather than being tempted to speak for the person.

Assessment tools such as Mini-mental State Examination (MMSE) (Folstein *et al.* 1975) and Alzheimer's Disease Assessment Schedule (ADAS) (Hodkinson 1973) rest heavily on verbal responses to a set of standard questions, which are then reduced to a single measure of 'cognitive impairment'. Sabat and Collins (1999) point out that information derived from tests of this kind may tell us very little about a person's ability to attach meanings to social situations, respond to them and express aspects of selfhood.

The shortcomings in standard measures of cognitive impairment in dementia have a number of implications. They may in some cases lead to misdiagnosis, and this is a particular problem in cases of depressive illness where the person is simply too apathetic to respond to a battery of questions. Beyond this, however, lie issues relating closely to the whole question of how personhood can be maintained or undermined through the quality of interaction with people who have dementia. Many items in standard assessment tests betray evidence of what Kitwood (1997b) has described as '**personal detraction**'. This term refers to brief examples of negative interaction with a person with dementia which, although easily overlooked, may have enormous power to undermine self-esteem and well-being. Kitwood refers, for example, to 'outpacing', 'treachery' and 'disruption' as three among the total of 17 types of personal detraction so far identified.

It is a sad fact that many items designed to test cognitive function in dementia seem calculated to baffle and bemuse. For example, in one widely used test, the person is asked to repeat the words, 'No ifs, ands or buts.' Should he or she take this as a prohibition on using the words 'ifs, ands or buts' – a reasonable interpretation – it will be impossible to give the 'right' answer. The three types of personal detraction mentioned above are clearly evident in this test item, as in many others. The anxiety and distress that may be caused by assessments of this nature are painful to contemplate once we begin to focus on the subjective experience of the person who is 'on the receiving end' of them.

Whitworth *et al.* (1999) propose an assessment tool that involves caregivers in 'managing the communication' of persons with dementia. This tool is undoubtedly a move forward in that 'professionals' would no longer be the sole group involved in assessing communication abilities. However, the person with dementia is not central to the process and the tool is therefore of limited use in enhancing personhood through their involvement. The tool does, however, lead to strategies for carers to communicate with the person with dementia which could enhance personhood.

If a person with dementia has already been labelled, as the result of a diagnostic assessment or simply from routine observation, as having 'no verbal communication skills' or 'very little ability to communicate', care workers will tend to base their own interactions with the person on that label. (See Chapter 3 for further discussion of 'labelling'.) It has often been noted that 'social speech', for example greeting people and 'passing the time of day', is preserved for a considerable time even when a person with dementia appears to have lost the ability to hold a more sustained conversation. Research indicates that the typical interaction between care workers and those with dementia lasts only a few seconds, and tends to lack meaningful content (Bowie and Mountain 1993). The vast majority of interactions tend to be along the lines, 'Hello, Mrs Brown, how are you today? Nearly lunch time.' It is unsurprising that social speech is preserved if this is the only opportunity for interaction the person is offered. It is important that care workers learn the skills to extend their own repertoire for communicating, on both verbal and non-verbal levels, with people who have dementia.

HEARING THE VOICES OF PEOPLE WITH DEMENTIA

It is somewhat ironic that despite the current postmodern discourse (see Chapter 3) that has led to researchers attempting to 'hear the voice' of people who are the subject of the researchers' interest, we do not hear the voice of the group we purport to hear. Instead we frequently hear the voices of care practitioners and researchers. The title of Goldsmith's (1996) work, *Hearing the Voice of People with Dementia*, is an example of this. This book describes ideas about *how* to hear the voice of people with dementia based upon interviews with a small number of people with dementia (six) distributed to a large sample of caregivers for their comments. Therefore, the voice of carers is clearly heard but not the voice of people with dementia themselves.

Goldsmith (1996) heads one chapter in his book 'Communication is possible'. This is clearly a positive message, and a significant step forward. However, there is a more sobering message that needs to be taken on board. *Communication has been happening all along and* we *have failed to recognize it*. Communication in the full sense of the word involves far more than a coherent, rational, verbal statement made by one person and immediately understood by another. The vast majority of human communication is not like this at all. It is essentially a two-way process of negotiating meanings, which involves not only verbal interaction but also all the subtle nuances of facial expression, eye contact, posture, touch and gesture. A person who has lost verbal skills as a result of dementia may still have an extensive repertoire of such communicative actions at his or her disposal.

An example of a recent attempt to hear the voice of people with dementia by service providers is reported in Dabbs (1999). The aim was to discover what people with dementia thought about their care provision. Unfortunately little attempt is made to interpret the words people use and to get to the emotive level of how people feel about their care provision. Dabbs (1999) recognizes the multiple techniques advanced by Goldsmith to try and communicate with people with dementia and discusses these in his report but does not succeed in applying them other than to present a rather bland representation of statements that would have been worthy of further interpretation and analysis. Thus, despite suggestions about how to hear the voice of people with dementia using a variety of communication techniques, there remains a dearth of accounts of the experience of dementia from people with dementia (see also Chapter 5).

COMMUNICATION AS AN ART

Killick (1997) uses poetic licence in recording the words of people with dementia. By spending time with them and 'editing' their words in various ways he has produced some moving poems. These poems convey a 'feeling' of what the person might be trying to communicate rather than focusing on the precise nature of the words used by the person. Thus we get closer to capturing what people with dementia are trying to communicate. If the aim of communication is to maintain personhood, which relates closely to notions of the self as perceived by the person, then we are in essence close to an emotional discourse where we are attempting to get close to the emotions of the person in order to ascertain his or her state of well-being. As Gubrium (1989: 266) has put it, 'what is important about poetry as emotional discourse is that it is poetic, more what poetry does than what it says, a means of making meaningful something that is otherwise altogether too mysterious for words'. Thus Killick is successful in helping readers think that they have come closer to feeling what the person with dementia may feel. When we take the poetry away words can appear bland and not tell us much about the self, personhood or well-being of those who have communicated verbally.

Killick's work is often very moving, as it illustrates how the speech of people who have dementia can be imbued with deep meaning. The resulting growth of awareness has perhaps fuelled current research interest in possibilities for interpreting the spoken language of people with dementia. Here, however, interpretation is not likely to be straightforward. As Kitwood (1997b) notes, meaning may be conveyed in several different ways. The words of a person with dementia may be concrete statements of fact but they may also be allusive, referring only briefly or indirectly to the person's true cause for concern. Communication may also have metaphorical significance, linking events, people or places somehow connected in the person's mind. In a general sense, metaphors are figures of speech with shared social meanings. In dementia it often seems that 'metaphorical' forms of expression have a deeply personal meaning. For example, Knocker (1998) reports the case of a woman with dementia who used the words 'I've been camouflaged' to describe her feelings about going into residential care. Her experience was, perhaps, that she had been put in a situation where she simply faded into the background, where she did not stand out as a person in her own right. Knocker notes that there may also be associations with the word 'sabotaged'. Interpretation of such forms of expression will inevitably require a close knowledge of the person's life history and circumstances, as well as an ability to 'go with the flow', responding to the 'sense' and the tempo of the interaction, rather than to literal meanings.

PRACTICALITIES OF COMMUNICATION

Although much has been written on this issue, it would appear that we still have a great deal to learn. It is recognized that we must allow time for effective communication to occur and that we need to give our full attention to the person. What does this mean though in relation to hearing and attending to 'the self' that the person with dementia presents? We may give our full attention to what *we think* people are saying rather than what *they are* trying to communicate. Sabat and Collins (1999) present a wonderful case study of Mrs F. as an example of ways in which the listener can attend to the self that the person in question is presenting. Mrs F. was an accomplished musician and key member of her family. The case study exemplifies the use of this knowledge of Mrs F.'s life history in communication with those around her. Mrs F. clearly benefits by others responding positively to 'the self' that she presents. There are, however, accounts which are classic examples of the listener interpreting the words of people with dementia in a way that denies their self and personhood (Fontana and Smith 1989). For example, 'Doug', a man with Alzheimer's disease, was observed interacting with his wife. When Doug 'uttered nonsensical statements' the observer labelled him as 'a victim'. Communication was difficult to understand, therefore the attempts of Doug to communicate were disregarded and in the process his personhood denied. It appears that the words of the person with dementia are often noted but the underlying meanings of the words are overlooked, and the effect that the response of the carer has on the person is ignored. Thus, Fontana and Smith discuss the 'unbecoming' of the self of the person with Alzheimer's disease, attributing this process to the disease and not to the actions of those listening to the words.

There are practical issues to consider when communicating with anyone for example; can the person literally hear you speak? Can the person see you? Is the person communicating discomfort non-verbally, for example shivering because they are cold, or grimacing because they are in pain? Factors such as these can be overlooked if the listener has a view of the person based on their own interpretations of the self. For example, if a person is perceived as bad tempered, a grimace of pain can be interpreted as an example of a person's bad mood or displeasure rather than an attempt to communicate physical discomfort.

Communication can be further complicated if one does not understand the cultural background of the person with dementia. Brownlie (1991) provides a series of case studies where the behaviour of the person with dementia is not understood by the majority culture. For example, a Chinese woman's attempts to communicate her severe headache were understood by the family, but were interpreted by care home staff as a 'bad mood'. Her dislike of wearing underwear indoors was misinterpreted by care staff as inappropriate behaviour, rather than as her cultural habit. The difference in well-being when the cultural background of a person with dementia is considered is illustrated by the case of Amos, an African–Caribbean man described by Tibbs (1996). A package of care was introduced providing structure to Amos's day taking account of his cultural and personal preferences. Thus his religious observances were continued and he was provided with his favourite foods.

Implications for personhood

There is, of course, a good case for keeping communication with people who have dementia as simple as possible, for example for practical purposes related to their care, or when it is necessary to gain basic information. At the same time it is often evident that the feelings and concerns that people with dementia are trying themselves to convey are very profound indeed. This means that caregivers need the flexibility to be able to communicate on a number of different levels. Facilitating communication for 'everyday' purposes requires a great deal of sensitivity and patience, and a determination not to give up on someone whose speech may be slow or difficult to comprehend. People with dementia are often confused by direct, open-ended questions, such as 'What would you like for lunch?', or by the rapid-fire presentation of a number of choices: 'Would you like x, y or z?' Using a series of prompts and an interrogative tone of voice may be more constructive in many cases; for example, 'You'd like this one? . . . this one? . . . this one?', while showing actual dishes or allowing the person to indicate by pointing.

When interaction – whether verbal or non-verbal – is initiated by the person with dementia it is important that caregivers try not to interrupt the flow by introducing questions requiring direct responses that the person is unable to give such as, 'What do you want?', 'Where are you going?', 'Why are you doing that?' The person's sense of self is likely to be undermined by the inability to explain what he or she is doing or why. Facilitating responses are those which take the form, 'Can I help you . . . ?', 'Would you like to show me . . . ?', 'Shall we walk together . . . ?'

When the person with dementia asks the same question repeatedly, this may be because it has some deep significance not recognized by caregivers. If a person is repeatedly asking the time, for example, he or she may not want a literal response such as 'four o'clock . . . five past four . . . ten past four'. Their questions may be a sign of boredom; a feeling that time is passing very slowly. A friendly conversation *about* the time of day, what is happening, what people are doing and what's going to happen later on may make all the difference. The person does not have to be able to participate in such a discussion actively in order to enjoy it and benefit from it. 'Difficult' questions can tend to trigger a negative response in caregivers who lack confidence in their own communication skills. This may take the form of 'blocking' further communication by withdrawing from the situation and becoming emotionally unavailable to the person with dementia. Alternatively, caregivers sometimes attempt to gain control of the situation by offering answers too complex or detailed for the person to cope with. One man in a residential home was constantly asking with evident anxiety, 'Is he going to get married to her?' The standard immediate response to this was, 'Is *who* going to marry *who*?' This simply increased his anxiety. Responses of this kind will make any further confidence impossible, even though the caregiver may have a genuine desire to help. An 'enabling/facilitating' response may require a series of gentle cues which enable the person to open up the discussion further; for example, 'Getting married

Table 9.2   Checklist for communication

In any communication with a person with dementia it is worth bearing the following points in mind:

- Make sure the person can see you.
- Make sure the person can hear you.
- Make sure the person is comfortable – look out for any obvious signs of discomfort and respond to these first.
- Reinforce your presence through reassuring physical contact (e.g. touch the person's arm before you speak).
- Take your time; be prepared to give your full attention and to wait until the person feels ready to talk to you.
- Learn as much as you can about the person's life history; for example, what is important to them, what they enjoy doing and their cultural beliefs.

... that's a big step', 'You're worried about that ... ?', 'You think they might get married ... ?' Interestingly this technique is one which is widely used in the form of humanistic psychotherapy pioneered by Carl Rogers and known as 'client-centred therapy' (Rogers 1965). In this form of therapy, the client's statements are never challenged, disputed or undermined – he or she is simply invited to elaborate further until the underlying concern becomes apparent.

Key points to consider in communicating with people with dementia are summarized in Table 9.2.

REFLEXIVITY AND COMMUNICATION IN DEMENTIA CARE

Our sense of identity, belonging and being effective is undermined when we are unable to understand what other people say and do. We may feel that the words and categories we use have to have fixed and stable meanings and when a person with dementia challenges this view it can cause a sense of anxiety and a sense of threat. Our own over-dependence on verbal communication means that we quickly become anxious and confused when others do not share our understanding of the structures and meanings of language. Exploring the reasons why caregivers find it difficult to respond to language and behaviour that they consider disordered, bizarre or inappropriate may be the key to developing new ways of working through interpersonal communication. Disordered and unorthodox modes of expression are perhaps less of a problem for the person with dementia than they are for caregivers.

Communicating with people with dementia requires care workers to reflect not only on what the person with dementia is expressing, verbally or non-verbally, but to reflect on what they themselves are expressing through their words and body language. Maintaining the personhood of each person with dementia, and recognizing and acknowledging the self with which the person with dementia identifies, requires caregivers to develop self-awareness skills, to recognize the power dynamic within the care relationship and to recognize how the person with dementia views others. Thus we arrive at the conclusion that reflexivity is required of caregivers.

If we can reframe both verbal and non-verbal forms of communication available to people with dementia as a positive resource in our thinking about dementia – and our working in dementia care – then the personhood or self of the person with dementia will stand a greater chance of remaining intact.

FURTHER READING

Goldsmith, M. (1996) *Hearing the Voice of People with Dementia: Opportunities and Obstacles.* London: Jessica Kingsley.

Killick, J. (1997) *You Are Words.* London: Hawker Publications.

Killick, J. and Allan, K. (2001) *Communication in the Care of People with Dementia.* Buckingham: Open University Press.

Kitwood, T. (1997) Personhood maintained, Chapter 4 in *Dementia Reconsidered.* Buckingham: Open University Press.

Sabat, S. and Collins, M. (1999) Intact social, cognitive ability and selfhood: a case study of Alzheimer's Disease. *American Journal of Alzheimer's Disease,* January/February: 11–19.

10

DAWN BROOKER

Therapeutic activity

KEY POINTS

- The range of therapeutic activity has increased rapidly over recent years particularly in the area of creative therapies, sensory therapies and person-centred approaches.
- There are many ideas for good practice but little hard evidence of effectiveness. A strong evidence-based practice model cannot be presented.
- Dementia care has undergone a radical shift in recent years. There will be a latency period before this is reflected in an evidence-based model, particularly given the problems of carrying out valid, reliable and meaningful research in this arena.
- Agreement on core outcomes of therapeutic activity for people with dementia is required, along with standard measures of these outcomes, in order for progress to be made in this research.
- The challenge for therapists is in deciding which therapeutic activity is likely to benefit which individual.
- The development of a general therapeutic environment in formal care settings for people with dementia, along with specifically tailored individual or group activity, is a challenge for service providers.

INTRODUCTION

Therapeutic activities in dementia care are inextricably linked to how dementia is construed. The current popularity for therapeutic activity is part of the **old**

culture – new culture shift (Kitwood 1995). Thirty years ago the
of people with dementia would have been seen as part of their
and no attempt would have been made to reverse it. Indeed, di
activity was seen by some as a fundamental part of the ageing p
given as an explanation of why older people did less than
(Cumming and Henry 1961).

During the 1970s and into the 1980s the pioneering wo
positively with people with dementia began to flourish. There was a backlash
against institutionalization and a wish to provide people with valued lives.
Approaches such as reality orientation, validation therapy and reminiscence
therapy (described below) gained popularity. In the 1980s and early 1990s the
trend in therapeutic activities became more focused on treating behavioural
disturbance, challenging behaviour and distress (Stokes 1996). Since the late
1990s, Kitwood's work on the link between the social environment and well-
being in dementia has had a major impact on therapeutic activity. The person-
centred approach is now very popular within the therapeutic literature for this
client group. This is reflected in the increase in therapeutic activities that aim
to validate individual experience and the express aim to communicate even
with those experiencing the most disabling stages of dementia.

This chapter will begin with a brief overview of the many therapeutic activities that are described in the current literature. Issues regarding the general
purpose of therapeutic activity and matching therapies to individuals will be
discussed. The chapter will conclude by considering what is known about
therapeutic process with people with dementia.

THERAPEUTIC ACTIVITIES: AN OVERVIEW

There are now more types of therapeutic activities available to this client group
than ever before. These are exciting times indeed, but they can also be quite
bewildering for newcomers to the area. Therapeutic activity for people with
dementia can be divided into five main groups. The first are those therapeutic
techniques that attempt to compensate for the level of disorientation associated
with dementia. The second group is those that use long-term memory as a means
of therapeutic **engagement**. The third group is a collection of therapeutic approaches that use elements of person-centred counselling. The fourth group
uses creative media as a means of helping people and the fifth use primarily
sensory interaction. Within each of these groups there are some activities that
have a group focus and others that have an individual focus. In practice many
activities draw on all five means of engagement, but most activities will name
one as being primary.

Orientation therapies

The rationale for reality orientation (RO) is to try to re-provide information
that people have lost through neurological impairment, primarily to orientate

the person to place, time and person. This can take place through all direct staff–client interactions throughout general care and orientation signage (24-hour RO) or through small structured group sessions (formal RO). The **Cochrane review** on RO (Spector *et al.* 1999a) concluded that there is evidence that it improves behaviour and cognition in people with dementia. Holden and Woods (1995) provide a useful review of RO practice and research.

RO has fallen out of fashion in recent years, mainly because of the abuses of the method, which could render it a rather mechanistic, and sometimes a pointless, confrontational therapeutic technique. Indeed, some writers (for example Jones 1995) actually see RO as counterproductive to well-being in dementia care. It is easy in hindsight to dismiss RO as simplistic and dehumanizing. Seen in its historical context, however, this was far from the truth. Much positive therapeutic work was carried out under the banner of RO. Providing orientating information with the aim of improving confidence and well-being appears to be common sense. There is much still to recommend a sensitive use of RO with some individuals particularly during the earlier stages when people are struggling to keep a grip on present reality.

Therapies recalling past experience

Reminiscence lends itself well to people with mild to moderate dementia. At this stage, new learning is difficult but well-rehearsed memories are still accessible and can be shared verbally. Many people, both with and without dementia, find reminiscing to be an inherently pleasurable experience. Reminiscence therapy involves the sharing of memories often evoked through the use of stimulating material such as old pictures, songs, household items and newspapers. Originally this was developed for use by elderly people without dementia to help them in reviewing life experience (Coleman 1986a). It was also often incorporated into RO groups but here the aim was to reinforce current reality. Woods and McKiernan (1995) provide an excellent review. The main positive outcome from group reminiscence for people with dementia appears to be in increasing contributions, enjoyment and engagement. Well-being has been shown to improve during participation in reminiscence groups over other types of group activity for people with dementia in day-care settings (Brooker and Duce 2000).

The research evidence for the benefits of reminiscence therapy to date is weak. The Cochrane Review (Spector *et al.* 1999b) on the subject found that no firm conclusions could be reached regarding the effectiveness of reminiscence therapy for people with dementia and highlighted the need for more systematic research in this area. In clinical practice, reminiscence therapy is now extremely popular with major conferences and networks firmly established (for example Schweitzer 1999). It may be, as with many of these therapies, that the outcome measures used have not been sensitive to change. Like all therapies there are particular skills to be learnt in its application, not least in the recognition that powerful negative emotions can be brought out as well as powerful positive ones.

The use of life histories and life-books has grown increasingly popular in practice in recent years and these can help to ensure that reminiscence can be individualized to maximize well-being. There is very little research in this area apart from a promising study by Gibson (1994). In her work, life history compilation was used to improve communication and relationships within the present environment. Individualizing reminiscence in this way can be a means of helping care practitioners recognize the person rather than the disease process, and can enable them to understand 'confused' behaviour better.

Cheston and Byatt (1999) provide an interesting single case report on the use of taped memories recorded by a husband of a lady with dementia (simulated presence therapy – SPT). It was noticed that although she was calm when her family visited her in a nursing home she would become very distressed after they left. She appeared to be comforted by the tape. SPT is presented as a way of helping decrease attachment anxiety caused by separation from a beloved person. Camberg *et al.* (1999) attempted to evaluate SPT in 54 nursing home residents, comparing it to usual care and to listening to a tape of a newspaper being read. Staff observations were that it produced a positive effect and in a rating of happy facial expressions, SPT was at least equivalent to usual care.

Therapeutic counselling approaches

Many therapeutic approaches recognize the importance of responding to the emotional needs of the person with dementia – particularly in helping people feel validated in their experience. Validation therapy works with the emotional experience of the client. It has its roots in a person-centred counselling approach (Rogerian counselling) although it was originally used in elderly care by Naomi Feil (1993). Disturbed behaviour is seen to have meaning in expressing unmet needs for human contact. The needs fall into three broad types:

* needs for nurture and love;
* needs for engagement in activity;
* needs for an understanding response to the expression of distressing emotions.

Validation therapy can take place one to one or in a group setting. Group validation sessions cover discussion topics with an emotional context such as separation from family or loss of role. Individual group members are given responsibility for specific group tasks such as giving out the drinks or leading the singing. There is very little in the way of published research into the usefulness of validation therapy although Finnema *et al.* (1998) report ongoing research. Feil's ideas have, however, had a direct influence on the development of the person-centred approach in dementia care.

There has been a growing interest in the use of individual and group psychotherapy and counselling with people with dementia. Cheston (1998) provides a review of the literature. Resolution therapy (Stokes and Goudie 1990; Stokes 2000) is described as a way of using basic counselling skills in order to clarify emotional responses, to validate them and to identify unmet needs. Care planning is used to try to meet these where possible. Bender (1999a, b) usefully describes counselling in practice.

Jones (1995) presents an interesting discussion about the application of Sullivanian psychotherapy with people with dementia. Sullivan saw one of the main functions of the self as managing or avoiding anxiety. In dementia, anxiety is increased early on because of awareness of cognitive impairment. Cognitive impairment also diminishes the individual's internal mechanisms for coping with anxiety. As cognitive abilities decline, the individual's threshold for coping with environmental stress lowers. Therefore, a therapeutic activity is one that becomes less challenging and more supportive over time, matching the cognitive powers of the individual. The main therapeutic task is to engage individuals without overwhelming them.

Positive person work (Kitwood 1997b) could also be regarded as being a counselling approach. Kitwood outlined a provisional list of 12 types of positive interactions which he proposed enhance personhood including:

- recognition of the person;
- negotiation of choices;
- collaboration on tasks;
- play experiences;
- timalation of the senses (refers to ways of working with sensory rather than cognitive pathways);
- celebration of joy;
- relaxation;
- validation of emotions;
- holding of vulnerability (refers to containing or holding people who may feel very anxious);
- facilitation of agency (refers to empowering people to make decisions or helping them to do things for themselves);
- creative expression;
- giving by the person with dementia.

In Kitwood's view, this sort of psychotherapeutic work would form the basis of the way people with dementia are cared for, whatever activity is being undertaken. Therapeutic activity in this context would not be seen as an add-on carried out by a visiting professional, but as something fundamental to the act of living. Johnson (1998) makes the same argument, albeit from a more practical viewpoint. She suggests that fundamental activities such as meal preparation, homecare, shopping, childcare and gardening should be primary vehicles for those with dementia and their caregivers working together.

Some intervention strategies draw on a number of different techniques. Haupt (1996) describes 'mediator-centred interactional therapy' in which care staff (the mediators) are encouraged to support four areas which threaten the self-worth of people with dementia. First, they incorporate RO strategies to ensure a linkage between past, present and future. Second, they encourage the clients to be active and they engender a feeling of helpfulness and usefulness on the part of the people with dementia. Third, they use validation-type techniques when responding to confused statements of reality. Fourth, they ensure communication is at a level that is appropriate to the person with dementia. Haupt claims that in his experience this strategy leads to a reduction or elimination of disturbed behaviour although this has not been systematically evaluated.

Creative therapies

These are now increasingly being used with people with dementia. Groene *et al.* (1998) report a comparison of music and exercise therapy for six individuals with dementia. In this small group study participants responded more purposely to exercises to music as opposed to singalongs. Jensen (1997) writes graphically about her experiences of running an art group over a period of years with older people living in a nursing home. Approximately 60 per cent of her groups were made up of people at varying stages of dementia. Her approach was to combine art, music, and movement. She began her groups with music and movement, usually from the Big Band era, which was culturally appropriate for her group. Drawing with oil pastels was geared towards aiding reminiscence and recall in an effort to improve self-identity and self-esteem. No formal evaluations were made but she presents two very interesting case studies. Ashida (2000) presents some group data that suggests a decrease in depressive symptoms in nursing home residents with dementia following a five-day reminiscence-focused music therapy. Batson (1998) writes very enthusiastically about his work as a drama therapist with people with dementia, with many useful insights for those who wish to work creatively. Again, no formal evaluation has been made of the work.

Sensory therapeutic activity

Activities based around sensory stimulation have a simple aim of increasing engagement in activity by using sensory rather than cognitive routes to contact. The rationale for using these therapies with this client group is straightforward. As cognitive abilities decline it becomes increasingly difficult for the person with dementia to communicate verbally. People with advanced dementia often appear distressed but, because of the barriers of cognitive impairment, the therapeutic approaches described above are seen as ineffective. Communicating at a more basic level through massage, sound, and aromatherapy seems to be common sense. The aim of such therapies is to relax, to decrease anxiety and to improve well-being.

Multisensory environment stimulation such as **Snoezelen** has grown in popularity. This sort of stimulation, which typically consists of clients experiencing multisensory input in the form of music, projected images, bubble-tubes, aromatherapy, fibre-optic sprays etc. set up in a specific room, has its origins in the field of learning disabilities and paediatrics. Hope (1996) provides a review of the limited literature that is available in the field of dementia care. Evidence available at the moment would suggest that such activity is enjoyable and relaxing for some and that staff often view it as positive. Hope makes the point that using the environment to make full use of the clients' senses in their everyday lives may be preferable to taking them off to a special room for a specific 'therapeutic' experience.

Brooker et al. (1997) evaluated the effects of aromatherapy and massage on disturbed behaviour in four individuals with severe dementia using a **single case research design**. Each participant received ten treatment sessions of aromatherapy, aromatherapy and massage combined, and massage alone. The effects on each individual's behaviour in the hour following treatment was assessed against ten 'no treatment' control sessions. The opinion of the staff providing treatment was that all participants benefited. On close scrutiny of the data, however, only one of the participants benefited from the aromatherapy and massage to a degree that reached statistical decrease in agitation. In two of the cases aromatherapy and massage led to an increase in agitated behaviour, although not to a statistically significant degree.

The use of modality specific stimulation, that is just using one sense such as sight or hearing, has also been reported. Burgio et al. (1996) reported using 'white noise', that is the sort of noise one hears when a radio is not tuned, to decrease verbal agitation. This paper reports using audiotapes of white noise delivered by headsets with 13 very dependent elderly people with severe dementia. It is difficult to assess the exact reduction in verbal agitation as the results were aggregated across many sessions. The definition of verbal agitation used in this study was very broad and included verbal behaviour which could have been seen as non-agitated by some observers. There is no discussion of whether participants were displaying less 'verbal agitation' because they found the white noise soothing or because they simply wanted it to stop. It may be that the method is worth further investigation but that attention needs to be paid to the factors that determine reduction for individuals. Lyketos (1999) et al. report on the usefulness of **bright light therapy** which appeared to help those with disturbed sleep patterns to achieve a better night's sleep.

McNamara and Kempenaar (1998) describe a pilot study and some planned randomized controlled research on sensory stimulation. Clients are assessed to discover their preferred mode of sensory stimulation. It is planned that relatives should then carry out the specific sensory stimulation at home. The results are not available at the time of going to press. This is also one of the few studies to investigate therapeutic activity within a domestic environment.

From this brief overview of current approaches it can be seen that the field of therapeutic endeavour with this client group is burgeoning. The gap between research and practice is wide. A strong evidence-based practice model does not (yet) exist. The field of therapeutic activity in dementia care is a rapidly developing one. Ideas on care culture and therapeutic outcomes have undergone a radical shift in recent years. There is bound to be a latency period before this is reflected in research, particularly given the problems of carrying out valid, reliable and meaningful research in this arena.

THE MEASUREMENT OF THERAPEUTIC OUTCOME IN DEMENTIA

The question arises as to why so much energy is being spent in developing therapeutic activity with this client group. This is in part a humanitarian response to the evident withdrawal and distress that can be seen in dementia care settings. Defining and measuring therapeutic outcome in dementia care is a difficult challenge. **Rehabilitation** of function to pre-morbid levels is not achievable within dementia. People with dementia have a disability that will, by definition, lead to an increasing degree of cognitive impairment. Perrin and May (1999) provide a comprehensive discussion of the sorts of outcomes that occupational therapists have traditionally striven for (such as rehabilitation and independence) and find these unhelpful in the arena of dementia care.

Some writers describe the reduction in number or frequency of challenging or distressed behaviours as a good outcome for example Burgio *et al.* 1996; Brooker *et al.* (1997); Doyle *et al.* (1997); Sival *et al.* (1997). A good outcome in dementia care has also been described as improving well-being (Haupt 1996; Kitwood 1997b; Coppola 1998; Hasselkus 1998) or decreasing anxiety (Jones 1995). It may be that challenging behaviours are an indicator of underlying **ill-being** or distress but experience would suggest that this is not always the case. There are cases of challenging behaviour which may be problematic for staff groups or family members but which are not indicative of distress in the people with dementia themselves.

In old culture-speak the sole purpose of therapeutic activity was to decrease disturbed behaviour or agitation. In new culture the main purpose is to improve well-being through improved communication. Kitwood (1997b: 58–69) cites some examples of 'rementia'. This is characterized by high levels of well-being in the face of high levels of cognitive loss. It can occur in formal care environments which pay particular attention to maintaining personhood. The vast majority of these examples are anecdotal or small-scale. Currently a larger scale UK longitudinal study is underway under the auspices of the Bradford Dementia Group. This seeks to describe the natural history of dementia for individuals who are being cared for in a person-centred care environment.

The definition and measurement of well-being in dementia is an important one in knowing whether therapeutic activities are achieving valid outcomes. Verbal reports of life satisfaction may not be reliable because of the problems that many people with dementia have with verbal expression and recall. Batson (1998) describes outcome in terms of the frequent occurrence of 'quality moments'. He defines well-being here as the behavioural indicators that one would be looking for within a Dementia Care Mapping evaluation (Bradford Dementia Group 1997). Indicators of well-being in this context would be recognized by the person with dementia demonstrating assertiveness, bodily relaxation, sensitivity to the needs of others, humour, creative self-expression, showing pleasure, helpfulness, initiating social contact, showing affection, signs of self-respect and expression of a range of emotions. Brooker and Duce (2000) used DCM formally to evaluate the effects of reminiscence therapy. The Bradford Dementia Group has developed a scale for assessing the profile of well-being and ill-being for individuals and this could prove to be a useful outcome measure (Bruce 1997, 2000).

At present the maintenance and improvement of well-being in people with dementia is the therapeutic outcome indicator which best fits with current thinking on dementia. There are a number of research papers on therapeutic activity that document staff comments on improvement in individual clients but no significant change in terms of the outcome measures used (for example Brooker *et al.* 1997; Doyle *et al.* 1997). This may be because, in an area such as dementia care, where practitioners are desperate to see clients improve, effectiveness tends to be overestimated. It could also be, however, that the outcome measures used were insensitive or inappropriate. Standardized measures of well-being in the arena of therapeutic activity in dementia care requires further development in order that practice can become evidence-based.

MATCHING THERAPIES TO INDIVIDUALS

People with dementia are an extraordinarily heterogeneous group of individuals who lead a wide variety of different lifestyles and who have a long life history behind them. In order best to promote well-being within dementia care there needs to be careful matching of type and style of therapeutic activity to individuals. The question addressed in this section is not, 'How can we engage people with dementia?' but rather, 'What should we do to engage Mrs Bloggs and why is that different to what we do to engage Mr Brown?'

Given that past behaviour is usually a good predictor of future behaviour, then knowing as much as possible about past likes and dislikes can help enormously in planning therapeutic activities. Likewise, knowing a person's history can be useful in trying to interpret current behaviour. It is often difficult to obtain this sort of information from the people themselves once the disease process has taken hold. Many care units have developed formal ways of collecting this sort of information from carers and relatives (see Oyebode *et al.* 1996). Knowing what activities people enjoyed is important. Also, the way in which they enjoyed things may be equally important. Strivers may need to continue to achieve, watchers may need to continue to observe, players may need to continue to mess about and gossipers may need to continue to chat.

It may also be that there are particular emotional issues that are more pertinent for people with dementia to work through at particular stages. At diagnosis, for example, there may be many issues around acceptance and fears for the future. Later on there may be issues about accepting help and dependency. Later still there are likely to be issues around emotional security and holding. Cheston (1998) suggests that different types of psychotherapeutic intervention may require different levels of 'cognitive competence'. Cognitive approaches may only be suitable early on where verbal reasoning skills are still comparatively intact. Behavioural interventions may be more suited to middle stages whereas contact through more physical and sensory means may be more appropriate in later stages.

Jones (1995) also emphasizes that therapeutic approach and goals need to be tailored to the level of dementia. Increasing degree of insight is a traditional goal in psychotherapy. As Cheston (1998) points out this may not be an appropriate aim for clients with dementia. The insight may simply intensify distress without leading to resolution because of memory problems and lack of support. Jones (1995) also recommends that insight-orientated interventions may be counterproductive in middle to late dementia.

As dementia is a disability of cognitive functioning, an assessment should be made of the person's relative strengths and needs in this area. Although general patterns can be attributed to length of time since disease onset, this is not reliable enough for planning some types of therapeutic activity. New learning will be difficult at all stages. Difficulty with perceptual processes, dyspraxias and communication problems will make a great deal of difference to how clients engage with the world and what practitioners need to do in order to support them in this (for more detailed discussions see Morris 1996 and Stokes 2000). Unless practitioners are aware of these specific disabilities they may ask their clients to engage in ways that they will find impossible, subsequently experiencing the loss of well-being that failure engenders.

A number of writers have looked at a reversal of the stages of childhood development as holding a clue to our understanding of decline in cognitive abilities in older people (see Stuart-Hamilton 1996). Perrin and May (1999) use the assessment of level of developmental ability as a starting point for appropriate engagement. They equate the traditional stage descriptors in dementia (early, early to middle, middle to late and late) to the stages of child development identified by the psychologist Piaget (reflective, representational, sensorimotor and reflex). Thus in the early stage of dementia there is little damage to major cognitive systems and people will probably enjoy goal-directed activities such as competitive games and quizzes (similar to the abilities of the reflective stage). At this stage they may well also enjoy tasks with end products such as in crafts and making things. As people enter the middle stage of dementia, their abilities become more like those in the representational period and reflective-type activities become increasingly difficult and anxiety-provoking. During this time the people can only be concerned with themselves, seeing themselves at the centre of the world and interpreting events from this perspective. Generally people will be happier being alongside each other or on a one-to-one basis rather than working cooperatively in a group. So called 'delusional' ideas are readily expressed during this stage which may have a function in maintaining the individual's sense of self-worth. Commonly heard ideas such as blaming others for accidents or mistakes, or claiming that one is expected home shortly, or that one is in day-care to help out with the old people, may have this sort of function. Perrin and May (1999) suggest that activities such as music, dance, drama and art may be particularly therapeutic during this stage, tapping into the freedom of expression that is part of this developmental stage.

As the disease progresses, in the later middle stage, working at this sort of symbolic level becomes much more difficult as the sensori-motor period becomes prominent. Thought becomes more concrete and people respond primarily to their physical senses and the pleasure of sensation in the here and now. Perrin and May (1999) suggest that Snoezelen, pets, massage, ball games, bubbles and dolls among other things will provide therapeutic benefit at this time. In the most advanced stages people are said to be in the reflex period. Their reflexes in response to the external world are all that may be left. Holding, stroking, rocking, singing and smiling form the basis of our human interactions. Perrin and May (1999) contend that these are as important at the end of life as they were in the beginning.

Perrin and May (1999) are at pains to point out that this approach is not to infantilize people with dementia but rather to guide our way of being with them. For example, they say:

> ... we approach a twelve-month-old rather differently to how we approach a seven-year-old. And we approach a fifteen-year-old rather differently again. Our expectations and our demands vary according to our understanding of their abilities and their perception of the world. Openness, consideration and courtesy can easily be a constant in our approach to all age groups, but unless our expectations are modified by our appreciation of level of ability in cognitive and social skills, our interactions are likely to be unproductive.
>
> (Perrin and May 1999: 42)

Whether the stage theory proves useful in helping us to individualize therapeutic activities for people with dementia needs to be verified by empirical research. It may simply be that we are seeing decline in abilities linked to patterns of damage to neurological structures rather than the development of psychological processes for dealing with a changing internal world. This may or may not follow the development in such structures at the other end of the lifespan. Nonetheless, the idea that we relate to people according to their level of ability is central to the establishment of any therapeutic relationship. It is key to providing therapeutic activities.

THE PROCESS OF THERAPEUTIC ACTIVITY

The attitudes and skill with which any therapeutic activity is undertaken is crucial to its success. A number of writers have described skills that are important within all therapeutic activity for people with dementia. Jones (1995) provides some useful pointers on therapeutic process based on his experience. He feels the physical context in which the therapeutic intervention occurs is much less important than the quality of the relationship between the person with dementia and the therapist. Perrin (1997a) in her study of persons with severe dementia found that very few of her sample were able to maintain any activity without the direct and sustained help of a care practitioner. The skills involved in this sort of work cannot be underestimated. The special skills of engagement and communication with people with dementia are key to any therapeutic activity.

Hasselkus (1998) and Coppola (1998) describe an 'occupational process model' that includes three phases of preparation, engagement and outcomes in engaging individuals with dementia in therapeutic activities. During preparation they describe staff using skills of persuading, redirecting, teaching, enabling and searching for the key that will unlock communication and lead to meaningful engagement. This is called 'meeting of the minds' by Hasselkus. This continues into the engagement phase. True engagement is seen as a fleeting experience for the person with dementia. The skill of caregiving here is to attend closely and connect with the client, using many levels of communication, to entice the person with dementia to remain engaged. Hasselkus stresses the importance of individually tailoring activities to the abilities and frame of reference of the client as well as the importance of providing a care environment that is rich in opportunities for engaging in activities and occupation. The outcomes phase is seen as striving for well-being for the individual with dementia which in turn leads to feelings of well-being for the care practitioner.

Following on from their developmental model Perrin and May (1999) draw on the literature of attachment theory to offer care practitioners a way of being with people with severe dementia. In order for people with severe dementia to feel secure in their attachments they suggest the following principles of caregiving:

- Carers should be easily accessible, and responsive to clients' signals and bids for attention.
- Carers need to be able to be free to express emotions in an overt manner.
- Carers should enjoy and actively solicit close physical contact with their clients.
- Carers should encourage their clients' exploration of and engagement with their immediate environment.
- Balanced care should be able to alternate soothing, holding and comforting, with playful, novel stimulation, as indicated by the clients' behavioural signals.
- Care should aim at consistency of long-term relationships as far as possible within the constraints of the institutional setting.

(Perrin and May 1999: 55–6)

Perrin and May emphasize the ability to be 'playful' and unselfconscious as being a key attribute in effective dementia care practitioners. As they say, this is not a trait commonly found in the average professional. This clearly has implications for staff selection, training, working practice and support.

The needs of maintaining emotional well-being for people with dementia are unlikely to be met through the traditional 'therapy hour'. Ways and means of providing this emotional support for people with dementia requires carefully documented case work in order to identify good practice in this area. There is very little evidence about the optimum frequency of therapeutic sessions with people with dementia. Common sense would suggest that a limited number of therapy 'sessions' are not going to sustain changes long-term. Cheston (1998) cites recommendations from earlier work that sessions should be shorter and more frequent than with non-cognitively impaired clients. The model of a therapeutic environment in formal care settings where the physical environment, the organization of care and each interaction with clients is aimed at improving well-being fits much more with what we know about the nature of dementia.

In all therapeutic activity there is a need to recognize the way in which distress is construed in terms of the client's culture and also to be aware of the cultural appropriateness of the therapeutic activity being offered. This is as true in dementia care as in any other arena (Yeo and Gallagher-Thompson 1996; Valle 1998).

Cheston (1998) in his review of psychotherapy discusses process issues that receive scant consideration by many care practitioners. The boundary around beginnings and endings is one such issue. Most therapeutic endeavours with people with dementia tend to be open-ended, mainly because of the difficulty of negotiating any other type of contract. The decision when to end working with someone is often based on agreement with care staff or family rather than with the clients themselves. As Cheston (1998) and Jones (1995) point out, however, the long-term and reliable involvement of a therapist through the repeated losses experienced during the dementia process may in itself be a positive intervention. Kitwood (1997b) is even firmer in his conviction that in therapeutic endeavours with people with dementia no end point is reached. Holding, validation and facilitation need to be ongoing and indeed probably increase as cognitive loss increases, if feelings of well-being are to be maintained. Bender (1999a) advocates the long-term involvement of therapists in counselling people with dementia. There appears to be a strong argument here for having the same care practitioners throughout the disease process. The reality is that these will usually change with each care environment.

As Midence and Cunliffe (1996) point out, there is very little published on the personal experience of dementia and still less on the personal experience of therapy for those with dementia. Gaining consent, particularly informed consent, for psychotherapeutic intervention with this client group is not possible to all intents and purposes. There are a number of papers that have appeared on the issue of consent (for example Fellows 1998) that offer some useful pointers to clinicians working psychotherapeutically with this client group. Bender (1999b) describes a peer supervision group for therapists providing direct counselling to individuals with dementia. Issues of confidentiality, consent, role conflict for the therapist and powerlessness are frequently discussed. In practice, care practitioners often struggle with these issues on their own. Gaining supervision in this area, particularly in view of the many difficult therapeutic process issues outlined in this section, would seem at least as important as gaining supervision with other challenging client groups. At present such supervision is the exception rather than the rule.

CONCLUSIONS AND FUTURE DIRECTIONS

Therapeutic activities can no longer be seen as something that are 'done to' people with dementia according to a timetable drawn up by busy professionals working Monday to Friday, 9 am to 5 pm. We have moved into an era now where it is seen as desirable that the whole environment (social, psychological and physical) is geared up to the promotion of optimal well-being. There is research that needs to be done in verifying the use of certain therapeutic activities particularly in determining which therapies at what stage improve well-being with which individuals. The way in which outcomes of therapeutic activity are measured requires much development. Despite all the different types of therapeutic activity written about here, the day-to-day reality of most people with dementia is an existence without any activity (let alone that which is therapeutic). How to turn this around is a major challenge for service providers, purchasers and researchers.

FURTHER READING

Perrin, T. and May, H. (1999) *Well-being in Dementia: An Occupational Approach for Therapists and Carers*. London: Churchill-Livingstone. Aimed primarily at occupational therapists, this has much to offer all care practitioners.

Woods, R.T. (ed.) (1996) *Handbook of the Clinical Psychology of Ageing*. Chichester: Wiley.

Woods, R.T. (ed.) (1999) *Psychological Problems of Ageing*. Chichester: Wiley. Provide many useful chapters for those generally interested in therapeutic approaches with older people.

Useful reviews of key therapeutic activities include: Holden and Woods (1995) on RO practice and research; Woods and McKiernan (1995) on reminiscence; Cheston (1998) on psychotherapy; and Spector *et al.* (1999a, b) on RO and reminiscence.

11

MIKE NOLAN AND JOHN KEADY

Working with carers

KEY POINTS

- A complete understanding of caring cannot be achieved unless satisfactions are also considered.
- Carers have a sense of their own expertise in providing care and they want this acknowledged.
- Realizing the person with dementia is not to blame for his or her situation is central to adaptive coping.
- Caring is an evolving process that requires skilled intervention appropriate to each individual's experience.

INTRODUCTION

The title of this chapter reflects the current emphasis in the policy and practice literature on forming partnerships between professional and family carers. Such a model of working has been actively promoted in recent years due both to the rising influence of consumerism on health and social care and to a growing appreciation of the complex and multidimensional nature of family care. This latter factor in particular has forced a reappraisal of the purpose and nature of support given to carers, raising questions about the bases for professional practice. Despite the rhetoric, however, a number of recent studies have suggested that carers' needs remain poorly addressed, with a need for a considerable reorientation of existing practice if well-intentioned initiatives are to be of genuine benefit. While a range of complex factors require attention including funding and resource issues and the challenges of genuine multi-agency working, there is a more fundamental need for a clear framework to guide interactions between professional and family carers. This chapter outlines a model for assessment and intervention in family care, with particular reference to carers of people with dementia. It is beyond the scope of this chapter to review the extensive literature on family care in dementia and to describe the model fully (for a more detailed account see Nolan and Grant 1992; Keady and Nolan 1994a; Nolan et al. 1996, 1998; Keady 1999). We therefore highlight the essential elements of the model and their implications for policy and practice.

The major focus will be on the implementation of a multidimensional approach to assessment which recognizes both the difficulties and satisfactions of caring and which tailors interventions to individual circumstances and stages of care.

Family carers receive support from a diverse range of agencies and staff, both qualified and unqualified, and we believe that working in partnership is essential. However, despite the diversity of service provision, the underlying philosophy we suggest is relevant across agencies and groups. Furthermore, although our focus here is on the needs of family carers these cannot be considered in isolation from the needs of the person with dementia who should, wherever possible, be an active agent in all discussions (Keady 1999). Moreover, while there is now greater appreciation of the complexities of family care, significant gaps in understanding remain, for example, on the needs of carers from differing ethnic groups and of young carers. We cannot assume that the important issues are necessarily the same and there is a need for further research and practice development in a number of areas.

SUPPORTING FAMILY CARERS: REALIZING THE RHETORIC

The response of virtually all developed countries to an ageing of their populations has been to initiate a policy of community care, both to reduce costs to the state and maintain older people in their own homes (B. Davies 1995). In reality community care is family care with approximately 80 per cent of all the support needed being given by the family, usually spouses or children and most often women (Walker 1995). Therefore if community care is to work there have to be adequate support mechanisms for carers which can respond rapidly and flexibly to their needs. Evers (1995) argues that any intervention should primarily complement and supplement, rather than replace, family caring. Conversely it is also important to recognize when it is inappropriate to expect a family member to care and when interventions should be aimed at helping a carer to give up his or her role (Nolan et al. 1996). Recent developments in policy and practice reflect such an orientation.

The implementation of the Carers (Recognition and Services) Act 1995 gave family carers in the UK a statutory right to an assessment of their needs. But a number of recent studies suggest that the Act has had little impact, with many carers being unaware of their rights, receiving little information and advice, and being poorly prepared for their role (Henwood 1998; Warner and Wexler 1998; Banks 1999). In recognition of these limitations the UK government launched the Carers' National Project in 1998, which resulted in the Carers' National Strategy being introduced in early 1999 (DoH 1999a). This strategy was intended to mark a 'decisive change' in policy and practice with family carers, giving carers a right to:

- choose to care (or not);
- be adequately prepared to care;
- receive relevant help at an appropriate stage;
- be enabled to care without detriment to their inclusion in society or to their health.

The strategy places particular emphasis on providing support at key transition points, notably at the beginning and end of care, and on helping carers develop skills and competencies. Perhaps most fundamental of all is the notion of choice, with the stated intention of the strategy being to 'support people who choose to be carers' (DoH 1999a).

While stating such aims is deceptively easy, achieving them is quite another matter. As Twigg and Atkin (1994) have noted, most agencies and practitioners lack a clear rationale for intervening in family care, beyond maintaining carers in their role and thereby implicitly using them as resources. Furthermore, most research has focused on the stress and *burdens* of care (see Nolan *et al.* 1996 for an extensive review), with interventions having tended to concentrate mainly on the physical act of caring. Consequently decisions about whether carers are eligible for services are based primarily on the amount of help that the carer has to provide to the cared-for person.

Recently many studies have suggested that, while not unimportant, such factors are of limited value and that a full appreciation of carers' needs will not emerge until there is a clear understanding of the multidimensional and dynamic nature of family care. Indeed, a focus on the physical aspects of care potentially disadvantages many carers, as captured by Lévesque *et al.* (1995: 352):

> Because the level of the care receiver's functional impairment was not significant (in predicting carer stress), and because that is currently the most frequent criterion for assessing the need for formal assistance for the caregiver, the latter may be deprived of much needed services unless a broader range of stressors is examined.

According to Lévesque *et al.* (1995), greater consideration should be given to the coping efforts carers employ and the role of satisfactions in reducing perceived burden. This calls for a rethinking of the goals and type of support that carers receive.

In summarizing the results of a symposium on supporting family carers given at the World Congress of Gerontology in Adelaide 1997, Askham (1998) argued for a broader definition of the purpose of interventions with carers which more fully reflects an empowerment model. According to Askham, support is any action which helps the carer to:

- take up, or decide not to take up, a caregiving role;
- continue in the caregiving role;
- end the caregiving role.

She also stressed the importance of providing a variety of interventions ranging from training and preparation for caring through information and emotional support, in addition to more traditional services such as home help or respite care. Implementing this more holistic approach requires a framework for assessment that is sensitive to the dynamic nature of caregiving and a mechanism for collecting the information needed. It is to this area that attention is now turned.

ASSESSING CARERS' NEEDS: TOWARDS A MORE HOLISTIC MODEL

As noted earlier, Twigg and Atkin (1994) argue that service agencies and professionals lack a clear rationale for work with family carers and that they tend to adopt one of four largely implicit models. These are:

- carers as resources – where the aim of support is instrumental, that is to maintain carers in their role;
- carers as co-workers – where despite greater involvement of the carer the main aim is still mainly instrumental;
- carers as co-clients – where it is difficult to distinguish the needs of the carer from those of the user;
- the superseded carer – where the aim is for services to entirely replace the carer.

It has been argued that, while some of these models might be appropriate in given circumstances, none is adequate as a primary basis for intervention (Nolan *et al.* 1996), as they fail to reflect the ethos of empowerment, partnership and choice noted above. Underpinning such notions is the belief that all parties bring something of value to an encounter and that this provides a common basis for establishing and agreeing shared goals. The literature suggests that this rarely happens, and that professional and family carers often have differing and not necessarily complementary goals and sources of knowledge, which need to be reconciled for partnerships to develop. For instance, Harvath *et al.* (1994) argue that professionals have what they term 'cosmopolitan' knowledge, that is generalized understanding of a condition, for instance dementia, whereas carers have 'local' knowledge, in other words a unique understanding of a particular case of dementia. Research by Askham (1995) reinforces this suggestion. In her study she found that carers constructed numerous and diverse accounts of dementia which were often at odds with a professional understanding. For example, a quarter of carers attributed dementia simply to 'old age'. In the absence of a shared understanding of the basic issues it is difficult to begin to develop a sense of partnership. Harvath *et al.* (1994) contend that it is essential to blend cosmopolitan and local knowledge so that a more complete understanding emerges. A further example of the differing perspectives held by professional and family carers was highlighted by Clarke (1995). She found that professionals focus primarily on the problems that carers face, and that professionals are mainly concerned with dementia and its future impact. Carers, on the other hand, adopt a much more person-centred approach and are concerned with preserving the 'essence' of the individual with dementia.

THE 'CARERS AS EXPERTS' MODEL

What is required is a model that helps to develop a shared understanding of differing perspectives so that interactions more fully reflect a partnership and empowerment approach. One such model is the 'carers as experts' approach described by Nolan *et al.* (1996). Central to this are a number of basic assumptions, as follows:

- While it is important to recognize the difficulties of caring, greater attention must be given to the quality of past and present relationships, the satisfactions or rewards of caring and other resources, such as income, housing and social support, that carers can draw upon.
- The stress or difficulties of care are best understood from a subjective rather than an objective perspective. That is, the circumstances of care are less important than a carer's assessment of them.
- It is essential to assess both a carer's willingness and ability to care. Some family members may not really want to care but feel obliged to do so. Conversely, while many family members are willing to care they may lack the necessary skills and abilities.
- Although recognizing the importance of instrumental services such as respite care and in-home support, the primary purpose of the 'carers as experts' approach is to help carers to obtain the necessary competencies, skills and resources to provide care of good quality without detriment to their own health. In this context helping a carer to give up care is a legitimate aim.
- 'Carers as experts' recognizes the changing demands of care and the way in which skills and expertise develop over time. A longitudinal perspective is therefore crucial, and the degree of 'partnership' will vary depending on the circumstances of care. For example, in the case of carers new to their role, professional carers are likely to be 'senior partners'. They have important knowledge of a 'cosmopolitan nature' which is needed to help the carers understand the demands that they face, for instance, what dementia is and what carers might expect. Conversely experienced carers, many of whom have learned their skills and expertise by trial and error, often have a far better grasp of their situation than professionals, and acknowledgement of

this is vital to a partnership approach. At a later stage the balance may shift again, so if it is necessary to choose a nursing home carers may go back to a 'novice' stage. They have probably never had to select a home before and will therefore need additional help and support. Recognizing and achieving such a balance is the crux of the 'carers as experts' model.

Having identified the basic premises of the 'carers as experts' model the rest of the chapter will elaborate upon these, using both the literature and data collected by the authors. Particular attention is given to the satisfactions and coping efforts of carers and to adapting a longitudinal approach to supporting carers.

'CARERS AS EXPERTS': MAKING THE MODEL WORK

In order to help apply the 'carers as experts' approach three indices have been developed by the authors. These indices can be used as the basis for a holistic assessment of need. These are: the **Carer's Assessment of Difficulties Index (CADI)** (Nolan and Grant 1992); the **Carer's Assessment of Satisfactions Index (CASI)** (Nolan and Grant 1992); and the **Carer's Assessment of Managing Index (CAMI)** (Nolan *et al.* 1995). In order to illustrate how the indices can be used to help design interventions, data gathered from carers of people with dementia will be used. The three indices were developed over several years and are based on the **transactional model of stress** developed by Lazarus (1969). This approach is based on the belief that potentially stressful events are 'appraised' by an individual and consequently what one person finds difficult may not be a problem for another (see Nolan *et al.* 1996 for a fuller account). Appraisal involves a subjective judgement about whether or not a particular event is seen to pose a threat, harm or challenge. Therefore, the objective nature of a demand is less important than how it is perceived. This model underpins CADI which comprises 30 items, with carers being asked to rate how stressful each item is. In this way an individual profile of stressful events is compiled for each carer. This can then form the basis for discussing agreed goals.

The value of a transactional model and an individual approach to understanding stress has gained support from a number of studies in the field of dementia (Aneshensel *et al.* 1993; Jerrom *et al.* 1993; Brodaty *et al.* 1994; Lévesque *et al.* 1995; Picot 1995). Our own work with varying groups of carers suggests that the most difficult aspects of caring relate mainly to the quality of relationships, the help carers receive from their family and emotional reactions such as guilt, anger and so on (Nolan and Grant 1992; Nolan *et al.* 1996).

Such results highlight the importance of assessing the quality of the relationship between the carer and the person with dementia (Pallett 1990; Spaid and Barusch 1994; McCarty 1996). For example, Spaid and Barusch (1994) contend that the closer carers feel to the person with dementia, the less burden they experience. They argue that attention to quality of relationships should form a key part of all assessments and interventions. Taking a slightly differing approach, McCarty (1996) suggests that the way each carer approaches caring (termed a 'negotiation style') is significantly influenced by his or her prior relationship with the person with dementia. A reciprocal negotiating style, in which both parties have an equal say, is usually the product of a good prior relationship, with carers often finding gratification and meaning in what they do. A unilateral negotiating style, where the viewpoint of the carer dominates, is the result of a poor or neutral prior relationship. Here the carer finds little gratification. A conflictual style emerges from an ambiguous previous relationship, with the carer often emotionally detached and distant from his or her role. Prior relationships are also important in determining how a carer reacts to the diagnosis of dementia (Morgan and Laing 1991). When there has been a close and loving prior relationship then the usual response is one of sadness and grief, with caring unlikely to be seen as burdensome. Where there has been a less positive prior relationship carers are more likely to respond out of a sense of duty and responsibility, experiencing frustration and higher levels of stress.

The influence of prior relationships reinforces the importance of including the satisfactions of caring as part of the assessment process. Although studies in this area are still limited, research into dementia caregiving has often led the way in exploring the potential satisfactions of carers. For example, Hirschfield (1981, 1983) noted the importance of 'mutuality', that is the gratification and meaning carers find, and highlighted its role in reducing stress. Others such as Motenko (1987) and Jivanjee (1993) added to the growing body of evidence suggesting that a complete understanding of caring cannot be achieved unless satisfactions are also considered. It was the need to explore potential satisfactions further that led to the development of CASI (Nolan and Grant 1992).

EXPLORING THE SATISFACTIONS OF CARING

CASI contains 30 statements based on a detailed analysis of qualitative data from a large postal survey of carers and interviews with 50 carers. It has now been used in a number of studies, which demonstrate that finding satisfaction from care is the 'norm'. The sources of satisfaction that carers experience are illustrated in Tables 11.1, 11.2 and 11.3, with these data being taken primarily from studies of carers of people with dementia. We have organized the satisfactions under three headings: Giving good care (Table 11.1), Working for a positive outcome (Table 11.2) and Caring counts (Table 11.3). The figures in each table relate to the percentage of 200 carers who found this aspect of caring provided either quite a lot or a great deal of satisfaction.

Table 11.1 highlights the importance that carers place on being able to provide good care. This relates not only to the physical components, such as seeing the person they care for well turned out, but also includes more subtle aspects such as maintaining their dignity, seeing the person happy and giving them pleasure. As can be seen nearly 8 out of 10 carers feel that they are able to give the best care, based on the sort of intimate personal knowledge of the person with dementia described in a number of studies (Bowers 1987, 1988;

Table 11.1   Giving good care

	%
Maintaining dignity	96
See the person well turned out	91
Seeing the person happy	88
Giving pleasure to the person	87
Tending to the person's needs	79
I give best care	78

Table 11.2   Working for a positive outcome

	%
Expression of love	89
Overcome difficulties	78
Closer to cared-for person	49
See small improvements	48
Help reach potential	45
Closer to family	39

Harvath *et al.* 1994). It is essential that professionals are aware of those aspects that carers see as important, for carers often act as the 'arbiters of standards' (Twigg and Atkin 1994) and may reject services such as respite care if they feel they are not of suitable quality (Nolan and Grant 1992).

Table 11.2 illustrates how carers actively work to achieve positive results from caring, both in terms of their interpersonal relationships and by helping the person with dementia to remain engaged with the world. Elsewhere this has been termed 'maintaining involvement' (Keady 1997, 1999).

While some of the items in Table 11.2 are mentioned less frequently they are nevertheless important. For example, it is clear that caring is one way for carers to express their love (Morgan and Laing 1991; McCarty 1996). Moreover, caring can also bring people and families closer together. Other items in this table highlight differing aspects of maintaining involvement such as helping the person with dementia overcome difficulties, working for small improvements and helping them to reach their full potential. There is now growing awareness of the therapeutic benefits of helping family carers work actively with the person with dementia, especially while a tangible level of awareness remains (Keady 1999).

The items in Table 11.2 also have implications for service providers. For example, services such as respite and day care should provide some therapeutic benefit for the person with dementia. Second, and perhaps more importantly, we believe that poor relationships and an absence of satisfactions are key indicators of fragile, and potentially abusive, relationships. A number of studies note

Table 11.3   Caring counts

	%
Know I've done my best	90
Appreciation from cared-for person	59
Appreciation from others	56
Feel wanted	53
A challenge	48
Grown as a person	43
Widened interests	30
Purpose in life	25

that carers who experience satisfactions are less likely to be stressed (Hirschfield 1981, 1983; Given and Given 1991; Archbold *et al.* 1992), or to feel trapped in their role (Opie 1994; Aneshensel *et al.* 1995). Therefore, greater attention to the presence or absence of satisfactions can help to highlight caring situations in which there is a need for careful monitoring and support.

Table 11.3 shifts the focus away from the person with dementia to those aspects of caring that provide more direct sources of satisfactions for the carer. These items suggest that many carers want recognition for what they do and appreciation for their efforts. These data also illustrate that for a smaller, but by no means insignificant, number of carers, caring meets important personal needs such as feeling wanted, providing a sense of having grown as a person, or giving life greater meaning. This suggests that developing satisfactions may have a therapeutic role. For example, studies from the USA demonstrate that efforts actively to 'enrich' caring relationships, such as helping both carers and cared-for persons maintain or rediscover 'treats', can be very effective (Cartwright *et al.* 1994). This may take the form of either maintaining important personal routines or identifying new and stimulating shared interests. Certainly Keady's (1999) recent study drawing on data from carers and people with dementia highlights the importance of 'maintaining involvement' so that both parties remain engaged and active in their world. The nature of perceived difficulties and sources of potential satisfactions comprise two key elements of the assessment process. Appreciation of these factors is essential in helping to design the type of services and support that help carers to care more effectively. In addition, however, it is necessary to understand the type of caring strategies carers use and we now turn attention to this area.

HELPING CARERS TO COPE

According to Milne *et al.* (1993), helping carers to develop and improve their ability to cope is one of the most useful of all interventions. To do this effectively, however, requires a comprehensive and individualized assessment of the types of stresses carers face, the coping efforts they employ and how successful these are perceived to be (Lazarus 1993; Thompson *et al.* 1993; Burr *et al.* 1994). Although a number of general coping indices exist which look broadly at life stresses, it is recognized that these are of a limited use in helping to identify the specific stresses that carers face (Hinriden and Niedireche 1999).

It was our desire to have an index that could explore the ways in which carers cope. This resulted in the development of the Carer's Assessment of Managing Index (CAMI) (Nolan *et al.* 1995). As with CADI and CASI, CAMI was developed following a review of the literature and a series of in-depth interviews with carers, many of whom were looking after people with dementia. Since its development this index has also been used to collect data on carers of people with dementia and these provide useful information about how such carers cope. These data are presented in Tables 11.4, 11.5 and 11.6. Table 11.4 considers carers' problem-solving coping, Table 11.5 focuses on reframing the meaning of situations and finally Table 11.6 briefly considers efforts to deal with stress.

There is a strong tendency in the literature to see problem-solving coping as the most effective style (Braithwaite 1990; McKee 1994; Kiernan and Alborz 1995). But there is also growing awareness of the importance of having a variety of coping strategies on which to draw and on matching a particular strategy with the type of difficulty being faced (Lazarus 1993; Burr *et al.* 1994; Lévesque *et al.* 1995). Furthermore, the way a stressor, or potentially stressful event, is viewed is also important, so, for example, if a particular event is seen as a challenge, rather than as a threat or harm, then individuals are less likely to be stressed (Stoller and Pugliesi 1989; Turnbull and Turnbull 1993; Burr *et al.* 1994). Therefore, it is important to help carers not only to improve their problem-solving efforts, but also to look at their caring role in a differing light. Tables 11.4, 11.5 and 11.6 give an indication of the diverse coping efforts that carers employ. The figures relate to the percentage of 260 carers who used each strategy and found it helpful.

In terms of problem solving it can be seen that a number of coping tactics are used and seen as helpful by the majority of carers, with finding out as much information as possible being the single most useful. This is not a new finding but recent surveys suggest that carers still struggle to get the information they would like (Henwood 1998; Warner and Wexler 1998; Audit Commission 2000). This is as true in dementia as other areas (Keady and Nolan 1995;

Table 11.4 Helping carers cope: managing events

	%
Find out as much information as possible	85
Get as much help as possible	83
Talk over problems with someone you trust	82
Rely on own experience, expertise	82
Plan in advance	79
Establish a regular routine	78

Table 11.5   Helping carers cope: managing meaning

	%
Realize cared-for person not to blame	92
Take life one day at a time	88
Realize someone worse off	81
See the funny side of things	80
Ignore the problem, hope it will go away	4

Table 11.6   Helping carers cope: managing stress

	%
Keep a little of free time to self	79
Take mind off things	71
Maintain interests outside caring	70

Audit Commission 2000). Being able to get as much help as possible is also clearly important, but carers often find it difficult to understand the complex system of health and social care and they therefore need all the help and advice they can get (Turner and Street 1999; Audit Commission 2000). The value of having a confidant to talk over problems with is quite apparent, yet this can be particularly difficult, especially if the person with dementia was the carer's usual confidant. Certainly there is a need for carers to develop a relationship of trust with professionals and other formal service providers and this requires continuity over time. The data also illustrate carers' strong sense of expertise and, as stressed earlier, it is a central tenet of the 'carers as experts' model that this expertise is actively developed and acknowledged. The last two items in Table 11.4 highlight the value carers place on being able to plan in advance and of establishing a regular routine. This is often particularly important in dementia caregiving. It is therefore essential that services such as respite care try, as far as possible, to fit in with carers' existing routines.

Table 11.5 draws attention to the more cognitively orientated forms of coping, the main aim of which is to look at things in a differing light. While problem-solving efforts are very useful they are counterproductive when problems cannot be solved, as is often the case in caring for a person with dementia (Lazarus 1993; Burr *et al.* 1994; McKee 1994). It is therefore important that carers have other strategies on which to draw. As can be seen from Table 11.5, the single most used and useful tactic is realizing that the cared-for person is not to blame. This is particularly important in caring for a person with dementia when the potential for misunderstanding, especially prior to diagnosis, is considerable (Hutchinson *et al.* 1997). This again highlights the importance of information in helping carers and people with dementia establish a clear understanding of what dementia is (Keady and Gilliard 1999). The remainder of the terms in Table 11.5 are largely self-explanatory. It is encouraging to note that passive strategies, such as ignoring the problem and hoping it will go away, are rarely seen as being helpful.

Table 11.6 provides an indication of how carers manage the stresses of caring and, consistent with the literature (see Nolan *et al.* 1996 for a review), highlights the importance of being able to keep some time free from caring in order to maintain outside interests. This requires flexible respite care that reflects carers' existing routines.

RESPONDING TO CHANGING NEEDS OVER TIME

The other essential element of the 'carers as experts' model is its temporal dimension which recognizes that the demands of caring vary over time and that services must be able to respond in flexible and non-routine ways. Studies in dementia have a long tradition of applying a longitudinal perspective, in which data are collected from the same people at several different points in time, and these studies have added considerably to our understanding (for extensive reviews see Nolan *et al.* 1996; Keady 1999). Building on this tradition the recent study by Keady (1999) provides important new insights, highlighting how early intervention and support, both for the carer and the person with dementia, can have a potentially very powerful effect. Keady (1999) also presents a detailed consideration of the dynamics of caring in dementia and charts changing relationships over time, with an indication of how services can best provide support. For instance, in this study, which involved interviews with 64 carers and 10 people with the early experience of dementia, it was found that the early adjustment by the person with dementia was a secretive process, which could last for several years. Indeed, for an open disclosure and investigation of the early signs of (predominantly) memory loss by the carer and person with (undiagnosed) dementia, a number of steps were required (Keady 1999: 230–1):

- a good prior relationship;
- a willingness by the person with (undiagnosed) dementia to openly disclose their fears, concerns and coping behaviours with a trusted person;
- a willingness by the trusted person (carer) to hear these concerns, validate and act upon them;
- a mutual decision to do something about it, where both parties recognize and agree that 'this is (might be) serious';
- a reasonably quick decision to seek a medical opinion on the cause of the experienced signs;
- primary health care teams taking the reported signs and symptoms seriously, and having the necessary knowledge and skills to facilitate an early diagnosis of dementia. Alternatively, the primary health care team response may be to refer the person/couple to more specialized support services, such as a memory clinic, for a more detailed assessment;
- an early diagnosis being made and the person with dementia and the carer being informed of the diagnosis and prognosis;

- the person and carer understanding the implications of the diagnosis;
- an explicit willingness by the person/carer/family to work through the processes involved in living with the experience of dementia in a supportive manner;
- specialist services being available on a continual basis to help support 'the partnership' – and the family – through this transition; and
- ability of the carer to 'maintain involvement' even when the person with dementia may have a diminished awareness of their situation, i.e. the carer was able to gain satisfaction and meaning from the act of caring itself.

These steps form part of a basic social process in caring that the authors have termed 'Working together'. While the conditions require further testing, their presence seems essential if support, and a diagnosis of dementia, are to occur at an earlier point. Moreover, such conditions appear crucial to fostering the positive coping responses outlined previously in Tables 11.1–11.6. Thus caring is best understood as a process that involves changing relationships over time and that requires skilled intervention as the experience of dementia unfolds.

CONCLUSION

Although it is important to recognize that there has been significant progress in services for carers and people with dementia in recent years, there is no room for complacency. The Audit Commission review on health services for older people (Audit Commission 2000) highlights a number of areas of concern, not least of which is the relative neglect of the needs of people with dementia and their carers, particularly during the early stages. While not providing a panacea we hope that the model we have outlined here will open up new options for professionals and others interested in improving the support given to people with dementia and their carers.

FURTHER READING

Knight, B.G., Lutzky, S.M. and Macofsky-Urban, F. (1993) A meta-analytic review of interventions for caregiver distress: recommendations for future research, *Gerontologist*, 33(2): 240–8.

Nolan, M., Grant, G. and Keady, J. (1996) *Understanding Family Care*. Buckingham: Open University Press.

Taraborrelli, P. (1993) Exemplar A: becoming a carer, in N. Gilbert (ed.) *Researching Social Life*. London: Sage.

12 | **MARY MARSHALL**

Care settings and the care environment

KEY POINTS

- Person-centred care is the aim. It is not easy to achieve and many settings fall short of it.
- Residents need a purpose to their lives.
- Attention to physical health is crucial.
- Sex and death cannot be ignored.
- Good design is helpful.
- Conflicts of interest and power are inevitable and need to be dealt with.

QUALITY LIVING

What does quality living mean for people with dementia who cannot remain in their own homes, and for their relatives and friends? This is a question usually answered by one sentence, such as, 'It means achieving your full potential as a person', or by a list of quality indicators (Cox 1998). In terms of anything more specific, it does of course mean different things to different people. This chapter will walk a path between the general and the particular by focusing on aspects of the social and the built environment which are important for everyone who lives in a care setting. It will conclude with a commentary on some current issues and future trends.

CARE SETTINGS

We need first to consider the range of alternatives to home. This list grows all the time as expectations of what will suit people with dementia develop. At present the alternatives to home include:

- *Other people's homes.* The '**boarding out**' of people with dementia either for breaks or permanently remains unusual in spite of the fact that it has been happening in Liverpool since the 1970s. This is surprising since the importance of a familiar environment to people with dementia is now widely understood. If you cannot live at home there is, generally speaking, nothing more homely than someone else's home. There are probably several issues that contribute to the lack of development of this kind of project: recruitment of suitable households, the need for reliable round-the-clock support, the need for training, the bureaucracy of the health and safety requirements and the commitment of management required to make such a complex arrangement possible. One project has been recently written up (Allinson 1997).
- *Housing models.* These are on a continuum from the use of ordinary, everyday houses to housing models that look just like a modern residential facility; indeed the difference may be very hazy given the trend to small domestic-scale units in residential and nursing homes. Twenty examples of units for people with dementia, described in Judd *et al.* (1997), demonstrate this blurring. Moorside in Winchester, for example, was built as a residential home and Sidegate Lane in Ipswich was built by a housing association and yet they were built to almost exactly the same principles. Cox (1998) gives details of ten housing options, which include normal sheltered housing with round-the-clock help. St Leonard's in Edinburgh, for example, is a set of blocks of flats all linked to a resources centre by intercom. Among the flats are twenty tenants who are in effect being provided with residential care levels of support but in their own homes; many of this group have dementia.
- *Hotel models.* Many providers of long-term care clearly wish to replicate a hotel environment for their residents. The corridors, lavish reception areas, and style of furnishing and fittings represent nothing more clearly than a hotel, often more '2-star' than '5-star'. These models are a huge improvement on many old converted mansion houses and ward settings but they are far from homely.
- *Clinical models.* The persistence of the clinical setting can be hard to understand for those used to social care approaches. Some health settings have wrenched themselves away from it, such as Charter House in Trowbridge, but even there staff seem to be able to make it feel like a hospital ward in spite of a more homely design. This may be an issue of status. Nursing staff may feel that a clinical setting has more status than a homely one. It may reflect a preoccupation with clinical procedures with an insufficient appreciation of the struggle experienced by many people with an impaired brain to cope with such an unfamiliar environment.

There are no clear parallels between the type of organization running services for people with dementia and these four models. There are very homely models in NHS acute assessments wards for people with dementia, for example Stratheden in Fife where the units are in a couple of bungalows and are filled with old-fashioned furniture (Marshall 1997a). There are very clinical housing association models, and hotel models exist in every provider category. The four approaches do however form a useful classification since they describe the vision of the unit and thereby imply what they expect from the people with dementia.

CARE ENVIRONMENT QUALITIES

Social environment

Most people in dementia care espouse the principles of person-centred care (Kitwood 1997b). This means, in brief, that the care is tailored to meet the needs of the individual rather than the group or the needs of the staff. However, it is not unusual to find units where staff plainly see people with dementia as neither needing nor deserving even the normal rules of decent human interaction, let alone interactions tailored to their individual needs. Staff still stand and talk about people sitting only yards away from them. They still provide a largely activity-free environment beyond watching the television and occasional group outings or concerts. They still fail to interpret the non-verbal communication of the desperate, bewildered expression or the rage at the intrusion into private space. Person-centred care is difficult. It needs to be implemented at the most micro level of a glance as well as the relatively macro level of the regime. Dementia Care Mapping (Kitwood 1994) is a well-developed tool to assess the success with which it is being achieved.

A meaningful life

A purposeful and meaningful life is what most of us seek. Yet many people with dementia who are living in places which are not their own homes are denied any opportunity to live a life with purpose and meaning beyond survival. Barnett (1997) in her analysis of her conversations with long-stay patients and users of a day hospital with dementia found a preoccupation with three themes: home, loss and making a contribution. The day hospital patients, for example, recalled the time they had helped the bus driver reversing. Reed and Payton's (1997) research on sources of satisfaction for people without dementia living in residential homes found that friendship was very important. This is surely about relationships giving life meaning. We know little about the friendships between people with dementia in long-stay establishments beyond knowing that they can happen and that when they do they clearly bring a lot of satisfaction. This raises a dilemma about the need for homogeneity in units to which I will return.

Purpose and meaning in long-term care relate to the concept of autonomy, which has been identified as very significant in guidelines to improve quality in long-term care (see for example RCP 1998). We all need to feel some sense of control over ourselves and our environment and we achieve this by making decisions. These can be very small decisions, such as when to get up and what to eat. But opportunities to make this kind of decision are not always encouraged in care settings. As in so much of this work, activities provide useful opportunities for people to choose what they want to do, to what extent and with whom.

Allowing people with dementia to do things to help others is important. Sometimes it will be simply to stroke an arm; others can play the piano or sing all the words to a song. Some people with dementia are lucky enough to have the gift of humour and making people laugh is something they can do for them. One lady who had lost her teeth said to a friend, 'I've got nae teeth and nae brains' which made them both laugh. Many of us protect ourselves with our professional demeanour, which may be essential in some circumstances, but it can be very disabling for people with dementia who have no idea about our formal role. They can, however, sense when we are withholding ourselves from genuine interaction. We need to be able to have real conversations with people with dementia so they can offer us knowledge, opinions, jokes. In a sense we accept this gift in reminiscence work because it is then that we acknowledge that they have experiences we have not had. But this can be extended to ordinary interactions as well. It must be irksome if the only time staff take what you say seriously is when you are talking about the past!

Carers often experience a loss of purpose and meaning in their lives when they relinquish full-time care. Some wish to retain the role of carer and are not always given the opportunity. They can feel excluded by staff either because they perceive the staff to have greater expertise or because they are not encouraged to retain any of the responsibilities they had at home. Archibald and Murphy (1999) have produced a guide for staff to ways in which carers can be involved through activities.

The importance of health

A high quality of care includes making strenuous efforts to maximize health since poor health impairs coping with dementia. Perhaps the most frequently neglected illness that occurs in people with dementia is depression. Nineteen per cent of people living in residential and nursing homes were found to have depression and it can occur at any stage of the condition. Warrington (1996) has provided a useful guide to identifying the danger signs and seeking treatment. Another neglected health factor is sensory impairment. Hearing and visual impairment are common in late life but must be very difficult to cope with alongside impaired reasoning. It is important to ensure that people who will tolerate a hearing aid have it in and that it is clean; and spectacles may need to be constantly retrieved. Identifying people who have infections and other acute episodes is often difficult since people with dementia may not be able to give an account of pain, nausea or a raised temperature. There are some useful guides to delirium, which sometimes arises as a consequence of an infection. Pain is being identified as an issue in dementia care somewhat belatedly; Cook *et al.* (1999) have recently reviewed the literature. The increasing interest in palliative care links to this (Cox 1996).

Food and dementia is now receiving the attention it deserves. The VOICES (1998) publication on this topic provides an invaluable resource. It points out that eating is about more than nutritional levels, although these are important. Eating well for people with dementia is also a matter of mealtimes and helping people to eat. Some people with dementia can no longer bear to sit at a table, for example, and need to eat on the move.

Love and sex

Love, like sex, is not a word often used in dementia care. C.S. Lewis (1966) said, 'Grief is the price we pay for love.' This is especially true in this field. People die. Loving friendships and relationships between residents, between staff and residents, between staff and carers are all more likely to end in death than with other age groups. Yet the capacity to love does not diminish with dementia: feelings seem to remain intact. This must include the love of God that is so important to some people. We need to provide the opportunities to love that people want, and these will vary from person to person. But staff need support to avoid being burned out if they are willing to invest their feelings.

Sex is a closely related issue and is often seen as highly problematic in long-term settings. What it involves will vary from hand holding to sexual inter-course. The first question that needs to be asked is, 'For whom is it a problem?' We are not providing long-term care for innocent children. Yet some people with dementia can be very vulnerable. Archibald (1994) has provided a guide and a video to help staff take the first crucial step, which is being able to talk about it and to assess what, if anything, needs to be done. Sex between staff and residents cannot be condoned in dementia care, as in any other setting; the power imbalance is simply too great. However, all staff will have to confront the issue of sex if only because they will encounter conversations about sex and probably sexual advances. Sex and death are two topics that are commonplace in settings where there are groups of older people. Staff who are unable to handle these topics do people with dementia a disservice.

Past trauma

The impact of past trauma, such as childhood sexual abuse or wartime experiences, on the way people experience dementia, and thereby on their behaviour, is slowly gaining recognition (Hunt *et al.* 1997). Feil (1992) considers that a lot of what we see in the apparently irrational behaviour of people with dementia is 'unfinished business' from the past which can no longer be kept locked away. We need to be able to provide opportunities for people to tell their stories (Sutton and Cheston 1997). However, the experience of the psychotherapists who have contributed to the book by Hunt *et al.* (1997) suggests that trust is a prerequisite and that this can take quite a lot of time and effort to establish. Many staff are well aware that some people they care for have been sexually abused, for example, because they react so negatively to intimate care. There is a need for a great deal more work in ways of helping people with dementia to share and perhaps to resolve some of this past trauma if the present is not to be intolerable.

Reducing stress

One of the greatest gifts we can give to people with dementia is to reduce the stress they experience as a result of their efforts to cope with their diminishing mental competence. There are numerous ways we can do this. We can change the physical environment (see below). We can aim for a stress-free regime, which means first and foremost staying calm ourselves. This is very difficult and, like every other aspect of care, it is a responsibility of management. Stressed staff make stressful environments. There are numerous ways to reduce stress and we all do it for ourselves all the time. The challenge is to find the right technique for each person at the right time. When we are stressed we sometimes need a warm bath, we sometimes need music, and we sometimes need exercise. The fact that everyone is different is one good reason why groups in shared care should be small and why the one-to-one of a boarding-out arrangement can be so much less stressful. There are general principles. One is to reduce noise and to manage its level to provide the right amount of stimulation or relaxation. The right amount of music at the right time is relaxing for most people. Touch if soothing is often very relaxing: hand massage, foot massage, hair brushing and a manicure are relaxing for most people. Some smells are relaxing, notably lavender. Snoezelen rooms (see Chapter 10) provide a multisensory experience, which assists many people – residents, relatives and staff – to unwind. The literature on multisensory work is well reviewed in the *Journal of Dementia Care* (Ellis and Thorn 2000).

Activities

Activities can be relaxing if they are failure-free and build up self-esteem. Activities have many functions in any setting. Archibald and Murphy (1995) have produced a training pack to assist staff in thinking about the many reasons for undertaking activities. These can include:

- maintaining skills;
- relieving boredom;
- restoring confidence;

- opportunities to socialize;
- building self-esteem;
- exercise.

There can be a tendency to think of activities mainly in terms of formal input, perhaps provided by an occupational therapist, whereas they ought to be everybody's business. Archibald has produced two books of activities to give staff ideas (Archibald 1990, 1993). Life storybooks (Murphy 1994) can provide an endless source of stimulation for conversations. Anything happening in day-to-day living can be made into an activity: mealtimes, bath times, grooming, laundry and so on. It is a question of seizing the opportunity to involve the person in a positive way. Activities must be failure-free if they are to be therapeutic. Normal everyday activities are easier in some settings than others, for example baking and cooking are restricted to care settings with kitchens (Gresham 1999).

Spiritual needs

Finally in this section I want to look briefly at spiritual needs because they are sometimes neglected in care settings. Spirituality is discussed in detail in Chapter 4. For some people spiritual means religious; for others it may mean communing with nature, reading poetry or meditating. Spirituality is hard to describe but everybody benefits from some attention to activities that are on a different and more reflective plane. In the hurly burly of most people's lives opportunities have to be made for these activities. This is especially true of group care settings where just getting through the day with everybody clean and comfortable is very time-consuming.

THE BUILT ENVIRONMENT

This section is much shorter than the one above because while the built environment is important it is nowhere near as important as the care provided by staff. Person-centred care can exist in the most terrible buildings and institutional care in the most sensitive and enabling buildings. Poor care in a good building is better than poor care in a bad building because the residents do not have to cope with a disabling environment as well as disabling staff. A good building can make the best care easier; it cannot make it happen. Having said that, a building does reflect the attitudes and aspirations of the people responsible. Staff will quickly recognize a building where their needs have not been considered: where there is no decent staff room and they have to take incontinent residents down the corridor to the bathroom because there are no en-suite facilities; or they have to walk incredible distances to keep an eye on their residents.

At the start of this chapter I tried to divide places which care for people unable to live at home into four types: other people's homes, housing models, hotel models and clinical settings. The differences between these models are often initially expressed in the built environment. The hotel model, for example, is usually instantly recognized with its plush lounges and long corridors.

There are two ways of approaching the design of the built environment once its importance has been established (Marshall 1997b). The environment is important for people with profound disabilities because it has to assist them; it has to compensate for the disabilities. More often environments add to disabilities. Those of us fortunate enough to be fit can, generally speaking, understand and cope with our environments; we are usually able to do what we need and want to do. People with disabilities have endless frustrations: buildings with steps which mean they are unusable by people in wheelchairs; buildings with stiff doors and windows which are unusable for people with impaired grip; out of reach plugs which are unusable for people with impaired reach; and buildings that are disorientating which means they make people with dementia unnecessarily dependent.

The two ways of looking at design are in terms of principles and of a list of design features. Both approaches can be found in many books about design for dementia (Calkins 1988; Cohen and Weisman 1991; Netten 1993; Hiatt 1995). This literature represents an international consensus even if little of it is based on systematic research.

The consensus on *principles* of design is that design should:

- compensate for disability;
- maximize independence;
- enhance self-esteem and confidence;
- demonstrate care for staff;
- be orientating and understandable;
- reinforce personal identity;
- welcome relatives and the local community;
- allow control of stimuli.

The consensus on design *features* includes:

- small size;
- familiar, domestic, homely in style;
- plenty of scope for ordinary activities (for example kitchens in care units, washing lines, garden sheds);
- unobtrusive concern for safety;
- different rooms for different functions;
- age-appropriate furniture and fittings;
- safe outside space;
- single rooms big enough for lots of personal belongings;
- good signage and multiple clues where possible e.g. sight, smell, sound;
- use of objects rather than colour for orientation;
- enhancement of **visual access** (that is what you can actually see);
- controlled stimuli, especially noise.

These two lists need little elaboration but there are one or two factors which seem to raise constant difficulties. The first factor is size. The need is for as small a group of people as possible. The trend towards housing options is encouraging because there is a much longer tradition in housing services of having small units with all the attributes of a normal home. This is not some idealistic nonsense; it is logical if you think about dementia. People with struggling intellects need to have a managed environment. For example Davis (1989), in his personal account of the experience of dementia, lucidly describes how large groups of people exhaust him. It is much harder to manage an environment of large numbers of people and lots going on.

The second factor is familiarity. The concept of *familiar* is very important in dementia care. If we can provide a familiar environment we will help people who have difficulty learning new things. For example, Stratheden hospital in Fife has a rapid throughput as an NHS assessment unit and the staff have worked hard to make it familiar. It is full of huge bedroom suites from the 1940s and sitting room furniture of the same vintage (Marshall 1997a). Ideally people should be surrounded by familiar possessions. There are therefore advantages in letting rooms unfurnished so that people have to bring in their own things.

There is often an assumption that most people orientate themselves using colour, when in reality most of us do it by landmarks. Unless the colour is very conspicuous we are much more likely to remember our way by a picture or a plant than we are by the colour of a corridor. Landmarks can be very helpful to people with dementia. Also, and perhaps most importantly, it is worth remembering that noise is as disabling to people with dementia as stairs are to people in wheelchairs.

ISSUES

Conflicts of interest and power

People with dementia can make very considerable demands on those who care for them. This is not to say that there are not rewards in relationships and in the sense of a job well done. But there is nothing to be gained by ignoring the fact that care for people with dementia demands the highest level of skill, emotional maturity, creativity and patience; this is essential if they are to reach their potential and to have the best possible quality of life. Yet many settings employ care staff who cannot and do not put the interests of people with dementia first. It is very easy to fail to provide optimum care. People with dementia can rarely complain or explain what is going on. Failures of care, imagination and persistence can usually be attributed to the dementia. It is all too easy to find 'a malignant social psychology', Kitwood's (1994) term for negative interactions in care settings, since many families still feel shamed by the disease, many units are in impoverished buildings, many people including professionals consider this to be low-status work, and many carers are ignored and excluded.

There seems to be an inevitable momentum towards task-centred rather than person-centred care in any care setting. The needs of staff increasingly become paramount. It is easier, cheaper, and quicker to provide task-centred care. The best units are constantly pushing against this momentum through training, through reasserting and reviewing principles, through staff supervision and through care monitoring including the use of Dementia Care Mapping (Kitwood and Bredin 1992b). For broader discussion of quality management see Chapter 17.

Conflicts of interest exist in any relationship. Usually they are resolved by mutual agreement; a compromise is reached. However, in dementia care they are often resolved in a way that meets the interest of the stronger party. Thus residents are moved to new settings because units are closing; residents have to have a cold supper because the kitchen staff go home at 6 pm; residents' meals are so rushed that for many mealtimes are not pleasurable, and so on. The issue is how these conflicts of interest can be addressed and resolved. A major step has been taken if conflicts of interest are acknowledged. Once they are acknowledged there are options, but all involve the resident having an advocate of some sort to balance up the power relationship. Options might include negotiation, mediation or arbitration. Negotiation is the process by which both sides work to achieve a mutually satisfactory compromise. If we take the example above of an enforced move it might be possible to negotiate on the matter of timing or the quality of the new option. Mediation requires an external person to help both parties to hear each other's point of view. Thus a relative might be concerned that the person with dementia was not eating enough because he or she was rushed to finish meals before the cook–chill food became unsafe. The relative would be assisted to express these concerns and the management could explain its position in relation to costs and convenience. It might then be possible to reach a resolution, for example by providing the person with dementia with some finger food outside mealtimes to make up the nutritional deficit. Arbitration is the process whereby an outsider hears both sides and takes a view on the rights and wrongs. The arbitrator might consider it unreasonable for the unit to be unable to provide a hot meal in the evening for residents who had always had their main meal at night, in which case some special arrangement would have to be made. A range of people can hold the role of negotiator, mediator or arbitrator. Sometimes the commissioner of the service has this role, sometimes Registration and Inspection staff, sometimes a professional such as a community psychiatric nurse. It is very striking that the roles are rarely recognized as such and training provided for them.

Conflicts of interest also occur on a daily basis between residents. It can, for example, be advantageous for the group if a very disruptive resident is moved elsewhere but it may not be advantageous for the person who is moved. It may be advantageous for a couple to have a double room but disadvantageous for the widow who has to move out to allow the couple to have it. These situations would be helped by use of the conflict resolution approaches described above.

More difficult are the abuses of power that can exist in relationships between residents; those that cause most anxiety are sexual abuses. A great deal of openness and sensitivity is needed to resolve these issues.

Communal settings

It seems ironic that people with dementia, who are least able to learn, are required to make major adjustments at the end of their lives to a model of living which most of us would find very hard. Most residential settings, even most housing schemes for people with dementia, require group living. This means residents spend most of their time with a group of strangers and this is demanding. It is difficult to be on your best behaviour all the time and, not surprisingly, some people cannot manage it. There may be pressure to make 'small talk' all the time: a special skill that may be beyond many people with dementia. Communal settings can suit some people really well, particularly those who are highly skilled socially. Often they are the people who are the life and soul of the party, they relate well to the staff and other residents perhaps by having a special contribution such as a vivid sense of humour or skills as a raconteur. Some people really value the opportunities that communal settings provide for a social life. But it should never be assumed that the presence of other people necessarily leads to a social life.

Homogeneity

Whether or not establishments should aim at homogeneity is one of the hottest issues in dementia care. The literature on specialist dementia units (Peppard 1991) stresses the importance of having a group of people with the same levels of ability. This is based on the view that it is then possible to match the skills of the staff, the design and the regime to meet the needs of the residents. This links to the issue of behaviour. Should residents with very challenging behaviour be grouped together? They do require special skills from staff and consistency of response from the staff can be very important. The influential CADE units in New South Wales are psychiatric units designed for this group and every aspect of the environment is geared to their needs: the design, the regime which concentrates on constant familiar activity, the clear care plans, the outside space and so on. Patients are discharged when they no longer need this intensive help, usually because they have 'gone off their feet'. However there are always pros and cons of segregating the most challenging people. Specialist units can easily become bins for the most unpleasant patients, staffed by people who have no other choices, in buildings that would not be acceptable to any other patients. Conversely, they can be centres of excellence and best practice with lots to teach other units.

It is thought to be desirable for people from minority ethnic groups to have specialist units. In specialist units their needs in terms of religious observance, gender of staff, food traditions and activities can be properly attended to. However, there are not yet the numbers of people with dementia to make specialist units of this kind generally viable. There are good reasons for concern about the lack of sensitivity of staff to the needs of people from minority cultures (Anderson and Brownlie 1997). However, there is again a need to be alert to the possibility that specialist units might become isolated from the mainstream and deprived of resources.

There do seem to be strong arguments for a degree of homogeneity of resident population on the basis of lifestyle. This could be according to minority culture or to a whole set of other criteria such as hobbies, education and interests. It might speed up the possibility of making friends with like-minded people. In the UK this raises the spectre of class. This is rarely discussed. But for people with dementia who have impaired learning and reasoning skills it may be crucially important to be with people who are familiar, in a routine which is familiar.

Staffing

It is the staff who determine the quality of care and yet it is notoriously difficult to specify what it is that is important about them. Gilloran *et al.* (1995) looked at the quality of care in several long-stay psychiatric units and established that the quality of the leader of the ward – the middle manager – was the key determinant. The leader who was out and about, rather than in the office, who was good at communicating, and who lent a hand when necessary was the most successful.

Training is often held to be crucial for good quality care. This is not so much in terms of the qualifications of the staff and the skill mix, as the in-service training. However, it is well understood that training without commitment by management is not worth the effort. The lessons of training have to be constantly reinforced in practice if they are to stick.

Most documents about standards of care (Centre for Policy on Ageing 1984, 1996) emphasize the importance of staff supervision as a means of developing and supporting staff. In supervision staff can talk about their own needs and concerns while at the same time receiving support for work which is in line with the philosophy of the unit.

It is a truism that staff who feel cared for and respected are more likely to be able to care for and respect residents. The poor salaries and conditions of many front-line staff are for these reasons alone a concern in dementia care; they are a measure of how much staff are valued by their organization.

It is questionable how long even the best-supported staff can remain in the front line of dementia care. There are arguments that for full-time working the answer is probably three years before staff should go and work somewhere else, or take a break. There are strong arguments for staff working part-time although this may be confusing for people with dementia.

Compromises

It seems important to end this chapter on a cautious note, recognizing that most care environments involve compromises. The building design may have to be a compromise because of the site, the budget or the location. The staff may not be as experienced or as dedicated as required; the right staff may not even be available. The activities may be constrained by the building, the staff time available, and the skills of staff. The food may not be as imaginative or as individualized as it should be. The furniture may be uncomfortable and unable to support all shapes and sizes adequately; and so on.

   Yet there are lessons in compromising. One is to be candid about it. What is said in the brochure must be what happens in reality. Another is that some people rise to challenges and are forced into imaginative practice simply out of frustration with less than ideal circumstances. Another is the need to recognize the extent of these compromises and to compare them with those that are being made for other client groups. Another useful comparison is the rigid adherence to the rules of health and hygiene and to fire regulations while there is much less adherence to best care practice. As long as compromise is recognized and acknowledged then it becomes a first step to trying harder and aiming for higher standards. It is when it is accepted as reasonable, for perhaps the most vulnerable and socially excluded people in our communities, that it must be condemned.

FURTHER READING

Garret, S. and Hamilton-Smith, E. (1998) *Rethinking Dementia – An Australian Approach*. Melbourne: Ausmed Publications.

Kitwood, T. (1997) *Dementia Reconsidered: The Person Comes First*. Buckingham: Open University Press.

Marshall, M. (ed.) (1997) *State of the Art in Dementia Care*. London: Centre for Policy on Ageing.

Case Study
environmental impacts
on interactions

JILL MANTHORPE

13

Ethical ideals and practice

KEY POINTS

- Dementia care raises a host of ethical debates – for practitioners but also for carers and policy makers.
- The language of rights and individualism has been highly influential in welfare services – applying this to dementia is complex.
- Principles of 'doing good' or 'doing no harm' remain central to much care provision but can result in over-protective or paternalistic attitudes.
- Professional ethics may need to be revisited to see how well they fit with those providing the bulk of personal and practical care at home or in services.
- Thinking about ethics is likely to become more important and of higher profile in the context of intensive debates about new genetics, resource allocation and end of life decision making.

INTRODUCTION

This chapter provides an overview of some of the key ethical debates in dementia care related to service planning and provision. It is impossible to cover all ethical debates, theories and controversies so some general principles are outlined and discussed in the context of services. In many ways, however, almost all chapters in this book provide discussion and illustration of ethics although the words values and principles may be used instead.

ETHICAL IDEALS AND DEMENTIA CARE

Virtue theory derived from Aristotelian thought (Almond 2000) uses the idea that every object (humans included) has its own essential function: in the case of humans it is to fulfil specific virtues. The kind of society that will enable humans to flourish or to fulfil traditional virtues is morally good. The notion of flourishing is highly relevant to dementia care. A good care environment may encourage individuals to reach their 'ideal state', whatever this might be. For a person with dementia it might be that he or she could demonstrate courage, excitement, interest or pleasure through human contact, contact with objects or his or her environment. This philosophy has close associations with **normalization**, the influential ethical base which has traditionally been linked to care practice in work with people with learning disabilities.

The relationship between ethics and dementia is constructed at various levels. But at its heart lie the individual and his or her relationship with others. For some the ethical dimension of their feelings, thoughts and labour will remain undeveloped or instinctual; for others the discussion is more analysed and outspoken. Ignatieff (1993), for example, in writing the story of a family where the mother develops a dementia, presents an example of a self-conscious dualism:

> I suspected that the breakdown in her memory was a symptom of a larger disruption in her ability to create and sustain a coherent image of herself over time. It dawned on me that her condition offered me an unrepeatable opportunity to observe the relation between selfhood and memory. I began to think of my mother as a philosophical problem.
>
> (Ignatieff 1993: 53)

Warnock (1998) rejects a morality based on the concept of rights. She is hostile to the notion of 'personhood', seeing it to be a fundamental 'red herring' in developing a language about rights. If being a person is to be human and to be able to have and recognize one's own interests then:

> Everyone who tries to come up with factual or scientific criteria for personhood gets into difficulties over what we are to say about infants or those who, though they once satisfied the criteria, are no longer able to do so, such as those in a coma, or suffering from dementia . . . There is no way of looking at the facts about, say, a demented woman, and deducing whether she is a person.
>
> (Warnock 1998: 55)

Closely associated with the Hippocratic principle of beneficence (or doing good) is that of **non-malficence**, often referred to in the Latin, *primum non nocere*, and translated as 'above all do no harm'. Largely related to its medical origins it is a powerful motto for professionals who may seek to reduce risk of harm or danger but in doing so take insufficient account of other harms produced by action.

Sherman (1999) illustrates these ideals at the level of personal interaction. She provides an example of a difficulty which she says is commonly encountered, that of telling people with dementia about the death of their close relative or spouse. She has found that both staff and family members may argue that it is 'kinder' not to tell, that there is no point in telling or that the reaction of the person with dementia will be hard for them to deal with. Sherman, however, points out that it may not be 'kinder' not to tell because the person with dementia may, in the long term, react to the absence of the dead person and may need to be supported in any event. However, she argues that, for some people,

> not emphasising the death of a loved one is the most desirable path to follow . . . it is essential that careworkers learn to accept the 'reality' of the disturbed mind and try to step into and understand the confused world of dementia.
>
> (Sherman 1999: 135)

In effect this is a balancing of beneficence and non-malficence: a balancing of the right to know with the right not to be harmed. The right to ignorance has not been widely canvassed in respect of dementia services. The next section explores some of these new arguments.

The right to knowledge

The development of public knowledge about dementia, services such as memory clinics and knowledge about genetics have contributed to a growing movement to earlier diagnosis and recognition of dementia. As an example, a leaflet available to the public and produced by the drug companies Eisai Ltd and Pfizer Ltd (1998) is entitled *Is Someone You Care For Becoming Forgetful?* It advocates getting 'doctor's advice soon' and briefly outlines possible causes of memory loss, the signs of Alzheimer's disease, its assessment and sources of help for the person with dementia and/or carers. Outlining the 'tell or not tell' issue of diagnosis, the leaflet acknowledges: 'People with dementia may not want to hear that they have a problem but if the disease is in its early stages, they *can* benefit from being fully informed' (p. 5).

However, counselling or advice-giving in such contexts presents practitioners with a range of difficulties. They have generally assumed a moral stance of providing information in a manner which is 'non-directive' and 'value neutral', particularly influenced by principles developed in the field of genetic counselling (see Petersen 1999). However, with the increasing ability to locate and define individuals 'at risk' of inherited problems, for example early onset dementias, individuals may be pressurized to submit to tests and counselling as conditions of employment or insurance. The acceptance that people have a right to know their diagnosis, or their possible likelihood of having or acquiring a dementia, is clearly related to principles of autonomy and self-determination. Some individuals may argue that they have similar rights not to know and that genetic testing and counselling, by their very nature, appear to them to be value-laden and implicitly directive.

Other arguments arise from principles of 'best interests'. Iliffe (1997), for example, suggests that general practitioners need to work with the primary care team to produce a climate of optimism that much can be done to relieve stress and distress, either long-standing or at crisis. Early identification, therefore, needs to be combined with practical assistance and emotional support to avoid producing better informed but despairing individuals and families.

Rights and justice

The interests of people with dementia have become more closely identified with a rights-based approach. Rights of course are not new social goals but part of a language promoting individual freedom. Such philosophies can be applied to the example of dementia care.

Utilitarianism, for example, seeks to maximize the benefits for the greatest number in society and to permit individual liberty of action unless it harms others. These ideas can be applied in support of the notion that restraint and confinement are only defensible when there are grave concerns about the safety of others: in this way the liberty of the individual is morally valued. This philosophy, however, has drawbacks in respect of the importance it places on the greatest good. For example, a society might decide it was in the collective interest to practice active euthanasia or mercy killing of those without mental capacity (see the novel by P.D. James, *The Children of Men*, 1994, for an illustration). On a day-to-day basis commentators like Rawls (1972) have pointed to utilitarianism's tendency to equate efficiency with the optimal solution to social problems. This can also result in impersonal and managerial responses. In dementia care such an approach might stress safety and order to the detriment of creativity and well-being. Furthermore, utilitarianism finds it difficult to encompass the perspective of those who cannot articulate their own views of happiness or whose views are significantly different from those of other people.

An alternative approach based on rights, both specific and contextual legal rights, is associated with the concept of 'human rights'. Among professionals the rights theory has considerable currency. In the UK health care system patients have rights under 'Charters'; for example, they have rights to complain and rights to seek access to their records. The language of patients' rights has provided some counterbalance to notions that medical experts know best. It has been expressed in ideas about procedural justice, which emphasize that patients/service users have rights to:

- information;
- opportunities to make representation;
- knowledge of the decision-making system;
- consistency;
- reasons for decision making;
- access to appeal or similar.

In the UK a specific example of a rights issue in practice has been the development of Continuing Care funding. For example, a person with dementia who is deemed not appropriately placed in hospital care may receive funding for alternative care (thus crossing the traditional resource pattern that the NHS does not pay for 'social care' outside hospitals; see Malin 2000). Government guidance in this area of continuing care follows a model of procedural justice whereby information, representation and decision making are to be made public. Less emphasis is placed on the substantive decision, that is whether the experts make the correct decision about care. The emphasis is rather on the process of arriving at a justifiable decision. Patients (or their families) have been awarded rights within this process.

However, as carers' accounts sometimes reveal, the rights approach may be limited in practice. Grant (1998) presents a picture of the dilemma encountered by carers, and many professionals, in overriding a fundamental human right to liberty in her account of her mother's dementia:

> It is the story of how we made the crucial decision to take away her freedom and put her in a home, whether she wanted to go or not, in defiance of every democratic instinct which demanded human rights, even for the old.
>
> (Grant 1999: 30)

Acting in a person's best interests is thus practically and emotionally difficult. Ethically it sets competing principles against each other – human rights to self-determination and rights to protection. A best interests approach requires acknowledgement that in an imperfect world protection from harm may override other principles. As each individual's circumstances are unique it is difficult to create 'recipes' for action. In the next section we explore ways of negotiating conflicting ethical principles in practice.

Principlism

Chadwick and Levitt (1998) consider that **principlism** is the most popular approach to health care ethics. By applying principles to an issue, they argue that practical questions can be resolved or at least clarified. Chief among these principles is autonomy, a notion raised in respect of dementia care by a number of key writers. Associated with autonomy are respect for individuals' wishes and preferences as leading determinants of action. At the level of care planning this can mean listening to people at the early stage of memory impairment to seek their views about future action, such as whether they might wish to be involved in drug trials, how they might feel about residential care or what they wish to happen to their finances should they be unable to manage these. Such listening may be translated into formal agreements, such as Enduring Power of Attorney documents, or be recorded more simply for later reference. Recent government guidance on resuscitation (DoH 2000), for example, sets out the requirements for health care staff to consider a person's prior wishes when stated in documents such as living wills or **advance directives**.

Autonomy may also relate to the value framework exhibited by services, or by anyone supporting a person with dementia. Cox *et al.* (1998) outline five core values that centre on the person with dementia. These are:

- maintaining personal control;
- enabling choice;
- respecting dignity;
- preserving continuity;
- promoting equity.

(Cox *et al.* 1998: 30)

The first three may be included under the 'umbrella' of autonomy. They offer some of the essence of a highly prized status of independence but acknowledge that complete independence is rarely achievable. Operationalizing one element of these values, such as dignity, shows the relevance to the person with dementia in less abstract form. Thus dignity means:

- I continue to be in control of as much of my life as is possible for me.
- I have opportunities to make real and informed choices when I want and am able to choose.
- I am known, respected and valued as a unique individual in meaningful relationships with others.

(Cox *et al.* 1998: 32–3)

The value framework outlined by Cox *et al.* (1998) is useful in grounding principles, particularly as it sought to engage with people with dementia in developing the framework.

Chadwick and Levitt (1998) also consider the principle of beneficence: 'the obligation to do good to the patient (which) frequently conflicts with the principle of autonomy, where the pursuit of autonomy is thought to be injurious to the patient's interests' (p. 106). In illustrating this principle by reference to the question of whether suicide is morally defensible they employ an example which is common in mental health debates across all age groups.

As observed earlier, the motivation to protect can be applied to people with dementia, in respect of looking after their 'best interests'. This was clearly illustrated by the Law Commission (1995) in its report 'Mental Incapacity'. A brief discussion of the ethical issues around suicide in respect of people with dementia is relevant at this point for it is often heard that people express a wish 'to be dead' if they 'get dementia'. An ethical stance based on beneficence justifies thwarting this desire if one holds that death removes all possibility of improving the quality of a person's life or that it ultimately and forever removes the person's autonomy. In many circumstances the desire to commit suicide is seen as an indicator of irrationality or a symptom of mental distress and it is therefore in people's best interests to prevent them harming themselves. Behind such standpoints may lie the influential beliefs which hold that human life is sacred because it is in the image of God and God is the ultimate authority over matters such as life and death. Acceptance of what is 'God given' is a fundamental moral principle which permits some individuals to come to terms with their illness (see Kennedy 1990 for a rebuttal of this). A Christian-based ethic of dementia care of course can extend to far more than the issue of death (see Chapter 4). The ethical stance of other religions in relation to care has also been explored (see Dean and Khan 1998 for a discussion of the challenge to western professionals by the Muslim faith and Muslim minorities).

Some mental health service users have challenged the idea of beneficence, arguing, for example, that statutory powers to detain and treat cannot be concealed under the guise of 'protection' or 'best interest'. The appearance of Advanced Directives within personal plans may well challenge professional codes underpinned by principles of beneficence. Religious beliefs may well be articulated in such documents and professionals will have to explore whether they feel comfortable and equipped to venture into this field.

ETHICS IN PRACTICE

Risk and decision making

The rise of interest in risk among social scientists combines with long-standing concerns among professionals that dementia produces behaviour in which risk is miscalculated or ignored. Many research projects and professional accounts point to a common picture of 'risky' behaviour among people with dementia. In a study of community- and residential-based services for example, Walker and Warren (1996) report a son's concern about his mother, Mrs Kingman, who had dementia: 'She was losing keys, leaving the cooker on . . . She was dangerous to herself and everyone else' (p. 78). Although support workers visited her three times a day she was felt to need 'constant supervision' and so entered residential care, despite not 'liking' it and it making her 'upset'.

This portrayal of people with dementia as 'risky' is powerful in developing ideas that they need protection and that their community care can present dangers to others' community safety. Not all people with dementia, of course, are risky. Askham and Thompson's (1990) study of 104 individuals living at home found 27 displayed risky or dangerous behaviour frequently, 36 displayed such behaviour occasionally and 41 not at all. Only nine people demonstrated behaviour that was perceived to have a high level of serious consequence to themselves or others, such as leaving the gas on or starting fires, and thus necessitating 'continual guarding'.

For professionals the use of formal decision-making powers to control negative risks, such as those powers available under mental health legislation, has been varied. Some influential commentators take the view that people with dementia and without mental capacity are disadvantaged by professionals' reticence to invoke legal procedures (Marshall 1990).

The White Paper, *Reforming the Mental Health Act* (DoH/Home Office 2000) made a commitment to new provisions 'to protect the rights of people with long-term mental **incapacity** who need care and treatment for serious mental disorder.' The government noted that while such individuals might not resist care or treatment, they are not able to consent to it. Taking a 'best interests' approach explicitly, the government has identified such individuals as vulnerable to abuse or neglect (para 2.39). Making reference to the Bournewood case (R v Bournewood Community and Mental Health NHS Trust, Ex parte L (House of Lords 1998)) and its highlighting of the need for better safeguards in this area, the government has proposed that clinical supervisors (the medical consultant) will need to seek a second opinion when care and treatment lasts longer than 28 days.

Risk and decision making, however, do offer a conceptual framework both for practice and for those providing care for others informally. Practitioners are able, for example, to tease out the *benefits* of risk taking for individuals with dementia in maintaining their individuality and sense of pleasure. An example is given by de Villiers (1997) in respect of an individual with HIV-related dementia living in a supported home:

> His energy levels and demands for independence require negotiated risk taking, which includes a fall down the stairs with severe facial bruising as a result, but everyone, including his personal advocate and close family members agree that his overall quality of life would be poorer if he were more restricted.
>
> (de Villiers 1997: 202)

The positives of risk taking are one way of linking ethical strands about best interests and about protection. It is possible to accept that wandering for some individuals provides a high level of pleasure and that in certain circumstances it is not likely to lead to major harm. By accepting this risk the adult status of the individual is maintained and enhanced.

Ethics and interventions

Ethical debates around dementia often centre on the need for staff training and practice to be grounded in a value base. Claims are made that certain approaches to service intervention are ethical, often to counter doubts that people with dementia have been unable to consent to their involvement or resist the intrusion or activity. For example, Parker and Penhale (1998) outline four types of social work intervention that may constitute ethical practice and explain why. First they discuss cognitive behaviour or behavioural approaches (for description of this type of approach see Chapter 2). Despite the 'bad press' associated with these possible punitive and conditioning approaches, Parker and Penhale argue that environmental cues and stimuli may prompt learning. Moreover, behavioural approaches may be helpful in changing or modifying the behaviour of those closely associated with the person with dementia.

In stressing the ethical base of behavioural approaches the authors argue that they are appropriate to professional practice. 'Ethics' thus appears to be a key term in defining what is acceptable and professional behaviour. It is a prime construct perhaps because people with dementia are deemed to be unable to defend themselves.

Second, Parker and Penhale (1998) argue that crisis intervention is an ethically sensitive approach. In crisis intervention a social worker or other professional may manipulate the situation and operate judgementally. Their involvement may be time-limited and could be interpreted as minimalistic. However, Parker and Penhale consider that such interventions, encouraging problem solving and adaptability, are appropriate for people with dementia. They argue that practitioners need not take a naïve view of crisis intervention by sitting back and waiting for a crisis to precipitate. However, social workers will find, as will other professionals such as community nurses, that many initial contacts with services arise from a crisis and it is thus useful to recognize this for what it is. Using models of crisis theory can help offer a framework for dealing with immediate problems and resolving them by adaptive means within the existing systems of support of the person with dementia. As such they argue that crisis intervention is an ethical form of practice: 'Enabling a service user to employ a novel coping strategy may offset not only a crisis but also a permanent deteriorating in functioning' (Parker and Penhale 1998: 68).

Third, Parker and Penhale (1998) identify empowerment as a key element of professional practice. As a strategy it has combined social workers' beliefs in the necessity for socio-political change with intervention into the lives of those lacking power. Parker and Penhale discuss aspects of this at practitioner level, questioning the extent to which practice may be described as empowering if service users have not sought the involvement of welfare agencies or desired their 'interference'. Behind such questioning lies a 'best interests' approach which argues that involvement may ameliorate a painful, distressing or injurious situation for either the person with dementia or others. As we have seen, such an approach underlies much justification for intervention in the lives of those 'suffering' from serious mental illness or mental incapacity both in respect of legislation but also amorphously around services or support.

In this way empowerment may be legitimated on an ethical basis in that it prevents or diminishes harm or danger or reduces the likelihood of these. Linked to advocacy, however, the moral underpinnings become complex as advocacy in a pure form represents not best interests but the desires and expressed choices of an individual. Advocates working in dementia services have to resolve their basis for legitimacy – often striving to balance ideas of what a person did want, or might have wanted if current circumstances had arisen, with judgements about what seems to be in the person's best interests.

Fourth, Parker and Penhale (1998) discuss reminiscence work. They convey many of the typically positive responses to this type of activity:

> It shows a respect for the history of individuals, and acknowledges that people are social beings and have a need to share, teach and continue to review and experience aspects of their lives.
>
> (Parker and Penhale 1998: 156)

Much of the literature argues that it is possible to develop an ethical dimension to reminiscence by respecting individuals' involvement and contribution, by acknowledging people's rights to refuse to participate and by having resources available when strong or distressing reactions are elicited. The edited collection by Hunt *et al.* (1997) does not include 'ethics' in its index but from a variety of perspectives the principles of humanity, tolerance, sensitivity and acceptance are underlined. As many of the contributors illustrate, the possibility of early trauma surfacing in old age and perhaps causing extreme distress may challenge those on the receiving end of such accounts or behaviours to think very seriously about the most terrifying and depraved examples of human behaviour.

An ethical approach to dementia care has to encompass the support of carers and staff. Hunt (1997) points to the necessity for regular staff supervision to avoid staff being 'overwhelmed, unable to remain open to their clients' needs, preoccupied with their own feelings, and, consequently, liable to develop negative, uncaring attitudes' (p. 221). Supporting staff is possible through models of supervision, training and professional development. It reflects that staff too are people deserving of respect. In a context of limited resources where arguments are made that it is too expensive to raise standards in residential care there is evidence that staff are being expected to treat residents according to a different set of values than those applying to themselves. High staff turnover, poor wages, poor working conditions (Bornat and Chamberlayne 1999) characterize parts of the sector and seem antithetical to person-centred care.

These four examples of ethical practice are not confined to social workers or trained professional staff or those employed in care work. They also influence the experiences of informal carers who seek to balance a number of competing principles at times. The next sections move to consider debates about ethics in respect of decision making, starting with a discussion of research and concluding with an overview of professional ethics.

ETHICS IN RESEARCH

In recent years there has been growing recognition that people with dementia should be included in research, particularly among social scientists such as gerontologists. In part this draws on critiques developed by the disability movement that disability studies have to incorporate a social and political dimension and move beyond an individualized medical approach of illness and deviance. Despite the attempt within disability studies to 'unite the interests of all impaired people' (Abberley 1997: 41), many references and discussions of disability still fail to include dementia, and some only touch on ageing. However, the values of inclusion and listening to the voices of the 'subjects' of research are becoming an important influence in dementia research and follow many of the themes developed in disability and feminist studies (Oliver 1997; Ward 1997).

Moriarty and Webb (2000) provide an example of dementia research that presents the ethical reasoning behind a wish to include people with dementia as respondents in their survey. Their study explored the community care services provided to a group of older people with dementia over the period of a year. In their account of their methodology they outline the processes of making contact with people with dementia. It is clear that a range of filters operated in giving permission for people with dementia to be contacted. These included social workers, who asked for a small number of people to be excluded from the survey, and carers who refused access because they considered their relatives might be upset by questions 'designed to assess their level of cognitive impairment' (p. 19).

It is important to consider the issues of power in relation to such gatekeeping. For social workers the territory of research is far less constrained than for their health colleagues. In the UK there is a system of Health Authority Ethics Committees, procedural local bodies with both peer and lay involvement, which provides a watchful eye over research undertaken with 'patients' of the NHS. In contrast, service users of independent or social service provision may be unprotected or overprotected by those who have practical responsibilities. Within these areas there is considerable variance and much is left to the integrity of researchers, the interest of funding bodies and the vigilance of those with powers of access.

Moriarty and Webb (2000) debate another key area in their discussion of principles of informed consent and its application to people with dementia. They note that while the Helsinki Declaration (1964) outlines the necessity for research subjects to confirm their 'freely-given informed consent', it does provide for circumstances where subjects may be mentally incapacitated by outlining that reference to their legal guardian may be made for such consent. Within the UK context such a guardianship framework is undeveloped (Law Commission 1997). But *de facto* social workers, residential providers or relatives may be awarded such a role in recognition of their separation from the researchers' interests (in theory) and their espoused commitment (in theory) to the best interests of their client or relative. While such a model is paternalistic rather than legalistic it provides some measure of reassurance that the research relationship is ethically grounded. However, it also confirms the vulnerability of people with dementia and their potential isolation. Thinking around elder abuse has alerted professionals to the closed worlds of care and the ways in which people with dementia can be effectively silenced from discussion of their circumstances.

Moriarty and Webb (2000) argue that many people with dementia are able to provide opinions about services and that excluding their perspectives makes for a partial picture. They addressed a variety of concerns about potential distress from the interview process by recruiting and training interviewers who had experience in working with older people and carers and by equipping the interviewers with guidelines and advice. In their view, while exploration of a person's level of cognitive impairment might be a source of anxiety, it was better to establish some sense of the level in order to make sense of people's comments in relation to their disability. In fact, 40 per cent of their sample gave written consent to the interview and the remainder provided verbal agreement. To confirm this a proxy informant or carer was incorporated into the consent process. It was not possible to continue interviews with four out of the 122 individuals with dementia who had consented initially because of their reluctance during the actual interview. The interviews lasted about 30 minutes and carers were present with just over half of those interviewed.

Interviews are not the only means of eliciting the views of people with dementia. A commitment to thinking around the issues involved is but one step in developing an ethical stance to research that sees user views as important in assessing the outcome of any intervention or evidence. Other methods such as observation, most clearly articulated by processes such as Dementia Care Mapping (see Chapter 17), can engage with users' experiences. However, such methods need to acknowledge the sensitivity of occupying space in a person's home and to develop understandings with staff, carers and residents or service users in particular about the purpose and use of the research.

PROFESSIONAL ETHICS

For nurses the UKCC Code of Conduct (1992) establishes an explicit duty that the nurse should communicate concerns about identified needs that cannot be met, for example because of a shortage of resources. Clause 12 of the Code requires nurses to 'report to an appropriate person or authority any circumstances in which safe and appropriate care for patients and clients cannot be provided (UKCC 1992: clause 12). This should alert managers to unmet need and meet some of the dilemmas encountered by the nurse in attending to individual patient need and to resource issues. At the level of the individual practitioner the ethical responsibility may be satisfied: other decisions of course have to be taken by those who hold responsibility for allocating resources.

The moral responsibility to communicate concern has been taken up in a variety of spheres. Successful examples of 'whistle blowing' in the health and social care fields have created a more supportive atmosphere for the development of policy and legislation to enable staff to protect vulnerable people. The Public Interest Disclosure Act 1998, for example, enacts a framework for staff who consider that they should go beyond their duties of loyalty to their employers to bring their concerns to a wider audience. This audience might include managers, regulators, politicians or the media in a ladder of progression associated with the level and severity of the concern. The case of Judith Jones, matron of a nursing home for people with dementia, has been widely reported (Public Concern at Work 1998: viii–ix). Mrs Jones received information and herself witnessed behaviour by the owner of the home which appeared to be sexual abuse of residents who had dementia and who were blind. She alerted agencies outside her place of employment (not without difficulty), accepting that her duty of care and loyalty lay with the residents. Such whistle

blowing is upheld by the UKCC Code of Conduct and now by specific legislation: both encapsulate a moral duty to protect the vulnerable individual in the
context of the individual and public good. While the underlying principle may
be altruism, it is now increasingly perceived that to lay claim to professional
status means taking on accountability beyond the context of care.

Not all professionals or practitioners working with people with dementia
have the protection and guidance of a regulatory code. Social workers await
the new General Social Care Council and General Social Work Council to
provide a legislative framework for controlling and guarding the profession's
interests. The majority of people employed in providing support for people
with dementia, however, are not professionals but part-time, untrained (or
briefly trained) care staff working in residential or home-based services. Their
behaviour and moral codes remain relatively unexplored as an occupational
group but many of the discussions around professionalism are evidently relevant. The consultative document *Fit for the Future* (DOH 1999c), for example, proposes that residential and nursing home staff should see whistle
blowing not as a 'betrayal' of loyalty but as a means to protect residents.
This is a higher moral good.

CONCLUSION

While there are a number of different ethical standpoints from which philosophers and practitioners engage with dementia, there is a degree of consensus
that dementia matters. It matters more than in terms of finance and resources; it
matters on a higher moral plain how society and individuals treat people with
dementia. Giddens (2000) places such debates within a political framework:

> The question of what collective resources should be made available to the
> frail elderly is not just one of rationing. There are issues to be confronted
> here, including ethical ones of a quite fundamental sort.
>
> (Giddens 2000: 121)

FURTHER READING

Beauchamp, T.L. and Childress, J.F. (1998) *Principles of Biomedical Ethics*, 3rd edn.
Oxford: Oxford University Press.

Clark, C.L. (2000) *Social Work Ethics: Politics, Principles and Practice*. London:
Macmillan.

Hope, T. and Oppenheimer, C. (1997) Ethics and the psychiatry of old age, in R. Jacoby
and C. Oppenheimer (eds) *Psychiatry in the Elderly*. Oxford: Oxford University Press.

Kuhse, H. (1997) *Caring: Nurses, Women and Ethics*. Oxford: Blackwell.

Policy, organizations and research

14

CAROLINE CANTLEY

Understanding the policy context

KEY POINTS

- Dementia care is seldom treated as a policy issue in its own right.
- Policy and provision for dementia care are inextricably linked with policy developments for older people and for community care more generally.
- Current services for people with dementia are shaped by the community care reforms of the 1990s and a plethora of more recent government initiatives.
- Housing policy should be better integrated with health and social care policies.
- Policies should take account of diversity in the needs of people with dementia.

INTRODUCTION

This chapter begins by outlining the development of health and social care policy and provision as it relates to older people with mental health problems, including dementia. It deals with the period prior to the community care reforms of the 1990s. It then describes the main features of more recent community care reforms before examining six key themes in current policy development: planning and commissioning services; working together; primary care; **standards**; long-term care; and independence and empowerment. The impact of housing policy on dementia care is considered in a separate section. The chapter ends by commenting on the policy issues for groups whose needs have not been well considered in the mainstream of policy development.

Before embarking on this review of policy we must note that there is some variation in policy development across the United Kingdom (cf. Sharkey 2000). Although developments in policy and provision for care of older people have been broadly similar in England, Wales and Scotland there have been some differences in approach and in the pace of implementation (Hunter and Wistow 1987). The devolution of powers to the Scottish Parliament and the Welsh Assembly may well lead in the future to greater differences in policies and service organization across the three countries. Northern Ireland has a different administrative structure from the rest of the UK, with the integration of health and social services being a notable feature in the development of care in the community.

LEGACIES OF THE PAST

In the first half of the twentieth century, family care was the mainstay of support for physically and mentally frail older people. The main alternative was custodial care in institutions. Until the end of the 1930s older people with physical and mental health problems were considered for the most part to be outside the scope of medicine. Wilkin and Hughes (1986) attribute this lack of development of health services for older people to prevailing concepts of health and to stereotypes of old age:

> Ill-health continued to be seen as an inevitable corollary of old age. Even diseases which were considered treatable in younger patients were regarded as incurable when the patient was over 60 years of age. The best that could be hoped for was tender loving care – and even this was denied to many.
> (Wilkin and Hughes 1986: 168)

At the end of the Second World War, legislation was enacted that marked the end of the old Poor Law provision and the beginning of the 'welfare state'. This legislation set the framework for health services free at the point of delivery, for state pensions and for a 'safety net' of welfare benefits. It also gave local authorities the powers to provide home care for frail elderly people, although provision of domiciliary services was in practice mainly left to voluntary organizations. In the 1960s growing criticisms of institutional care led to a policy emphasis on a 'shift from hospital to community care'. National plans were drawn up to close large numbers of long-stay hospital beds and to transfer services to the community. Local authorities were given wider powers to provide services for older people and, through the Health Service and Public Health Act 1968, 'to promote the welfare of the elderly'. However, it was not until the late 1970s that local authorities were required to provide home care. Overall, in the postwar period, institutional care dominated service provision for the 'mentally infirm elderly' with few local authorities developing community alternatives (Phillipson 1982).

In the 1970s and early 1980s national plans set out principles and targets for 'priority groups' such as people with mental health problems, people with learning disabilities and older people. As Malin *et al.* (1999: 11) explain, 'Community care was an underlying goal of many of the plans but its presence was unremarkable and its objectives still rather vague.' Progress in developing community support services as an alternative to institutional care was generally slow although the overall commitment to community care for older people was affirmed in policy documents such as 'Growing Older' (DHSS 1981). A recurring theme during this period was the need for better collaboration between health and social care agencies in planning and implementing a shift in the balance of provision from institutional to community care.

Policy documents have until very recently used terms such as 'senile confused', 'senile infirmity' and 'elderly mentally infirm' rather than the term 'dementia'. Although the term 'dementia' did not feature in policy documents, the needs of people with dementia were still a policy issue (cf. Means and Smith 1998a). Early concern with the needs of older people with mental health problems is evident, for example, in work in the late 1960s that highlighted the maltreatment of older people in long-stay psychiatric hospitals (Robb 1967) and in Meacher's (1972) criticism of specialist homes for 'the confused elderly'.

The needs of older people with mental health problems were highlighted in *The Rising Tide*, a report by the Health Advisory Service (1983). This report drew attention to growth in numbers of older people with mental health problems and to increasing expectations of services. It warned that 'Unless the challenges are met, the flood is likely to overwhelm the entire health care system . . .' (p. 1). It also described the variation that existed across the country in services for older people with mental health problems. It argued for the development of comprehensive, specialized old age psychiatry services but noted that 'no one model for a psychiatric service for old age has yet emerged as preferable to all others' (p. 23). It emphasized that specialist old age psychiatry services 'do not stand alone' and drew attention to the need for multiprofessional and multi-agency working. Significantly it noted that in developing old age psychiatry services 'Both the organically impaired and the functionally ill are usually included since a dementia service alone raised a number of difficulties over staff morale, recruitment and work satisfaction' (p. 5).

The early development of services for people with dementia, as with other so-called 'Cinderella' groups, has been described as a history of neglect (Means and Smith 1998b). The reasons for this neglect are complex but Means and Smith identify the following contributing factors:

- The position of older people in capitalist society. Older people are excluded from the labour market. This leads both to their 'structured dependency' on the state and to their being low priority for the allocation of state resources. (For further explanation of this political economy perspective see Chapter 3.)
- The role of institutions in warning wider society against depending on state support. This means that admission cannot be seen to be a desirable option.

- Fears that the provision of services might lead families to abandon their responsibilities and their role in providing care.
- Negative cultural stereotypes of old age and the way that these stereotypes affect policy and service assumptions about what is desirable and possible in care for older people.
- The political complexity of implementing new policies and the slowness of change that results.

COMMUNITY CARE REFORMS IN THE 1990s

The roots of the 1990s community care reforms lie in the problems of service provision that were developing in the 1980s and in the 'New Right' thinking of the Conservative government of that period. An influential report by the Audit Commission (1986), *Making a Reality of Community Care*, identified serious problems with community care services for older people, for people with mental health problems and for people with learning disabilities. These problems included: slow build-up of community-based services; uneven provision of local authority services across the country; and rapidly growing numbers of people in private residential and nursing home care supported by social security benefits payments without an assessment of need. In response to the Audit Commission recommendations for a fundamental review of community care, the government commissioned the Griffiths Report (HMSO 1988) to advise on options for the future. Central to its recommendations was a new approach to community care founded on the view that the free market was a better mechanism than the public sector for delivering welfare provision. Many of the recommendations of the Griffiths Report were fed into the subsequent White Paper *Caring for People* (DoH 1989a).

Caring for People (DoH 1989a) heralded a major shift in the role of local authority social services away from direct service provision. Although local authorities were given the lead responsibility for community care, increasingly they would be expected to act as 'enabling authorities' purchasing services from independent sector organizations in a **'mixed economy'** of care. At the strategic level local authorities would lead on producing annual community care plans; at the operational level they would have responsibility for allocating resources through assessment and care management processes.

The main recommendations of *Caring for People* were implemented in the NHS and Community Care Act 1990. The Act was implemented in stages and from 1993 the funds that had previously been provided by the social security system directly to individuals to pay for residential care were transferred to local authorities in the Special Transitional Grant. This process served to put a limit on overall spending on residential and nursing home provision. It also aimed to encourage the development of alternatives to residential care by removing the perverse incentive of the previous funding system that promoted provision of care home places rather than services at home. Initially local authorities were required to spend 85 per cent of the funds transferred in the Special Transitional Grant on the independent sector rather than on funding places in public sector homes. Help with care home fees for individuals became dependent upon an assessment of need as well as upon a financial assessment.

Alongside the changes in social services there were radical changes in the NHS. The broad thrust of these changes, set out in the White Paper *Working for Patients* (DoH 1989b), was to introduce a so-called 'internal market' in health care and reinforce the role of general management. The NHS and Community Care Act 1990 created health authorities, to become the commissioners and purchasers of hospital and community services, and NHS Trusts, to become the providers of services. Trusts were expected to compete with each other. The Act also provided for the introduction of GP fundholding, a scheme that allowed general practices over a certain size to manage their own budgets for a range of services, drugs and practice costs.

Although it is beyond the scope of this chapter to review the full impact of these reforms, two major trends in provision for older people are important to note: a shift from public to independent sector provision in social care and a narrowing of the NHS role to that of provider of acute care (Audit Commission 1997).

It is clear that local authority social services varied in the speed and enthusiasm with which they introduced a functional split between purchaser and provider in line with market principles. Individual managers and front-line staff also varied in their response to the changes (Lewis and Glennerster 1996). Changes in the level of residential and nursing home placements by local authorities were similarly variable (Audit Commission 1997). Although the overall growth in placements in residential and nursing homes fell after 1993 the absolute numbers of placements did not. There were two reasons for this (Audit Commission 1997). First, local authorities, as we have noted, had to use 85 per cent of the Special Transitional Grant in the independent sector. But since there was little independent sector home care available this meant spending on independent sector care home placements. Second, even when there was no difference in the gross costs between home care and residential care, funding frameworks meant that for a local authority it was nearly always cheaper to place someone in residential care.

In response to a growing concern about the reduction in NHS long-term provision for older people, the Department of Health (DoH 1995b) issued guidance to health authorities on the establishment of eligibility criteria for the provision of free NHS continuing care. This explained that both the NHS and local authorities have responsibilities for providing continuing care. It required health authorities to develop eligibility criteria to be used as a basis for decisions about individual need for NHS-funded care. It also required them to develop policies about the range and type of NHS services to be provided to meet continuing health-care needs locally. However, the Audit Commission (1997) argues that resources to support implementation were limited and that 'The first legacy of the 1980s that needs managing is the change to the cut-off point at which the NHS stops providing care' (p. 13).

Lewis and Glennerster (1996: 206) suggest that 'In general, the community care changes have served to raise the profile of work with elderly people, which may in and of itself have a positive effect on the services offered to that client group.' Indeed, the changes in some ways may have served some people with dementia well. They have made explicit and legitimized the focusing of resources on those people deemed to be most dependent and at risk. People with advanced dementia may well have benefited. However, people in the earlier stages of dementia are likely to have been affected by the reduced availability of the type of support that aims to prevent or postpone the need for major service intervention. One of the much-cited benefits of the increased use of the independent sector is that it increases choice for service users. It is arguable to what extent this is the case for older people. For people with dementia there are additional issues to consider. People with dementia are more likely than other older people to need additional support in exercising choice. This support is seldom available. Neither are they served well if they have to cope with too many separate service inputs from different providers (DoHSSI 1997).

It is important to note one other significant development in community care in the late 1980s and early 1990s: the emergence of carers as a major focus of attention for policy and service provision. Twigg (1998) describes the reasons for a shift in policy:

> ... new emphasis was placed on the positive support of carers. This was largely justified on the grounds of cost effectiveness – supporting carers to support older people – but it did contain some recognition of the interests of carers themselves.
>
> (Twigg 1998: 131)

The problems of carers of people with dementia came to the fore in several research studies in the 1980s (see for example Levin *et al.* 1989) and carers have been important in stimulating service development in dementia care (Barnes 1997). There is a substantial social policy literature on the nature of informal care and its role in the context of state welfare (see for example Twigg and Atkin 1994). It is beyond the scope of this chapter to develop this theme further but carers' issues are taken up elsewhere in this book (see particularly Chapters 3 and 11).

CURRENT POLICY DEVELOPMENTS

Since the change of government in 1997 there have been some significant changes in the health and social care context in which dementia care is developing. The Labour government describes its approach to health and social services as a new 'third way'. The White Paper *Modernising Social Services* (DoH 1998a) criticizes the previous '**New Right**' policy emphasis on privatization as having led to fragmentation of services. It also makes clear that there will be no return to earlier models of local authority provision, which are viewed as inflexible and unresponsive to individual need. Thus *Modernising Social Services* states: 'Our third way for social care moves the focus away from who provides the care, and places it firmly on the **quality of services** experienced by individuals and their carers and families' (para. 1.7). Similarly the White Paper *The New NHS: Modern, Dependable* (DoH 1997c) describes 'a third way' for the NHS. This puts an end to 'the divisive internal market system of the 1990s' but rejects a return to 'the old centralised command and control systems of the 1970s [that] . . . stifled innovation and put the needs of institutions ahead of the needs of patients' (para. 2.1).

In July 2000 the government published both the *NHS Plan* (DoH 2000) (which set out its intentions for substantial additional investment in NHS services and staffing) and its response to the Royal Commission on Long Term Care (see below). A major thrust of the *NHS Plan* is to reduce unnecessary hospital admissions of older people and to prevent delays in hospital discharge. Specific commitments in the *NHS Plan* that are relevant here include:

- national standards for caring for older people to ensure that ageism is not tolerated in health care;
- single health and social care 'personal care plans' for elderly people and their carers;
- nursing care in nursing homes to become free;
- new intermediate care services to allow older people to live more independent lives, particularly to provide help for them to remain at home immediately after or during an acute illness.

This section has summarized current policy developments in community care. These developments do not constitute a radical overhaul of community care but they do introduce significant changes with important implications for dementia services. We can identify six main policy themes that are shaping current dementia services: planning and commissioning services; primary care; interagency working; standards; long-term care; and independence and empowerment. We discuss each of these below.

CURRENT POLICY THEMES

Planning and commissioning services

In a survey of health authorities, the Alzheimer's Disease Society (1997) found that there was no consistent approach to assessing needs for dementia services. Seventy-nine per cent of health authorities were unable to identify the resources spent on dementia care. The report concludes that there is 'a fundamental lack of recognition of dementia as a specific area of need' (p. 11).

Since the above report there have been changes in the way in which health authorities and social services are required to produce plans. The *Better Services for Vulnerable People* initiative (DoH 1997a) requires health authorities and local authorities to produce annual Joint Investment Plans (JIPs). These must, among other things, cover the development of services to avoid unnecessary admissions to hospital or care homes. JIPs are part of wider Health Improvement Programmes (HImPs), local strategies for improving health and health care and for delivering better integrated and user-centred care. Each health authority is required, with the involvement of partner agencies, to have a HImP and JIP in place. For JIPs the initial emphasis was on services for older people including people with mental health problems.

Analysis of the early JIPs suggests that the new planning arrangements have not yet addressed the limitations identified in the Alzheimer's Disease Society (1997) report. Thus the Audit Commission (2000) found: 'Most of the plans for mental health care for older people were underdeveloped, so special attention needs to be focused on this group' (p. 97).

One of the key issues for planning and commissioning dementia care relates to how it should fit within broader planning frameworks. National planning guidance has at times dealt with dementia care as an integral part of older people's mental health services and argued that these services have much in common with mental health more generally. For example, the Department of Health (1997b) argues that 'The principles of effective joint commissioning and working in mental health services for older people are no different to those in other areas of mental health' (p. 21). Yet in the context of the National Service Frameworks (see below) dementia care is considered within services for older people rather than mental health services. Dening (2000) suggests that, while links with mainstream psychiatric services are important, the rationale for including dementia with older people is that 'the separation of policy along the lines of age means that the needs of older people are not forgotten amidst the headline issues of younger patients with psychotic illness and severe personality disorders'. And it is the involvement of old age psychiatry services in provision for people with early onset dementia that provides the rationale for their inclusion in the National Service Framework (NSF) for Older People (see below). At local level, health authorities (Alzheimer's Disease Society 1997) and social services (DoHSSI 1997) also vary as to whether they plan and provide services within their programmes for mental health or older people.

Primary care

It is particularly important that we understand the changes that are shaping primary care since primary care services are so central to the provision of effective dementia care. Primary Care Groups (PCGs) were introduced nationally from April 1999. They have responsibility for commissioning services devolved to them from health authorities. They also have responsibility for the development of primary care provision. They have a cash-limited budget with which to commission and provide services giving them '. . . the opportunity to deploy resources and savings to strengthen local services and ensure that patterns of care best reflect their patients' needs' (para. 5.17). There is also provision for Primary Care Trusts (PCTs) which take on responsibility for the provision of community health services. The first wave of PCTs became operational in April 2000 and the *NHS Plan* (DoH 2000) expects all PCGs to become PCTs by April 2004. The *Plan* notes that PCTs '. . . provide a suitable means for the commissioning of social care services, using the Health Act flexibilities, for older people and people with mental health problems' (para. 7.8).

In the early stages of their operation PCGs and PCTs have been preoccupied with a huge management development agenda. Rummery and Glendinning (2000) provide a good overview of the changes in primary care and their implications for collaboration between health and social services in planning and providing services for older people. The impact that the new primary care organizations will have on dementia care is not yet clear. Iliffe (1999) suggests that the input to PCGs from social services and community nursing may be a crucial factor in creating better understanding of dementia in primary care. He concludes that 'the opportunities offered for more coherent and effective working for people with dementia are as great as the risks that dementia will remain a low priority for primary care' (p. 15). There is a risk that medical perspectives will dominate service commissioning through PCGs and PCTs. Such a development would be at odds with much current thinking about dementia care. However, there are substantial benefits in the opportunities that PCGs and PCTs provide for new ways in which primary care, community health and social care can work together. Early indications about the operation of PCGs suggest that there are grounds for optimism (Glendinning and Coleman 2000).

Working together

It is hard to overemphasize the degree to which agencies are exhorted to work jointly in community care generally and in care of older people and people with dementia more specifically (for example, DoHSSI 1997; Audit Commission 1997; DoH 1997b; RCP/RCP 1998; Audit Commission 2000). But achieving this is difficult and the factors that inhibit joint working are complex and powerful (for further discussion of the professional and organizational issues involved see Chapter 14).

For example, social services and health care have struggled to work jointly at the strategic level in planning dementia care (DoHSSI 1997), and Barnes (1997) identifies the following factors as contributing to the slow development of joint health and social care policies for older people with mental health problems:

- Within the NHS older people with mental health problems are generally the management responsibility of mental health services whereas in social services management responsibility is generally located in older people's services.
- Health and social services often have different geographical boundaries.
- There is a shortage of old age psychiatrists in some areas.
- These have been extensive and fast-paced organizational changes affecting services.
- The planning and resource base is at a low level.

It is not clear to what extent achieving joint working is a structural issue. Is the creation of a single agency the answer to better joint working across health and social care? The Audit Commission (1997) concludes that while structural solutions might help they can also create another set of boundary issues. Joint working towards shared priorities and procedures may be just as effective, and clarification of the roles and responsibilities of the various agencies involved in community care for older people may be the key to success.

The government's approach to promoting better joint working across health and social care has generally steered clear of structural solutions. We have instead seen the introduction of a variety of measures aimed at addressing the problems of joint working. These include the new planning arrangements described above and financial incentives such as the Partnership Grant to promote rehabilitation services. Measures also include legislation to permit use of a number of 'flexibilities' set out in *Partnership in Action* (DoH 1998c). The 'flexibilities' relax the rules about how health and social services can use their funds and make it easier for them to work together through: pooled health and social care budgets; lead commissioning by one agency; and integrated provision.

The *NHS Plan* (DoH 2000), however, indicates that structural change has not been dismissed as a way forward. The *Plan* announces that provision will be made for agencies locally to opt for the establishment of a new level of PCT, Care Trusts. These organizations will commission and deliver health services as well as social care for older people and other user groups. The *Plan* does not provide any details about the governance of these organizations although it does anticipate that some could soon be operational. Commentators have expressed doubts about whether the NHS has the ability to take on social care commissioning – given the extent of its preoccupation with internal reorganization in creating PCTs and with restructuring community health and mental health trusts (for example, Hudson 2000b).

Standards

Improving standards and making them explicit is a central theme in recent government policy. For example the national charter, *Better Care, Higher Standards* (DoH/DETR 1999), covers the standards that anyone requiring long-term care or support can expect from local housing, health and social services. As part of the policy drive to raise standards *Modernising Social Services* (DoH 1998a) introduces a National Care Standards Commission which aims to ensure greater consistency in care standards across the country. It also sets up eight new independent regional Commissions for Care Standards (CCSs) which from 2002 will be responsible for new arrangements for the registration and inspection of care homes, both residential and nursing, and which will also regulate domiciliary social care providers.

Central to concerns about standards is the issue of the variation that exists in service availability, eligibility criteria and charging policies in different areas of the country (see for example DoHSSI 1997; Audit Commission 1997, 2000). One specific concern in dementia care has been the variation across the country in prescribing new anti-dementia drugs. The government initiative called *Fair Access to Care Services* has been launched to improve the way in which local authorities define and apply their eligibility criteria for adult care services. In similar vein the *NHS Plan* indicates that statutory guidance is to be issued to councils to reduce variations in charges for home care services.

As a first step in developing national minimum standards for residential and nursing homes, the government commissioned advice from the Centre for Policy on Ageing. Following consultation on the resultant standards set out in *Fit for the Future* (DoH 1999b), the government has published *Care Homes for Older People. National Minimum Standards* (DoH 2001a). These standards will provide a foundation for the work of the new National Care Standards Commission and they will apply to all care homes from April 2002. The standards relate to: choice of home, health and personal care, daily life and social activities, complaints and protection, environment, staffing and management and administration. The standards are very broad but recognize that some groups of residents, including people with dementia, have particular needs for which there will be a requirement for 'additional specific knowledge, skills and facilities . . . in order for a care home to deliver an individually tailored and comprehensive service' (DoH 2001a:vii).

National Service Framework for Older People

The Government has introduced National Service Frameworks as a means of improving the quality of services and reducing local variations in services. A National Service Framework (NSF) for Older People (DoH 2001b) sets national standards and defines service models for the care of older people. It includes strategies to support implementation as well as performance measures to assess progress. The NSF builds upon a broad range of health and social care policies. Much of the NSF therefore addresses the broad policy and service issues that we discuss throughout this chapter as having a significant impact on dementia care.

More specifically related to dementia care, the NSF summarizes the requirements of a good mental health service for older people as follows:

> Mental health services for older people should be community-orientated and provide seamless packages of care and support for older people and their carers . . . The hallmark of good mental health services is that they are: comprehensive, multidisciplinary, accessible, responsive, individualised, accountable and systematic.
>
> (DoH 2001b: 91)

The standard that the NSF sets for mental health services is that:

> Older people who have mental health problems have access to integrated mental health services, provided by the NHS and councils to ensure effective diagnosis, treatment and support for them and for their carers.
>
> (DoH 2001b: 90)

The NSF describes the important elements of the early recognition, diagnosis and treatment of both depression and of dementia and it sets out a model for mental health services for older people. It requires health and social services to review current service arrangements and, by 2004, to ensure that:

- there are local plans developed by the NHS, local authorities and independent sector partners for an integrated mental health service for older people;
- every general practice is using a protocol, agreed with specialist services, health and social services, for the diagnosis, treatment and care of people with dementia or depression;
- there are protocols agreed by the health and social care systems for the care and management of older people with mental health problems.

There are other more specific points in the NSF that are significant for the development of dementia care, including:

- the requirement to establish a new single assessment process by 2002 and the impact of this on early recognition of dementia and on holistic responses to the needs of the people with dementia and their families;
- the recognition that action needs to be taken to improve acute hospital care for people with dementia;
- the recommendation that the NHS and local authorities should work with independent care home providers to develop services including specialist residential care places for older people with dementia;
- the recommendations for better management of medication including anti-dementia drugs and the use of neuroleptic medication in care homes;
- the attention paid to staff education and training as a foundation for service development;
- the commitment to NHS Research and Development addressing gaps in knowledge about health and social care services for people with dementia;
- the recognition of the importance of responding to the needs of particular groups of people with dementia (see below).

More general issues related to standards in services are discussed in Chapter 17.

Long-term care

The Royal Commission on Long Term Care (1999) was set up to produce recommendations for a sustainable system of funding long-term care for older people in their own homes and in other settings. The Commission's summary of the key element of their task provides a useful overview of the issues. There was a need to:

- assess current funding arrangements and their adequacy in the light of demographic change;
- take account of the expectations of older people;
- ensure fairness, effectiveness and efficiency;

- recognize the dignity of people requiring long-term care and their hopes of 'a just and socially inclusive provision';
- take account of the economic circumstances of individuals and of the state.

The Commission's first conclusion is important: 'For the UK there is no "demographic timebomb" as far as long-term care is concerned and as a result of this, the costs of care will be affordable' (p. xviii).

A key recommendation of the Commission's majority report was that there should be a split between living costs, housing costs and personal care costs in long-term care and that personal care should be available free to the individual and according to need.

The government's response (DoH 2000) is the introduction of legislation to allow full NHS funding of nursing care in nursing homes from October 2001. This applies to 'registered nurse time spent on providing, delegating or supervising care in any setting' (para. 2.9). Individuals will still be required to contribute to the costs of personal care on the basis of a financial assessment. Some measures are to be introduced to alleviate the effects of the means test, particularly to reduce the pressure on people to sell their own home when they enter residential or nursing home care.

Although aspects of the changes are welcomed there remains widespread concern about the new arrangements and the difficulty of determining what is nursing care and what is personal care. Many people with long-term conditions such as dementia, who have extensive needs for help with a whole range of essential basic activities such as eating and toileting, do not receive that care from trained nurses. Harding (2000: 23) summarizes the problem: 'We have a two-tier approach here – greater and more determined help for those with a prospect of recovery, but no resolution for those whose more mundane needs are not dignified with the name of nursing care.'

Independence and empowerment

An emphasis on independence and empowerment for older people runs through many policy initiatives. The government has established an inter-ministerial group to coordinate government policy for older people (Dening and Brown 2000). One initiative, *Better Government for Older People*, led by the Cabinet Office, involves older people in pilot projects to improve access to services and to improve links between agencies. A second initiative, *Building a Better Britain for Older People*, brings together a number of government departments to promote productive or active ageing, health and good quality care, and consultation and involvement. There are also financial incentives for health and social services. The Partnership Grant is to support the development of rehabilitation services. The Prevention Grant is to support the development of early intervention and low-level support services for people at risk of losing their independence.

At a more individual level there are efforts to empower older people through the extension of the 'direct payments' scheme to people aged over 65 years.

This enables local authorities to make payments to people assessed as eligible for services so that they can then make their own decisions about how they use the money to shape the care they receive. Also to assist individuals, the *NHS Plan* proposes that by 2002 a new Patient Advocacy and Liaison Service (PALS) will be set up in every NHS Trust. It will take over the Community Health Councils' role of supporting people in making complaints.

This policy focuses on independence and empowerment is welcome for most older people. However, it does give rise to concerns that people with dementia, and others who require continuing care, will be accorded low priority. Special efforts will need to be made if people with dementia are to participate in initiatives of this type and derive the benefits of empowerment that are being advanced for older people more generally. Chapter 18 discusses in more detail some of the ways in which people with dementia and their carers can be better empowered.

HOUSING POLICY AND PROVISION FOR PEOPLE WITH DEMENTIA

There has been no coherent policy approach to the integration of housing policy and provision with broader health and social care policies and services for older people. As Peace and Johnson (1998) explain:

> At present older people are faced with combinations of accommodation and care which have either evolved through housing policy in the form of sheltered housing or through social welfare and health care policy in the form of residential care homes and nursing homes.
>
> (Peace and Johnson 1998: 62)

Franklin (1996) similarly argues that the separate interests of the different agencies involved have dominated our approach to housing and care provision. She advocates more holistic, person-centred approaches to thinking about housing and support including a range of initiatives in 'ordinary living' and in communal settings. Support for people with dementia who live 'at home' in ordinary housing environments is discussed in Chapter 8.

One area of housing policy that is increasingly important in the care of people with dementia is sheltered housing. Since the 1960s, local authorities, specialist housing associations and commercial companies have provided sheltered housing. Since the 1980s, local authorities have substantially reduced their building of new sheltered housing and in the 1990s most of the growth in sheltered housing has been in the private sector. Peace and Johnson (1998) report two different trends in the development of the warden's role in sheltered housing. One trend is the use of high-tech alarm systems to enable wardens to cover a number of schemes. The opposite trend is for wardens to take on an expanded care role. The model of 'extra care housing' or 'very sheltered housing' has grown over the past two decades. It can involve provision of care, meals, and additional warden support and communal facilities. There is growing interest in exploring the potential of this 'extra care housing' model as a means of providing support for people with dementia.

Petre (1995) argues that sheltered housing will become a major form of accommodation for people with dementia. She gives several reasons. There are increasing numbers of very old people in sheltered housing and hence increasing numbers of people with dementia. Sheltered housing is attractive to carers as an alternative to residential care for people with mild to moderate dementia. Relatives of people with dementia in sheltered housing will want them to remain there as long as possible.

However, sheltered housing can have limitations as a setting for caring for people with dementia. Petre (1995) identifies the following problems:

- Wardens and other tenants often lack knowledge and understanding of dementia.
- Tenants with dementia can be socially isolated either because they withdraw from communal activities or because they are rejected by other tenants.
- The built environment, often with long corridors and rows of identical doors, seldom facilitates orientation.
- Tenants with dementia can pose risks or create disruption for other tenants.
- There are organizational issues such as lack of appropriate training and management support for wardens in dealing with dementia.
- Other services have unrealistic expectations of what wardens can provide.

Her research concludes that sheltered housing can provide a good environment in which to maintain the well-being and personhood of tenants with dementia and that its success is not related to cognitive measurement of the severity of the tenant's dementia. Rather, as Kitwood et al. (1995: 58) point out, 'The quality of social services support will determine in many respects the success of sheltered housing as a community care resource for people with dementia.'

The Audit Commission (1998) found that many local authorities provided sheltered housing without sufficient regard to changing needs and demands. As a result, current patterns of sheltered housing do not fit well with the needs of frail older people. This report advocated greater collaboration between housing, social services and health and clarification of the role of sheltered housing. It argued that better use can be made of resources by ensuring that personal support is available to people at an early stage rather than as a crisis response. It also highlighted the need for local action and for a national framework to address the role of housing in the support of increasing numbers of vulnerable people.

Cox (1998) provides examples of different types of housing-based initiatives that provide care for people with dementia. These initiatives adopt a variety of approaches: support in the person's own home; support in a shared house; specialist dementia support with communal facilities; sites which provide different types and levels of support; schemes to adapt people's own homes to enable them to stay there; and housing and support for people from ethnic minority communities. Although some early work has identified the potential for achieving high-quality care in ordinary housing environments (Svanberg *et al.* 1999; Cantley and Smith 2000), research in this field is limited and we know little about the advantages and disadvantages of different housing models.

One of the key issues in developing housing-based models for the care of people with dementia is the complexity of financial arrangements in relation to charges for accommodation, charges for servicing of the accommodation and charges for care. Further complexities arise in the benefits system where the level of financial support through Housing Benefit can vary in different parts of the country because different local authorities interpret the regulations in different ways (Cox 1998).

SPECIFIC SERVICE USER GROUPS

People with dementia in minority ethnic communities

It is only recently that the populations of the UK and other European countries have begun to include significant numbers of older people who belong to minority ethnic groups. Health and welfare provision for these groups has not been high on the policy agenda (Atkin 1998) and the specific needs of people with dementia have received even less attention. Askham *et al.* (1995) surveyed health and social services for older people from minority ethnic communities and Atkin (1998) provides an overview of issues from which we can extrapolate the following as being important issues for dementia care:

- Differences in the numbers and age structures of different minority ethnic groups will affect the numbers of people with dementia.
- Substantial growth in numbers of older people of Afro-Caribbean and Asian descent over 10 years will give rise to increasing numbers of people with dementia.
- Our knowledge of the extent of disability and chronic illness in minority ethnic populations is limited and that of dementia particularly limited.
- The distribution of different minority ethnic communities varies. For the most part they are focused in large industrial conurbations, often in inner city areas where service resources are frequently poorest. But there are some very dispersed populations where small numbers in any locality will present particular challenges to services.
- People in minority ethnic populations have enormously diverse social histories (including the timing and reasons for coming to the UK), life experiences and socio-economic circumstances. Understanding this will be crucial if services are to be person-centred.
- Minority ethnic groups frequently lack knowledge about health and social services and it is clear that they underuse services. Enabling access to services must be a key concern.
- Service responses are inadequate for a variety of reasons: structural barriers such as language and lack of attention to dietary requirements; misrepres-

entation of needs through cultural stereotypes; organizational practices that segregate and define minority ethnic groups as more of a 'problem' than the white majority population; racist attitudes and behaviour among staff.

To the above we can add a range of dementia specific points highlighted by Patel *et al.* (1998) in a recent report about dementia care in the UK and a number of other European countries. Patel *et al.* emphasize that:

- dementia has received little attention in mainstream work on ethnic minority health;
- current services for people with dementia are generally 'blind' to the needs of people from ethnic minority groups;
- many cultures fail to recognize dementia as an illness;
- there is a need for improved diagnosis of dementia in minority ethnic communities;
- funding for specialist care services, often provided by voluntary sector organizations, is inadequate and frequently short-term;
- there is a need for support for specialist minority ethnic organizations to develop their capacity in dementia care.

Research on dementia in minority ethnic communities is limited. Adamson (1999) highlights the diversity of carers' circumstances and experiences and their generally low use of formal services. Barnes (1997) recognizes some of the difficulties of planning services for older people with mental health problems from minority ethnic communities and particularly the diversity of needs that exists in different communities. She argues that agencies can plan and develop their services by working with community leaders, by setting up specialist projects and by employing development workers from these communities. She warns, however, that it is important to ensure that services respond to the views of older people, rather than the younger more articulate group who may be representing them.

People with early onset dementia

Younger people with dementia have not featured at all in policy discussions until very recently. Their cause has been taken up by the Alzheimer's Disease Society (1996) in a 'Charter for Younger People with Dementia'. One of the important features of the Charter is that it identifies service needs that extend beyond health and social services to issues that must be tackled by social security and employment services. Williams *et al.* (1997) in a Health Advisory Service report set out recommendations for comprehensive service approaches to meeting the needs of younger people with dementia, people with Huntington's disease and people with acquired brain injury. Specialist services for younger people with dementia have only recently begun to develop, often in an *ad hoc* way with no standard model of patient care (Barber 1997). Much of the discussion about specialist services for younger people with dementia centres on the importance of 'age-appropriate' provision. Tindall and Manthorpe (1997) identify the following as important factors in the arguments for specialist provision:

- the inadequacy of existing services;
- criticism of 'fitting' younger people into services designed for older people;
- perceptions that it is 'normal' and appropriate to be with one's own age group;
- the opportunities provided for services to develop expertise in working with this group of service users.

They point out that discussion is often underpinned by feelings about equity, justice and blame (including, for example, the 'tragedy' or 'unfairness' of early onset dementia as compared with dementia in old age). These feelings can be understood in a broader theoretical context as reflecting normative images of adulthood and ageist assumptions about older people. They conclude:

> Rationally the arguments . . . focus on the potential utility of a separate service to deal with problems of employment or mid-life relationships. They exist, however, in the context of other social beliefs, emotions and structures.
>
> (Tindall and Manthorpe 1997: 247)

The *NSF for Older People* (DoH 2001b) makes it clear that standards and service models relating to dementia apply for all service users regardless of age. It also specifically requires that for this group of users, health and social services should review current arrangements and implement local protocols for care across primary care, specialist services and social services.

People with learning disabilities and dementia

Our knowledge about the needs of older people with learning disabilities is limited (Hudson 2000a). People with learning disabilities who develop dementia have until recently received very little attention from policy makers and service providers. This is beginning to change as increasing numbers of people with learning disability, particularly people with Downs Syndrome, are surviving to an age when dementia becomes relatively common (Holland 1997). Their needs are recognized both in the learning disability White Paper (DoH 2001c) and in the *NSF for Older People* (DoH 2001b). The issues for policy makers, planners and service providers is how best to respond to people who, because of their age and their needs, cross the boundaries of a range of services.

CONCLUSION

This chapter has summarized the development of health and social care policies as they affect dementia care. It has also discussed some current policy themes: planning and commissioning services; primary care; working together;

standards; long-term care; and independence and empowerment. It has high-lighted the importance of housing as a policy issue in dementia care and it has commented on the needs of some specific service user groups.

Many of the current policy concerns affecting people with dementia have been long-standing policy issues (cf. Wilkin and Hughes 1986; Means and Smith 1998a, b; Twigg 1998). These include: concerns about the relative responsibilities of the individual, the family and the state; concerns about controlling costs, particularly of institutional care; concerns about managing the boundaries between health and social care; and concerns about eligibility and equity in service provision.

It is clear from the review of policy development in this chapter that people with dementia are seldom the subject of policy statements *per se* (cf. Barnes 1997). It might be argued that people with dementia should be treated as a special and separate group for policy purposes. This would no doubt bring some benefits by raising the profile of people with dementia and focusing attention more closely on their needs. But there are also potential risks. If people with dementia are treated separately their needs, and those of their carers, might also be excluded from the many wider policy debates that concern them.

FURTHER READING

Bernard, M. and Phillips, J. (1998) *The Social Policy of Old Age: Moving into the 21st Century*. London: Centre for Policy on Ageing. For a good overview of a wide range of policy areas.

Means, R. and Smith, R. (1998) *Community Care: Policy and Practice*, 2nd edn. Basingstoke: Macmillan. For an overview of the history of community care and more recent developments.

Sharkey, P. (2000) *The Essentials of Community Care: A guide for Practitioners*. Basingstoke: Macmillan. For a basic introduction to policy and practice issues.

Spicker, P. (1995) *Social Policy: Themes and Approaches*. London: Prentice Hall, Harvester Wheatsheaf. For a broad introduction to concepts of social policy and the organization and delivery of social welfare.

15

CAROLINE CANTLEY

Understanding people in organizations

KEY POINTS

- Dementia care is shaped by a wide range of professional and organizational influences.
- The organizations providing dementia care are socially and politically complex.
- Between the professions in dementia care there are important differences in status, knowledge, values and accountabilities.
- Successful multiprofessional and multi-agency working must be based on an understanding of the occupational and organizational factors involved.

INTRODUCTION

Dementia care is managed and provided by people in a wide range of occupational groups working in a wide range of organizations. Dementia care is also organized in different service settings: residential; day care; home-based; acute hospital and so on. To understand dementia care provision, and to understand how to improve it, we need to understand how staff and organizational factors influence service delivery.

This chapter begins by describing briefly the main characteristics of the different organizations involved in providing dementia care before discussing some key concepts for understanding organizations. It then discusses the nature of professionalism and how the main professions involved in dementia care shape practice. It ends by examining how people and organizations work together to ensure coordinated care for people with dementia and their carers.

ORGANIZATIONS PROVIDING DEMENTIA CARE

We begin by outlining some key features and differences in the main organizations that provide dementia care.

General practice

General practice often serves, more or less effectively, as the gateway to dementia care. General practitioners are in an unusual position in the NHS: they are generally independent contractors, often working in partnerships, rather than employees of the health service. This arrangement encourages a small business **culture** in which general practices tend to operate in line with criteria drawn from the interests of the practice rather than the interests of the general population or the NHS as a whole. There are some signs of change to this pattern with the introduction of the option of salaried status for GPs under new contractual arrangements and with the advent of primary care groups (PCGs) and primary care trusts (PCTs) (see Chapter 14).

In understanding the general practice response to the needs of people with dementia the following factors are important:

- General practices deal with a huge range of health problems of which dementia care is a relatively small part. A GP is likely to have an overall patient list of between 1500 and 2000 patients of which between 12 and 20 people will have dementia (Alzheimer's Disease Society 1995a).
- GPs' interest, experience and skills in the care of people with dementia vary considerably (Downs 1996; Iliffe 1997).
- There is considerable variation in referral patterns between general practices and secondary care services for people with dementia (cf. Audit Commission 2000).
- General practice is undergoing substantial change and dementia care development is only one relatively small component of an extensive agenda of organizational development.

Specialist health services

Specialist health services are provided by NHS Trusts. The principle is that Trusts provide services to meet local population needs. The commissioning of these services is the responsibility, in a variety of ways, of health authorities, PCGs and PCTs (see Chapter 14). Both Trusts and commissioning bodies work within policy determined by central government. One of the most important forms of specialist health care for older people with dementia has been the development of old age psychiatry services.

The Report of the Royal College of Psychiatrists and Royal College of Physicians (RCP/RCP 1998) notes that while specialist old age psychiatry services have been developing over the past 25 years, there are still areas of the country where there are no specialist services for older people with mental health problems. For the most part specialist health services deal with all serious mental health problems in old age and do not focus solely on dementia care. As the Royal Colleges Report explains, 'A few services have limited their responsibilities to people with dementia. This has not been popular and in many instances has not proved viable, although some services include specialist dementia teams' (p. 22).

There are advantages and disadvantages in creating specialties within health care for older people, and for people with dementia more specifically (Wilkin and Hughes 1986; Jolley 1997). The advantages include:

- facilitating more appropriate care;
- providing a clear focus for developing skills;
- providing a clear focus for use of resources;
- offering a solution, if only a partial one, to 'blocked beds' in acute hospitals;
- holding out the potential of moving people to lower cost beds;
- providing 'progressive patient care' by moving people through assessment, treatment and continuing care as their needs change;
- fostering multidisciplinary working.

The disadvantages include:

- difficulties in maintaining staff morale in specialist dementia teams;
- the problems that can arise from being isolated from mainstream services;
- problems of having too narrow a skills base among staff;
- the risk that holistic conceptions of care are lost as problems are seen in component parts as relevant to different specialists;
- the risk that specialization is less to do with clients' interests and more to do with professional interests in establishing a specialized knowledge base which brings status and power.

There are similar debates about specialization in the organization of services for people with early onset dementia (see also Chapter 14). Ferran *et al.* (1996) suggest that with services for younger people with dementia there are important questions about whether the extent of the problem warrants specialized services, about who should be responsible for diagnosis, and about the nature of the service. Central to these debates is the question of the relative roles of neurologists and old age psychiatrists in caring for this group of service users (Allen and Baldwin 1995). Specialist services for this group are beginning to develop but Barber (1997) found considerable variation in provision across the country.

Social services

Social services are provided by local authorities. Much policy making is therefore the responsibility of the elected members to whom officers are accountable. Local authorities also implement some central government policies. Within local authorities, social services may be provided in a single department, in combination with other functions such as housing, or in 'neighbourhood services' (Hill 2000).

In the 1970s there was a strong move towards generic social work services although some informal specialization tended to emerge (Smith 1980; Lewis and Glennerster 1996). In a small number of departments this included specialist social work for older people, especially in the field of psychogeriatric social work (Ogg *et al.* 1998). Fuller and Tulle-Winton (1996) found some benefits of specialist services for older people, including: better assessment and care planning; client-related activities consistent with use of specialist knowledge and skills; and more developed relationships with other agencies. However, they found little evidence that these benefits resulted in better outcomes for service users. This may be because of difficulty in measuring outcomes, it may be because of the intractable nature of many users' problems, or it may be because of lack of resources for implementing care plans.

The Social Services Inspectorate (DoHSSI 1997) suggests that social services for people with dementia are better where there is either specialist provision or specific consideration of the needs of people with dementia within generic provision. It recommends that: 'Attention needs to be given to the circumstances in which it is most appropriate to provide for older people with dementia within generic services for older people or separately. This may vary in different services and localities' (p. 5).

The structure of social work services is important for dementia care. However, we need to remember that it is home care services, day services and residential services that provide most of the social care for people with dementia. These services are generally organizationally separate from fieldwork, have fewer qualified social work staff and have a rather different identity and culture (Balloch *et al.* 1995).

Independent sector services

Chapter 14 explains how voluntary and private sector organizations have become increasing important in dementia care. With this has come growing interest in the organization and management of the voluntary sector (for an overview see Billis and Harris 1996). The key feature of organizations in the independent sector is their diversity (Taylor *et al.* 1995). They include: private or 'for profit' organizations; voluntary organizations; and 'not for profit' organizations including housing associations and trusts or companies 'floated off' from public sector organizations. Taylor *et al.* (1995) point out that there is also a continuum from small, simple, locally controlled organizations to large complex organizations with central policy and resource functions distinct from local service units. As organizations grow and develop, their position along this continuum may change.

Voluntary sector organizations have various functions: service provision, self-help, mutual aid, campaigning, and 'intermediaries' providing coordination, information and support to groups and organizations in the sector (Deakin 1998). In dementia care we see these different functions in, for example, residential and day care service providers, the work of the Alzheimer's Society and the work of regional Dementia Services Development Centres.

ORGANIZATIONS: SOME KEY CONCEPTS

There is a vast literature on understanding organizations from a variety of theoretical perspectives. This section focuses on some key concepts which help us to understand how organizations shape the provision and development of dementia care: structures and cultures; the formal and informal; goals; boundaries and permeability; control and influence; and change and development. This section argues that the simple picture of organizations that we get from charts showing structures and roles is inadequate, and can even be misleading. Organizations are complex social constructions (see Chapter 3) in which those involved are constantly interpreting and negotiating meanings.

Structures and cultures

The imperative of 'changing the culture of dementia care' requires us to understand the nature of culture in service-providing organizations. Organizational culture 'encompasses shared beliefs, values and norms insofar as they drive shared patterns of behaviour – "the way we do things here" ' (Egan 1994: 77). Handy (1993) describes four types of organizational culture and the organizational structures that are associated with them. We outline these below showing how they relate to different types of organization in dementia care.

First, there is role culture or what is often termed bureaucracy. It is common in dementia care particularly in social services and the health service. This type of culture is founded on order and rationality. It operates through rules and procedures. Individuals work to job descriptions and power is mainly related to the individual's position in the organization. There is scope for expert power in defined circumstances but little scope for personal power. The work of different functions or specialties is coordinated by a small overarching senior management team.

Second, there is power culture. We see this, for example, in some independent sector organizations such as specialist dementia care homes where an influential and charismatic manager shapes practice. Organizations with power cultures have strong central power sources. In power cultures there are few rules and procedures. The emphasis is on the centre choosing the right people and allowing them to get on with the job. These organizations are of course heavily dependent on the quality of people at the centre. Power cultures tend to judge success by results.

Third, there is task culture. We see this in innovative projects such as some new, multidisciplinary teams for people with early onset dementia. The focus here is on the job or project and on bringing together the right people, at the right level, with the right resources to complete the job. Influence is based on expert power but this is a team culture in which individual status and style is less important than pursuing the shared objective.

Fourth, there is person culture. Among providers of dementia services, general practices come closest to this culture. The individual is central to this culture and structure is as limited as possible. Control is by mutual consent, influence is shared and power is usually expert. This culture is rare in its pure form but individuals with a preference for this type of culture can often be seen within other organizational types. Typically they are specialists who pursue their own interests with limited attention to the interests of the wider organization or to its efforts to control them.

A key cultural issue in dementia care concerns the differences in the underlying values and motivations of organizations in the public, private and voluntary sectors. There are some important differences between public and private sector cultures related to their different accountabilities, different financial imperatives and consequently different relationships with service users (Flynn 1990). However, it is important not to make simplistic assumptions that the profit motive is the only, or main, driver in private sector organizations and that altruism is the only driver in public sector organizations (Flynn 1990; Taylor *et al.* 1995). Cultures and values are more complicated than that in all service sectors and as Taylor *et al.* (1995: 22) observe, 'there is likely to be "good" and "bad" in all types of organisations'.

The formal and informal

The culture of an organization may or may not be stated explicitly. Often statements about culture are made in an idealistic form and they may bear variable relationship to the reality of organizational behaviour. Organization cultures also vary in strength (Egan 1994). A strong culture is one in which the beliefs, values, and norms of the organization have a strong and consistent influence on behaviour. The culture may be overt or covert and impact either for good or ill. For example, the cultures of the old psychiatric institutions that provided care for people with dementia were strong but emphasized a warehousing model of care that failed to respond to the individuality of people with dementia. Other organizations, like some care homes, may have clear statements about individuality of care but staff within them know well that in practice the norms of working are task-centred rather than person-centred. A weak culture has limited impact on practice.

When beliefs, values and norms are unstated, or where there is a gap between cultural aspirations and reality, we need to examine what Egan (1994) calls 'the shadow side of the espoused culture'. This draws our attention to the distinction between the formal and informal aspects of organizations. The importance of understanding these differences is well illustrated in a study by Alaszewski *et al.* (1998) of the way health and welfare organizations manage risk, an aspect of practice that is central to much dementia care.

Alaszewski *et al.* (1998) found that professionals in many of the organizations in their study described their organizations as hierarchical and bureaucratic and as having a defensive approach to risk management. Thus the organization placed a higher priority on protecting its interests as compared to empowering the service user to take appropriate, calculated risks. Even in the organizations that claimed to have a more flexible management style and client-centred risk management policies, the staff tended to report that the organizations were bureaucratic and defensive. However, the study showed that professionals could act to counter the bureaucratic approaches and formal policies of their organizations. Alaszewski *et al.* (1998) found that no matter what management style was adopted by the organization, the professionals described their practice as altruistic, client-focused and not concerned with the protection of their own or their agency's position. In effect the service providers exercised their discretion about when and how to use agency policy in the interests of their clients.

As Alaszewski *et al.* (1998) point out, these findings are particularly interesting insofar as they contrast with the findings of some earlier classic studies of the relationship between formal and informal working in services. Thus, for example, Goffman's (1961) study of psychiatric care (see below) stressed how the informal culture served to meet the interests of staff at the expense of the agency's formally espoused therapeutic goals. Alaszewski *et al.* (1998) suggest that the difference in findings in their study is related to the extent to which the organizations were professionalized (see below). In earlier studies such as Goffman's (1961), the staff were largely unqualified whereas in the study by Alaszewski *et al.* (1998) the staff were largely professionals pursuing their own 'therapeutic' objectives.

Goals

A simple rational model of organizations suggests that they have clear goals that drive their activities. But this does not reflect the reality of organizational life. Smith and Cantley (1985) explain:

> . . . ambiguity and confusion of purpose are *typical* and not at all unusual features of most agencies. A good deal of research in hospitals and other organizations . . . has shown that objectives vary between and within significant groups. Goals of service are complex, multiple, conflicting and vary over time and between contexts. They are variously interpreted, notoriously ambiguous, and are sometimes difficult to locate at all.
>
> (Smith and Cantley 1985: 5)

Smith and Cantley's detailed study of a day hospital for older people with mental health problems shows how various interest groups (consultant, GPs, nurses, social workers and so on) pursued a range of goals including: maintaining a flow of patients through the service system; achieving clinical 'cure' or improvement; improving teamworking and service integration in the day hospital; assisting related services such as GPs; supporting relatives; and improving quality of care. Smith and Cantley's study also shows how different groups in the day hospital interpreted each goal in different ways and used different tactics to pursue the goals in line with their particular interests. So, for example, in 'patient turnover', the consultant had a particular interest in using the day hospital to prevent bed blocking. GPs on the other hand were most interested in using day hospital places for those patients who made demands on their time and energy. For the social worker the need to maintain patient throughput was markedly tempered by concern for the needs of the family; in that respect the social work perspective was rather different from that of other staff groups. And, as is so often the case, the concerns of carers were often at odds with those of service providers.

This study demonstrates the importance of understanding the interpretations and meanings that different groups place upon the operation of the organization of which they are a part. By drawing on the theories of political **pluralism** the study shows how different groups, with different power bases, interact in a system of checks and balances to shape the services that are delivered by the organization.

Boundaries and permeability

Goffman's (1961) classic study of institutions is much cited in drawing attention to negative aspects of institutional care. Goffman used the term 'total institution' to describe institutions in which:

- inmates live their whole life (working, sleeping, eating and playing) in one setting and have restricted contact with the outside world;
- there is 'batch living' in which people are managed in groups and there is a strong daily routine imposed on inmates;
- there are clear boundaries between inmates and staff who inhabit separate social worlds which coexist but with limited interaction;
- inmates experience a loss of identity and social roles;
- there is a distinctive environment with its own rituals, rules, privileges and so on.

The 'total institution' is essentially a theoretical model of one end of a continuum ranging from totally closed institutions to totally open or permeable organizations. The value of Goffman's work is not as a direct criticism of institutional care (for more general critique of institutional care see Jones and Fowles 1984; Peace *et al.* 1997; Jack 1998; Stanley and Reed 1999). Rather Goffman (1961) helps us to identify negative aspects of care settings such as hospitals, care homes and day centres and to identify measures for countering their adverse effects (cf. Fennell *et al.* 1988). This is particularly important in dementia care because, as compared with other older people, people with dementia '. . . are much more at the mercy of their physical, social and inter-personal surroundings' (Woods 1996: 372).

Although institutions in dementia care are not the 'total institutions' as described by Goffman, some features of **institutionalization**, that is the depersonalization of residents by limiting their privacy, dignity and ability to exercise choice, are evident in many settings. Innes (1998), for example, has demonstrated how care staff categorize or 'label' people with dementia. Also Peace *et al.* (1997) more generally draw attention to the impact of the organ-izational environment in residential homes:

> In delivering a service to large groups of people, the influence of the organ-isation is relatively stronger than that of individuals and can overwhelm the capacity of residents and staff to individualize and protect key features of a personal life-style. Such imbalance needs to be constantly checked.
>
> (Peace *et al.* 1997: 46)

Thus Goffman's ideas underpin much current thinking about good practice in institutional care for people with dementia, for example that:

- we need to avoid batch living and lack of privacy if we want to maintain personal identity;
- we should reduce the negative effects of group living by breaking down institutional routines and by caring for people in smaller groups;
- homes should be as open as possible to the wider community, encouraging people to visit and residents to go out.

Some dementia care services are much more open and permeable than others. In day centres and day hospitals, for example, staff and service users move between the different social worlds of home and care setting. Sheltered hous-ing too is more permeable as are organizations providing care in the client's own home. This permeability is important in ensuring that wider social influ-ences, rather than narrow sectional interests, shape dementia care.

Control and influence

The ways in which an organization exercises control over its staff, and the ways in which staff influence organizational functioning, vary with organiza-tional structure and culture. A distinction is often drawn between 'top-down' and 'bottom-up' management styles. Top-down management is typical of bureaucratic organizations. It is based on senior management drawing up policies and procedures to be implemented by staff in the organization. 'Top-down management' has been the dominant management approach in much of social services and in health service administration. However, the advent of greater **managerialism** in health and social care has brought more decentral-ized control involving local managers working more autonomously within strategic, financial and quality frameworks (see for example Flynn 1990).

'Bottom-up' approaches are typically less hierarchical, more participative and involve a wide range of people in decision making. Although 'bottom-up' management exists to varying levels within the statutory health and social care sectors, as an organizational approach it is more often, but not always, found in voluntary sector organizations. Taylor *et al.* (1995) suggest that this style is typical of devolved, federal organizations in which local branches typically have considerable autonomy while operating under the name of the parent organization which lends credibility and also a range of practical support.

The picture of control and influence in dementia care organizations is further complicated when we take into account the fact that many services operate as 'front-line' organizations, with staff working individually in settings where direct supervision by management is difficult. The concept of '**street level bureaucracy**' (Lipsky 1980) helps us to understand the functioning of front-line staff who deal directly with service users in health and welfare bureaucracies. Workers in these settings typically have to manage demand for services that exceed the resources available, have to cope with uncertainties in what they should be doing as well as unpredictability in the outcomes, and see themselves as relatively powerless implementers of organizationally defined policies or rules. However, paradoxically, workers in these organizations often have considerable discretion in their decisions about what services to provide and how to provide them.

Lipsky (1980) uses the term 'street level bureaucracy' to describe how workers in these circumstances adopt routine approaches to processing clients in ways that make life manageable for the workers themselves. This is often at odds with both organizational policies and the commitment and service ethos that brought people into this type of work in the first place. The key conclusion from this analysis of street level bureaucracy is that 'difficult work environments lead to the abandonment of ideals and to the adoption of techniques which enable clients to be "managed"' (Hill 1997: 204).

This account of street level bureaucracy, and research such as the study by Hunter *et al.* (1988) of policy making and service delivery in care of older people, demonstrates that policy is not simply transmitted from the top of the organization down to the front line. Instead, policy is mediated through the work of front-line service providers as they make numerous discretionary decisions in coping with the complexity and individuality of cases.

The complexity of the social processes involved in organizational control and influence are well illustrated in a classic study of a psychiatric hospital by Strauss *et al.* (1973) who demonstrate that order is not maintained rationally by a clearly defined and enforced set of rules. Rather, rules are often unclear and they are interpreted and used differently by different people in line with their particular interests. Order is maintained not simply by the imposition of rules or exercise of power in occupational hierarchies, but by a process of ongoing negotiation between and within different groups of professionals, other staff and service users.

Understanding these features of control and influence is important for thinking about how we initiate change in dementia care.

Change and development

Staff training and development is widely advocated as being one of the keys to improving dementia care (Chapman 1997; Sheard and Cox 1998). However, recent research (Lintern *et al.* 2000) has shown that training in individualized, person-centred care does not in itself ensure that a care philosophy will be translated into care practice. Lintern *et al.* (2000) argue that effective change requires attention to the organizational and management context of training and care provision. Others too have recognized the importance of organizational factors in changing dementia care (Bowe and Loveday 1995; Gilloran *et al.* 1995; Kitwood 1997b). Bowe and Loveday (1995) explain:

> If the new practices relating to care given to individuals are not reflected in the policies and procedures of an organisation, the occurrence of such changes at individual level is left to chance, and ultimately may not be consistent or sustained.
>
> (Bowe and Loveday 1995: 75)

So if dementia care is to change substantially it is necessary to go beyond training and take into account organizational structures, cultures and policy implementation processes. We have seen above, for example, that policies and procedures are not implemented in a simple and straightforward way. The different organizational cultures described above also alert us to the ways in which organizations will vary in their management of change.

Drawing upon the ideas of Handy (1993) we see that role cultures or bureaucracies function best in a stable environment but tend to be less successful at adapting quickly to a changing environment. Many people working in dementia care will be well aware of how long it can take to introduce service changes through the managerial structures of health and social services. Power cultures, in contrast, can adapt quickly to environmental change. But size can be a problem for power cultures in that it is difficult for the centre to maintain its influence if the organization grows too large. So, for example, a voluntary sector dementia care provider may struggle to maintain an innovative, person-centred and high-quality service as increasing size makes it difficult for the original small, central management team to maintain personal control and influence on everyday activities. Task cultures are particularly suited to change and we can see their widespread use in launching new services and new ways of working. However, there are difficulties for organizations in maintaining control in task cultures and often the task group is disbanded when the project is completed or it is incorporated into mainstream management structures. While person cultures can easily accommodate change at the level of the individual, their capacity for broader organizational change is limited by their lack of experience of corporate thinking and management. Thus general medical practices, in moving to PCGs and PCTs, are not only managing changed responsibilities and organizational structures, they are also undergoing a substantial cultural shift.

Egan (1994) warns that cultures can be too strong for the good of an organization and can inhibit change. Cultures need to be flexible to respond to a changing world. Egan suggests that this involves:

- constantly scanning the environment for changes that will require an organizational response;
- being proactive rather than reactive;
- letting go of the past;
- continually adapting and developing.

Egan's advice is apt in thinking about dementia care where development is taking place in a complex and changing technological, policy and organizational environment. The theme of developing dementia services is expanded in Chapters 16, 17 and 18 from the different perspectives of organizational development, quality development, and involving service users in development.

PEOPLE IN ORGANIZATIONS

Health and social care professions play a major role in providing and developing dementia care. This section examines the nature of that professional input and also comments on the roles of managers and care staff in dementia services.

The professions

The terms 'profession' and 'professional' are commonly used in discussions about dementia care. But there is often little clarity about what is meant by these terms other than that 'to be professional' in actions or judgement is generally seen to be a good thing. There is an extensive literature on the nature of 'the professions' and on the processes of **'professionalization'** (for discussion in the context of health and welfare see for example Wilding 1982; Cousins 1987; Abbott and Meerabeau 1998b). Early ideas about professions focused on the 'traits' or characteristics that identified an occupation as a profession. The traits included such features as a body of knowledge, service ethic, control over recruitment and education and autonomous practice. This approach to understanding what constitutes a profession was not very fruitful. A more productive approach is to consider professions as groups that have secured a dominant position in the division of labour (Wilding 1982) and to examine which groups make claims to be professions, how they do this and the extent to which they succeed (Abbott and Meerabeau 1998a).

Abbott and Meerabeau (1998a: 9) argue that: 'Key elements in any claim to professional status seem to be autonomy or control over work, a clearly defined monopoly over an area of work and a knowledge base.' They cite nursing and social work as occupations that have both claimed, but failed, to achieve full professional status on these counts. Indeed, the term 'semi-profession' is often used to refer to these occupational groups. Although nursing and social work have sought professional status, within these occupations there are different views, held by different groups, about the desirability of professionalization (Abbott and Wallace 1998; Hugman 1998; Rashid 2000).

One of the key features of professionalization is establishing that other groups have a subordinate position in the division of labour (Saks 2000). Saks cites as an example nursing's delegation of 'dirty work' to lower status auxiliaries (now nursing assistants). Abbott and Meerabeau (1998a) also note how both social work and nursing have tried to draw a clear distinction between their activities and those of unqualified care staff and informal carers. Volunteers would be similarly distinguished from professionals. Professionals also assume a position of power in relation to service users; this power is in part based upon having expertise that is not available to clients and in part on clients being dependent on professionals for access to services.

Ashburner and Birch (1999) identify several key boundary issues for professions in health care. We can extrapolate from this to social care. First, there is the definition and control of boundaries within individual professions. Second, there are struggles between professions over contested areas of work. Third, there are the boundaries between professions and outside groups such as managers. Fourth, there are the effects of the external environment on boundaries; for example policy changes, public expectations and technological developments. We can see below how these boundary issues are played out in dementia care.

Health and welfare professions have been the subjects of varied and increasing criticism focusing particularly on the tendency of professions to protect their own interests at the expense of the interests of their clients (cf. Wilding 1982). Some have challenged the nature of professional practice itself (for example Schön 1983). Thus there are debates about whether professional practice involves rational application of a knowledge base or whether it is more about artistry in dealing with complexities and uncertainties using 'a mixture of professional judgement, intuition and common sense' (Fish and Coles 2000: 292). The stance we take on this has substantial implications for the way we approach practice development (see Chapter 6 for further discussion). Other challenges to professional practice have come from increasing managerialism and increasing consumerism in health and welfare (Kelly 1998; Butcher 2000). Chapter 18 discusses further the extent to which people with dementia and their carers are able to challenge professionals in influencing service development. Abbott and Meerabeau (1998a) summarize the criticisms:

> What is common to all these challenges is their dissent from the view that professionals can define problems and solutions to them, that professional practice is disinterested and client-centred, and that caring professionals have a scientific knowledge base that enables them to be objective and value-free.
>
> (Abbott and Meerabeau 1998a: 13)

While the professions have come in for much criticism there are arguments in their support. Kelly (1998), for example, cautions against too simplistic an analysis of the conflicts between managers and professionals. She argues that the professions potentially play a significant part in promoting the cause of the service user and countering excessive commitments to managerial objectives.

The next section examines how some of these general issues affect the professions involved in dementia care.

Professions in dementia care

The professional groups involved in dementia care include doctors, nurses, social workers, psychologists, occupational therapists and other 'professions allied to medicine'. Malin *et al.* (1999) draw our attention to the differences that exists between professional groups in community care not only in their knowledge bases but also in their values, ethics, employment positions and accountability structures. We look now in more detail at three key professional groups in dementia care.

Medicine

Biomedical knowledge underpins doctors' work in dementia care but groups such as general practitioners and old age psychiatrists tend to have a rather broader approach than other medical specialties. For example, Malin *et al.* (1999) describe GPs as having a 'biographic and holistic approach'. Also, central to the development of old age psychiatry as a specialism has been the ability of a subgroup within medicine to claim a specialist knowledge base by developing an approach with an emphasis on functional assessment and rehabilitation (cf. Wilkin and Hughes 1986). This emphasis on rehabilitation, however, has tended to mean that continuing care for people with dementia has been viewed within the profession as a relatively uninteresting area.

Within medicine it is widely recognized that general practitioners are less powerful than their consultant colleagues in secondary health care (Malin *et al.* 1999). Also secondary care specialties have a hierarchy in which old age psychiatry ranks well down the ladder of status and influence. However, the advent of new diagnostic techniques and anti-dementia drugs is producing new areas of professional expertise. There are, therefore, new questions about internal boundaries within medicine, for example about the relative roles of general practitioners and consultant psychiatrists in controlling access to the new drugs.

Nursing

Any understanding of nursing as a profession must be founded on an understanding of nursing's relationship with medicine. Nursing is widely recognized as being subordinate to medicine (Abbott and Wallace 1998) and, within nursing, as in medicine, there are status hierarchies. Nursing people with dementia has low status because it is perceived as an area involving much routine 'care' and little technological expertise. Abbott and Wallace (1998) trace the development of adult nursing, pointing out that because 'cure' became the preserve of the medical profession, nurses were left with 'care' for which there is no established expert knowledge base. Nurses have therefore struggled to achieve status as autonomous professional practitioners and one response to this has been to emphasize the role of qualified nurses as managers of trainees and unqualified staff.

Community psychiatric nurses (CPNs) have developed as a specialty within nursing although Bowers (1997) notes that there is little organizational or professional clarity about what constitutes 'a CPN'. Adams (1999) describes how community psychiatric nursing with older people developed in the context of emerging specialist teams in old age psychiatry. He points out that the number of CPNs specializing in the problems of older people is low compared with the numbers in other fields of psychiatry. He argues that this low number is linked to social services having a lead role in providing services for older people. However, we might also consider two other possible factors; first, the effect of the low status of work with older people, and second, other priorities in community psychiatric nursing whether for more 'therapeutic' work with people with mood disorders and less serious forms of mental illness (cf. Bowers 1997) or, more recently, for work with people with severe and enduring mental illness.

Adam's (1999) research on the work of CPNs in dementia care suggests that their focus has tended to be on work with the main family carer rather than people with dementia themselves or with the family more generally. He identifies two factors as being important in promoting the role of community psychiatric nurses in dementia care: first, the development of the Admiral Nurse service, a service developed by a voluntary organization to undertake work with carers of people with dementia, and second, the findings of a study that demonstrates the benefits of advanced nurse practitioners in dementia care.

Keady and Adams (2001) set out a case for the broader development of the community mental health nurse role, and the role of the nursing profession as a whole, in dementia care.

Social work

Traditionally, work with older people has been viewed as low priority within social work and suitable for allocation to unqualified staff rather than qualified social workers (Bowl 1986). It is only comparatively recently, as social work has moved from psychologically oriented individual casework to broader approaches taking account of socio-political factors (Phillipson 1982; Phillipson and Thompson 1996), that work with older people has been seen as more rewarding. Current professional social work in dementia care can also best be understood in the context of care management bringing a much stronger managerial dimension to social work practice as care managers have to work within budgetary limits, and sometimes even as direct budget holders (see Chapter 7 for further discussion). The impact of the introduction of care management on social work has been profound as Ogg *et al.* (1998) explain:

In this climate, the values which have underpinned the social work profession in the past (values which saw social workers as agents of empowerment, enabling individuals to take control of their lives and to help them achieve their goals), are quickly receding into the background as the bureaucratic demands of the new structures take hold.

(Ogg *et al.* 1998: 117)

The introduction of care management has also raised significant boundary issues for social work. Although care managers for the most part have a professional social work background, some joint working arrangements between health and social services have opened up this role to other professions.

Care staff

From the perspective of service users, the advantages of receiving care from a professional rather than an unqualified service provider are not always self-evident. For example, Abbott (1998) found that clients expressed greater satisfaction in receiving personal care from home helps than from district nurses. She explained that 'this was in part because home helps were seen as friendly and approachable, whereas the district nurses were seen to keep a professional distance' (p. 203).

In general in dementia care the service providers who spend most time with people with dementia are not the professionals but the unqualified care staff. Herbert (1997) argues that it is staff attitudes rather than particular qualifications that are important in providing good dementia care. Gilloran *et al.* (1995) report, on the basis of their research in long-term hospital care for people with dementia, that feelings of work satisfaction among care staff are closely related to the quality of the care provided. This echoes the observations by Fennell *et al.* (1988) that

Depersonalizing the people cared for, disaggregating them into a series of tasks is a way whereby staff can protect themselves from confronting the pain of people-processing organisations where both carers and the cared-for alike are devalued by and unsupported in their social context.

(Fennell *et al.* 1988: 144)

Thus if better dementia care is to be promoted, more attention must be given to ensuring that care staff are valued through proper pay, support and recognition of their expertise.

Managers

Managers in dementia care work at different organizational levels and in different service contexts. Some managers have a career background entirely in management, some have moved into management from a professional background and some have 'come up through the ranks' of care practice. We do not know a great deal about managers in dementia care although there is some relevant research on managers in long-term care for older people (Johnson *et al.* 1999). We do know that the style and approach of first-line managers is a significant factor in determining the quality of dementia care practice (Gilloran *et al.* 1995).

Perhaps the most important observation to make here relates to the increasing managerialism in health and social care and the tendency to assume that private sector management approaches can solve the problems of community care. Harding (1998) points out that these assumptions are based on the misconception that management is a 'science' that can provide the means for the rational control of organizations. But as we have seen, health and social care organizations are too socially and politically complex to be amenable to simple, rational control.

Specialization in dementia care

A number of commentators have noted the overlap and blurred boundaries that exist between different professions in community care and some have raised questions about whether realignment may occur (Kelly 1998; Malin *et al.* 1999). We have seen in this chapter how different professional groups have developed specialisms in the care of older people with mental health problems. But we also now see some further specialization in the narrower field of dementia care. So, for example, developments such as 'advanced practitioner' posts within nursing enhance the claims of this particular profession to expertise in dementia care. There are also trends that cross professional boundaries; for example, the development of multidisciplinary advanced education programmes. The impact of these developments should be welcomed by those concerned with this client group. However, an understanding of the nature of professionalism alerts us to the risks that such specialization may not be entirely driven by the interests of service users with dementia. Professional interests in claiming expert knowledge and, through this, enhanced professional standing may also drive specialization.

WORKING ACROSS PROFESSIONS AND ORGANIZATIONS

Working across professions and organizations in dementia care is necessary for interagency planning and service development (see Chapter 14). It is also important in delivering services. This next section examines professional and organizational aspects of services working together to deliver holistic and coordinated dementia services. Such service delivery involves overcoming a range of difficulties rooted in the different ideologies and vested interests of professional groups and organizational 'tribes' (Dalley 1989).

Successful collaboration between health and social services requires managers and front-line staff to address a range of organizational, professional and interpersonal issues. Different groups of staff and managers have different perceptions of the issues involved in collaboration. This is illustrated well in Rummery and Glendinning's (2000) analysis of the different perspectives of managers, GPs, nurses, social workers and patients in collaboration between primary care and social services in caring for older people.

Teamwork

Teamwork is often invoked as a means of providing coordinated care. However, different people in different circumstances make different assumptions about what 'teamwork' entails; and there are indeed many different models of teamworking (Øvretveit 1993; Payne 2000). Payne (2000) advocates **'open teamwork'**. He uses this term to combine traditional ideas about teamworking with ideas about networking. In traditional models of teamworking the 'team' is a relatively closed group that fosters internal cooperation and works towards shared objectives. Networking on the other hand entails looser linkages in the broader organizational and community context of service provision. 'Open teamwork' aims to combine these approaches.

Teamwork in dementia care is often associated with community teams, but teamwork also takes place in acute hospitals, continuing care and day care settings. Each of these settings has distinctive features that affect the ways in which people work together. For example, in residential and day care settings much of the staff's work is carried out in the presence of others and generally involves an intensity and continuity of relationships that is not typical in community teams. Herbert (1997) discusses how professionals and front-line care staff should work together in dementia care. She argues that: 'It is the collective impact of the team which manages, advises and supervises the workforce in day-to-day contact with the person with dementia which determines the experience of the person cared for' (p. 115). Payne (2000) makes the case for extending the open teamwork approach to care homes and day care:

> Residential and day care settings might offer the classic group-based teamwork analysis, but this neglects the role of residential and day care in linking residents with outside relationships, agencies and the community and ensuring the participation of residents in their own living arrangements. We need to develop thinking about residential care practice beyond the staff team to understand the many links it has in wider networks.
>
> (Payne 2000: 194)

Collaboration in community services

There are many accounts of community teams providing dementia care (see for example Challis *et al.* 1997; Sheard 1997; Sturges 1997; Sheard and Cox

1998; Reed *et al.* 2000). The Audit Commission (2000) examined community mental health teams for older people in 12 locations. They found that the range of professions in the teams varied as did the nature and extent of joint working. The Audit Commission identified the following factors as being important in ensuring an effective joint service response:

- a mix of professions working from the same office;
- shared information and ideally shared case files;
- appropriate distinction between tasks that can be done by all team members and specialist tasks;
- ready access to practical and therapeutic resources with all specialists being able to access the resources of each agency without too much bureaucracy;
- consultants as team members although not automatically as the first point of contact for referrals;
- joint training across professions and agencies.

One of the crucial areas of collaboration in dementia care is that between general practice and social services. Rummery and Glendinning (2000) review a range of schemes, including some involving colocation of social workers in general practices, for improving joint working between primary care and social services in caring for older people. They identify the following as being the key factors for successful collaboration:

- commitment of key managers and budget holders in both organizations;
- gains for both parties and a sharing of any costs;
- realistic and achievable goals;
- clarity about the roles and responsibilities of the participants from the outset;
- involvement of community nurses;
- acknowledgement that interorganizational and interprofessional barriers exist and must be tackled;
- involvement of service users to ensure arrangements reflect their needs and priorities.

Involving service users and carers

Different professional groups use different terms – patient, client, customer, service user – to refer to the people with whom they work. Øvretveit (1997) argues these differences in terminology are significant and need to be debated in multidisciplinary teams in order to clarify the team's approach to person–practitioner relationships and more specifically to clarify how power, rights and responsibilities are balanced between the person and the professional.

In dementia care, different professions, drawing upon different models of the nature of dementia, take different approaches to involving service users. So in many multidisciplinary teams there will be substantial differences between professionals in how they view the triad of relationships between professional, service user and carer. One of the areas of dementia care in which these relationships are particularly important is in handling the provision of information about diagnosis, prognosis and treatment. Another area is in involving people in decision making; this is complicated in dementia care by the fact that the abilities of the service user will decline over time. Øvretveit (1997) argues that good communication is the key to addressing issues such as these. But communication will only be successful if it is based on an understanding of the complexity of the professional and organizational worlds that we have been discussing throughout this chapter.

CONCLUSION

This chapter describes some of the main features of organizations that provide dementia care. It outlines some important concepts that help to explain how organizations work. It looks at different staff groups and comments particularly on how professional interests play a part in shaping services. It discusses some of the organizational and professional factors involved in 'working together' to achieve comprehensive and coordinated dementia services. It concludes that if we are to succeed in developing better dementia care we must understand and work effectively to change the organizations in which care provision takes place.

FURTHER READING

Abbott, P. and Meerabeau, L. (1998) *The Sociology of the Caring Professions*, 2nd edn. London: UCL Press. For an introduction to ideas about professions and professionalization.

Handy, C. (1993) *Understanding Organisations*, 4th edn. London: Penguin. For a good, easily understood overview of organizational theory.

Payne, M. (2000) *Teamwork in Multiprofessional Care*. Basingstoke: Macmillan. For a theoretical overview and practical guidance on teamworking.

Developing service organizations

KEY POINTS

- Successful care providers have to be efficient, effective, and provide an appropriate quality of service. To achieve this the organization must have the capacity to respond quickly to changes in the external environment.
- From an organizational perspective the 'appropriate quality' is the one that best meets the customer's needs, represents 'value for money' and can be provided within the available budget of the provider.
- An effective organization will have developed ways of keeping close to its customers.
- The staff of a service organization are the most important and the most expensive asset.
- Implementing change is always difficult and must be planned for.
- Organizational development should never stop – complacency leads to poor services and ultimately to organizational suicide.

INTRODUCTION

For a considerable number of years people have argued about how transferable the skills of management are between different settings. On one hand there is the 'specialist' argument that says that a good manager needs to have an in-depth knowledge of the product or service; on the other hand are those who support generic management and believe that a good manager can 'manage anything'. This argument was particularly prevalent in health settings during the late eighties and early nineties when the introduction of the internal market in health care (see Chapter 14) and an increased emphasis on cost-effectiveness led to a more managerial culture. Many clinicians were dismayed at this development, believing that it was dangerous to give non-medical staff control over budgets because 'they wouldn't understand the issues'. Whatever one's views on this debate it is difficult to argue that health and social care organizations are so very different to any other organization that general management theories do not apply. However, compared to many other kinds of businesses the provision of care for people with dementia is a very complex operation. It may involve intermittent contact with service users, as in domiciliary or day care provision, or it may involve a 7-day-a-week, 24-hours-a-day service in a care home. It always involves providing for a diverse group of '**customers**' whose very different needs and expectations keep changing.

There is very little written about the theory of management of care services, let alone about dementia care services. However, all organizations that provide care can be defined as 'service organizations'. As such they share some key characteristics with other service industries such as hotels, shops and garages. There is a wealth of literature about these kinds of 'industries' which can inform our thinking about service development in health and social care. In using this literature we must take account of the variation in the nature of health and welfare organizations providing dementia care (see Chapter 15) and how this might affect the applicability of management concepts from other service sectors.

With the considerations above in mind, this chapter will examine some key management theories that can be related to dementia care organizations in order to try to establish the factors that appear to be critical to success. We shall also look at ways of assessing the current performance of an organization and at ways of planning for and implementing change. For the most part we illustrate these ideas with examples from the care home sector – but the ideas could equally be adapted in other types of dementia care services.

WHAT IS 'SERVICE DEVELOPMENT'?

From an organizational or management perspective, service development is best described as a process intended to increase the organization's effectiveness, efficiency and general 'fitness for purpose'. Development can take place as organizations grow in size, as they consolidate and even as they shrink (Hanson and Lubin 1995). It may include a change to the quality of the service provided, but it would be wrong to assume that service development always leads to a raising of the standard of service. There are circumstances in which an organization may reduce the standard of its service since from an organizational perspective 'fitness for purpose' means having a product of appropriate quality for the market, or in other words one that is affordable within available resources. While this may most obviously apply to the private care sector, voluntary and statutory service organizations also have to operate within a variety of resource constraints. What is vitally important for any service organization is that it is '. . . meeting or exceeding the customer's expectations at a price that represents value to them' (Harrington 1987).

THE NATURE OF SERVICE ORGANIZATIONS

The customers

It will become apparent throughout this chapter that all service providers should be aware of, and take seriously, the views of their customers. It is worth pausing for a moment to consider the range of potential 'customers' of a dementia service. Some will be potential service users themselves, some will be relatives and friends negotiating on behalf of the potential service user, some will be care managers working on behalf of a purchasing organization such as a local authority or health authority. Each of these types of customer is likely to have very different expectations about quality and about **'value for money'**. The majority of care service providers have to manage a mixed customer base and address a diverse set of expectations. So, for example, it is not sufficient to provide an excellent residential service that satisfies people with dementia and their families, only to send inaccurate invoices repeatedly to their care managers. Similarly, a quality day care service will need to provide appropriate amenities and activities at the centre and also a safe and timely transport service that relatives can rely on.

Customers in general want value for money and reliability. Anyone with sufficient resources can (though not necessarily will) provide a high-quality service; the knack is to be able to produce appropriate quality, time after time, at an affordable price. In this context an inefficient and poorly managed organization may be able to produce a quality service occasionally, or at a very high price, but it takes a quality organization to produce a consistent, appropriate quality service that represents 'value for money'. Appropriate quality, rather than low cost, has been proved to be a more effective way of increasing market share (that is attracting more customers) and a better way of differentiating the 'product' (that is demonstrating to the customer how the service is different from other similar services).

Typical features of service organizations

In our introduction we mentioned that there are different types of care service provider – this includes local authorities, NHS Trusts, charities and the private sector. These different organizations do have very different cultures and values but increasingly all of them are having to become more 'business-like' and the differences between the way they operate have narrowed. Rather than look at what makes specific types of care providers 'successful' it may be more instructive to look at the factors that typify flourishing service organizations.

Service organizations can vary enormously, even those concerned with the same need; think for a moment, of the differences between the operation of an exclusive restaurant and a hamburger bar. In the former, the emphasis is on meeting each customer's individual needs, in the latter, the emphasis is on standardization. In spite of this kind of variance there are at least five main characteristics that are shared by all service industries (Schmenner 1986; Jones 1989). All of these characteristics are relevant to dementia care providers.

Labour intensity

All service industries rely heavily on staff; they are labour intensive in terms of both the number of staff and the amount of staff 'effort'. Frequently the staff remuneration budget for a service industry will exceed 50 per cent of the total budget, and in care services staff costs may account for 55–70 per cent of the annual revenue.

Good service providers will appreciate that staff care, staff training and development, and the ways in which staff are deployed, are particularly important factors in the effectiveness of their business. They will also understand that the morale of the staff is critical to business success and will agree with the proposal that you cannot have customer satisfaction without employee satisfaction (Thompson 1995). Care organizations that develop new purpose-built, high-quality premises will confirm that while the building may attract customers initially, the quality of the staff group remains the single most important factor in determining the service's reputation.

Complexity

Managing a service is usually more complex than managing a production industry; there is no mass production, no automated technology, no single product, no steady **demand**, no simple measure of productivity (Thompson 1967). Instead there are customers, all with different requirements, wanting an individualized service and a tension between individual treatment and the managers' need to standardize the service as much as possible to reduce costs. For example, in a dementia care setting staff have to be able to undertake all of a very wide range of caring tasks (from personal physical care to facilitating social activities) and no two service users or days will be the same. At the end of their shift, the staff in the care setting can neither easily count how productive they have been, nor easily measure their success.

Service providers who are successful will appreciate the complexity of their organization's operation and ensure that their staffing resource is appropriate. They will also try to find ways of providing feedback to staff about their performance and recognition (and rewards) for their efforts.

Visibility

Management theory talks of 'front of house' operations and 'back of house operations'. 'Front of house' activities are those that the customer can see or be involved in. Organizations can be located along a spectrum according to the extent that their operations are 'front of house'. Near one end of this spectrum is the residential home where customers can see the operation all around them, all day. In fact, they are participants as well as observers of many of the processes – although there remain 'back of house' areas in which residents are seldom involved. The more customers are involved in 'front of house' operations, the more potential there is for them to collect evidence which will assist them in judging the **efficiency** and **effectiveness** of the service.

A care provider striving for excellence will ensure that all of the staff, including domestic and administrative staff, appreciate that they are a visible part of the service. They will also ensure that all of the premises are of a good standard. In dementia care settings it can be all too easy for staff to work on the assumption that service users with dementia cannot judge, and will not report on, the service that they are receiving. Good service organizations will ensure that expectations in dementia care are not lowered as a result.

Perishability

Services cannot be stored; they are 'perishable' and, if not used, are wasted. For example, the dementia care home or day centre will be staffed to manage the service hour by hour through the day. If some parts of the day are unexpectedly busy there is no stock of 'care' made earlier that can be called on. This characteristic emphasizes the need for careful planning around staff deployment. It also highlights the need for staff morale to be maintained so that they will be prepared to 'go the extra mile' when necessary; for example on the day when there are extra visitors, when the Environmental Health Officer turns up unannounced or when the house pet needs to be taken urgently to the vet!

Intangibility

It is much more difficult to describe a service than a product. The benefits derived from a service are often associated with emotions and feelings (Jones 1992) rather than just the more concrete aspects of provision. So, for example, a dementia care home will usually be described in subjective terms such as 'homely and welcoming' or 'institutional and cold'. Care providers need to ensure that they are aware of the image that the service projects. Picture a relative kept waiting outside a residential home on a cold night, because no one will answer the doorbell. Anyone with experience of care provision will know that this is likely to be because all of the staff are busy attending to residents. But the cold relative is unlikely to reach this conclusion and is more likely to imagine the care staff chatting in the staff room.

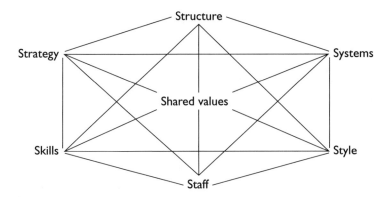

Figure 16.1 McKinsey 7 'S' Framework

IDENTIFYING DEVELOPMENT NEEDS

Determining the health of a service organization

The starting point for service development is generally a clear picture of 'where we are now'. There is a variety of tools that have been developed by management theorists that are designed to evaluate effectiveness, or organizational health. One of the better known and most respected is the 'McKinsey 7 S' **framework**, which was elaborated in *In Search of Excellence* (Peters and Waterman 1982). Peters and Waterman suggest that there are seven key inter-related variables in any organization: **strategy**, structure, systems, shared values, **style**, staff and skills. The seven elements are depicted in Figure 16.1.

They argue that in a healthy organization each of these elements is properly addressed and each of the components is in harmony with the others. A systematic evaluation of the health of a service organization can be undertaken by formulating questions that are based on each variable. A sample set of questions for a dementia care organization might include:

Strategy
- Does the organization have a strategy that seeks to meet both current and future needs of people with dementia?
- Does every member of staff know what the strategy is; are they involved in its preparation and review?
- Is the strategy reviewed regularly and adjusted as the external environment changes?

Structure
- Does the structure suit the organization's purpose and its size?
- Is the structure based on a historical view of what worked or does it look to the future?
- Is the structure organized for optimum performance, are roles and responsibilities of different staff clear and distinct?

- Is there the least possible number of management levels?
- Is the 'chain of command' as short as possible?
- Is the structure as simple as possible? How long does it take new members of staff to understand it?
- Does the structure assist in the development of new managers of the future?
- For multi-site organizations: Is there an appropriate relationship between 'head office' and individual sites?

Systems
- Is there a complete set of effective **systems**? Are these focused sufficiently on quality issues or are they solely concerned with financial processes?
- Are customers ever asked about their views on the systems used?
- Do all parts of the organization use the systems in the same way?
- Are the systems regularly **audited** and their continuing appropriateness reviewed?

Shared values
- Are the values of the organization made explicit? How?
- Do all members of staff know what these values are?
- How do senior managers check out whether staff share these values?
- Does the behaviour of managers in the organization reflect the value base?
- Is there any system in place to check out a person's 'values' during recruitment?
- Do senior managers adequately address tensions between values and efficiency and effectiveness? (For example, members of staff working for a dementia care-providing charity are likely to take issue with senior managers who tell them to become more businesslike and specifically to seek out self-funding customers who can be charged a premium rate.)

Style (or culture)
- Can staff describe the style of the organization?
- Would staff and managers share the same view?
- Is style ever discussed?
- Are customers' views on style ever elicited?
- Does the style fit with the values and the actual practice?

Staff
- Are recruitment processes fair and robust and are they adhered to?
- Is enough attention given to strategies to improve retention?
- Does every member of staff get an appropriate induction? How is the effectiveness of this monitored?
- Is there any evidence that the organization has thought about what motivates staff?
- Is there a formal process for the assessment of the performance of individual members of staff?
- Do personnel policies take account of the gender and age mix of the frontline workforce?
- Are policies 'family friendly' and do they take account of some staff's role as family carers?

Skills
- Are job descriptions based on competencies?
- Do staff know what skills they are expected to have?
- Is there any mechanism for auditing the training requirements of the service?
- Do the keenest staff get to go on courses or are the places given to staff who need the training?
- If staff attend training courses are they encouraged to feed back their learning to colleagues?
- Are training and development opportunities spread fairly across the different grades of posts in the organization?

Assessing a dementia care organization against the 7S framework should give a number of clues to the health of the organization and some idea of where change is needed most. However, for service development to be best achieved, it is important not only to promote the health of the organization but also to minimize any external hazards.

Assessing the impact of the external environment

In order to assess external risks to the operation or development of the service, an assessment of the environment in which the organization operates should also be undertaken (Perren and Webber 1998). This type of analysis is often referred to as a **PEST analysis**, referring to the four areas that it covers: political and legal; economic; social and cultural; and technological (Johnson and Scholes 1993). Table 16.1 illustrates the type of questions that might be posed for a residential care provider in relation to changes in each of these four environmental areas.

By undertaking an analysis of this kind, service providers may be alerted to environmental changes that would affect their plans for organizational development. For example, the providers of a residential home could have a comprehensive plan to make their business more effective. They could be planning to change the culture within the home, improve staff training and retention and update some critical administrative procedures. All of this effort would be severely undermined if they had not paid attention to the possible impact on their organization of, for example, changes to registration standards or to local authority community care payments.

Clarifying the kind of provider the organization wants to be

Before finalizing any plans for organizational change it is essential to get agreement from key **stakeholders** in the organization about the preferred end point. Senior managers, directors and, in the private sector, owners will have views about the direction they want the organization to take. In reaching this view they should have considered the following questions.

Table 16.1   PEST analysis: Elmwood Residential Care Home

	Aspect of the environment	Factors to be reviewed	Examples
P	Political and legal	Any political or legislative changes that could impact on the business	Changes to registration standards and structure of registration units Working time directive Extension of direct payments system
E	Economic	Any change that could impact on the financial viability of the business	Interest rates Unemployment rates Local wage rates Changes in the way LA allocates community care money Future number of full fee payers Change in number and quality of competitors
S	Social and cultural	Any change in local/ national social trends that could impact.	Growth in 85+ population Decrease in number of school leavers Availability of training opportunities Availability of public transport
T	Technological	Any development that could improve the efficiency of the business or change the style of the service	Improved computer-based admin. packages Use of CCTV to improve security of building Use of tagging by competitor

- *What market should the organization be in?*
  Services for people with dementia are already in a 'niche', or specialized, market but it is possible to specialize further by customer type. For example, an organization might choose to gear its service to particular groups of people with dementia, for example, early onset dementia. It might focus on service users funded through local authorities or it might opt to try to attract private customers. The style of the service, its price and the way it is marketed to its different customers will vary according to this decision. Where organizations sell their services directly to service users, factors such as location, cost and style may be critical. Where they sell to other organizations, contract value, company size and reputation may be more important. For example, local authority staff may value a dementia service because of its ability to 'cope with anybody', no matter what the presenting problem. The private paying customer on the other hand may value a service that is much more selective about the type of resident it admits.
- *Is the organization a 'bed for life provider'?*
  Many quality residential care providers have been staunch advocates of the 'bed for life' principle and have used this message in their marketing. While

the philosophy is admirable, there are operational consequences. Given the variation in rates of deterioration seen in dementia and the different manifestations of behaviour, a 'bed for life' policy can lead to a home having a very mixed resident group, both in terms of mental and physical ability. This, in turn, can impact on the staff mix and the staffing ratios required to manage the service safely. Consider a nursing home established to care for the physically fit person with dementia. Its expertise relates to the management of challenging behaviour and it charges a premium for this. Over time, it is likely that the profile of the resident group will change with an increase in the levels of physical frailty and a decrease in challenging behaviour. There may be a need for a change in the staff mix, particularly for more generally trained nurses in place of psychiatric nurses. It may also get increasingly difficult to justify the premium fee as care managers perceive the home as becoming 'less specialist'.

- *Does the service need to achieve financial viability?*
  Providing a dementia service is more expensive than the provision of 'normal' frail elderly services because of the requirement for enhanced staffing. In addition to the staffing costs there is likely to be heavier wear and tear on the buildings. While there is frequently a premium associated with the price charged for the service, most providers would agree that this does not cover all of the additional costs. An organization must therefore decide how it is going to compensate for this shortfall. The first option will normally be to try to negotiate a more appropriate premium rate. However, particularly for care home providers, this is becoming ever more difficult as local authorities find themselves with tighter budgets. If this option is tried and fails, the organization can explore ways of cutting the cost of providing the service or choose to provide larger scale services in an attempt to achieve some economies of scale. In the case of a small number of organizations, mainly in the 'not-for-profit' sector, they may have the additional options of bearing the loss, or cross-subsidizing the dementia service from other more profitable areas of operation.
- *Is the service in high demand?*
  Depending on the location of the service the provider may be able to be very selective about the customers it provides for. This selection could be in terms of the profile of prospective customers in terms of ability and behaviour or it could be in terms of their ability to self-fund. Where there is over-provision, the provider will have to find ways of differentiating itself from other providers. This could be in terms of the service definition, the quality of service or the price of the service.

Thinking about competitors

Competition is not only relevant to private sector providers. For example, voluntary sector providers often need to compete for service contracts and local authority services are increasingly required to demonstrate '**best value**' (see Chapter 17). Knowledge about 'the competition', both current and potential, is therefore vital for all services and should inform the development of service strategies, service specifications and individual services' marketing plans. Obtaining this information will usually require some 'mystery shopping'. This involves staff contacting competitors, pretending to be potential customers or employees. Organizations need to be able to answer the following questions:

- Who are we in competition with?
- How well are we doing in relation to the competition? Why?
- What makes us different from the competition? This difference is the service's 'USP', its 'unique selling point', which should feature in all marketing activity.
- What are the gaps in service provision?
- Are any competitors planning to fill this gap?
- Could we fill the gap?

In order to answer the questions it may be helpful to carry out a simple **SWOT analysis**. SWOT stands for strengths, weaknesses, opportunities and threats and a completed SWOT analysis for a care home is shown in Table 16.2.

The home owner who completed the brief SWOT analysis summarized in Table 16.2 decided to investigate the demand for respite and rehabilitation services by talking to his primary health care team. As a result, they decided to dedicate one wing of the home to this type of service and launched the service by having an open day for the local care management team.

Table 16.2   SWOT analysis: Greenpastures Rest Home – developing a five-year plan

Strengths	Weaknesses	Opportunities	Threats
New building	Hard to recruit staff	Cottage hospital closing shortly	New home opening in town centre
Large single rooms	Out-of-town site	No respite care locally	LA fee levels not likely to rise next year
En-suites	No private payers	No dual-registered home in area	New contract officer in LA
Good reputation	Small home	No rehab. nearby	
Large garden	Not in touch with many care managers	Manager now NVQ assessor	
Good GP service	Four empty rooms	Four empty rooms	

MAKING CHANGE HAPPEN

Planning for change

In recent years there has been much discussion about 're-engineering' businesses. This process starts by looking at all of the processes involved in a business and redesigning them from scratch (Hammer and Champy 1993). This usually involves major change in every aspect of the organization and has been criticized as a 'kill or cure' option. It may be an appropriate approach in a failing operation but its application in an already successful business has yet to be proved. An alternative approach, that will be more familiar, is to look at a more incremental and evolutionary approach to change.

If an organization addresses the questions based on the '7S' framework (above) and the questions asked about the external environment (above), it should identify areas of the service that need attention and improvement. It is tempting at this point to want to rush into action without adequate planning but it is well worth being disciplined and assessing all the possible actions that are needed against the following set of criteria (Perren and Webber 1998):

- Is this the most important change?
- Is this the most urgent change?
- Will the change alienate or disappoint important stakeholders or will they support and welcome it?

For example, a dementia care home may decide to use some monitoring technology to improve the supervision of residents and minimize risks. It may discuss and agree the change with registration officers and successfully install the equipment. However, in the months following, it may find that referrals from the local care management team 'dry up' because no one has taken account of the negative view they have about this use of technology.

- *Will there be a financial benefit to the organization?*
  The improvement may be 'intangible' but still have a significant beneficial impact on the budget. An example of this would be an improvement in the morale of staff through better training opportunities. This is likely to save an organization money through better staff retention, lower recruitment costs and a decrease in absenteeism.
- *What is the risk associated with this change?*
  Although difficult to measure, some assessment of risk is helpful when deciding on priorities for action. The risk may be financial or may relate to image and reputation. A decision to start offering care to people with challenging behaviour may result in an increase in income from fees but there will be costs associated with additional staff training and the potential to attract bad publicity if things go wrong.
- *Is this change compatible with the general stance of the organization?*
  Consider the problems that could be in store for a charity that has always provided a subsidized respite service to carers of people with dementia.

Imagine that it decides to open a service in a new locality that will charge the full market rate for the service, in spite of successful fundraising.

- *Are the resources available to make this change?*
- *What degree of resistance will there be to this change and from whom?* Every organization has a number of people who can affect the business. These 'stakeholders' will have varying amounts of power and influence. A successfully planned programme of change will have taken account of this by undertaking an analysis of their reactions. In the example in Table 16.3, the owner of a private specialist day centre is looking at a range of options. This simple analysis indicates that local care managers would welcome service development. However, the neighbours are likely to resist any development and without some input are likely to oppose any change of use. The option to provide a service to people whose behaviour challenges looks as if it would lead to the greatest resistance. This kind of analysis is not meant to stop any initiative but should be seen as an aide in planning, a way of ensuring that any resources used to encourage support are targeted on the right people.
- *Is this the right time to make this change?*
- *Is an attempt to make this change likely to succeed?* It is particularly important that the first action planned in any programme of change is one that is almost certain to succeed. One way of assessing this may be to use 'force-field analysis' (Lewin 1951). In this long-established technique the 'current situation' is envisaged as a vertical line which is subject on either side to pushing and pulling forces. The pushing forces are trying to move the service on, the pulling forces are holding the service back. If a development is planned, then, in order to achieve progress, one or more of the following must happen: the pushing forces must be strengthened or increased; the pulling forces must be weakened; or, the end vision must be rethought along more modest lines. Examples of 'pushing forces' in care services could be motivated staff, pressure from customers, the impact of training or the result of a high-quality supervision programme. 'Pulling forces' could include demotivated staff, poor processes and procedures, poor accommodation or poor team relationships.
- *Is there an actual or potential 'champion' for this change?* A champion is someone who will 'head up' the process and 'fight your corner'.

The answers to these questions should give an indication of both the order in which changes ought to be made and the negotiations that might be needed before commencing. There are still four things that remain to be done before starting the change process: clarify the time-scales; establish the criteria for measuring achievement in meeting the objectives; obtain senior managers' agreement to the plan; and share the proposal with the wider staff group.

Ensuring successful change implementation

No programme of change will be 'pain-free'; the discomfort that most people have with change is proportional to the scale and the rate of the change. All

Table 16.3   Stakeholder analysis: Whitefields Day Centre

Option	Internal stakeholders		External stakeholders		
	Staff	**Current users**	**Neighbours**	**Care managers**	**Bank manager**
Open seven days a week	✔✗	✔✔✔	✗✗✗	✔✔✔	✔✔
Enlarge premises	✔✔✔	✔	✗✗✗	✔✔	✗✗✗✗
Extend service to people with challenging behaviour	✗✗✗	✗✗✗	✗✗✗	✔✔✔	✔✔✔
Offer service to people with dementia who are wheelchair-dependent	✗✗	✔✗	✔✗	✔✗	✔✗

Note
✔ indicates strength of support
✗ indicates strength of negative feeling
✔✗ indicates mixed reactions

changes will require employees to 'unfreeze' existing behaviours, learn new ways of working and 'refreeze' these new behaviours (Lewin 1947). Many people's automatic reaction to change will be to resist; they may be fearful of a loss of status, of losing expertise and of having to relearn tasks and processes. The amount of resistance displayed will usually be greater in an organization that has experienced little change. It is possible to develop a culture that sees constant change and innovation as a way of life, necessary to the organization's continued viability. Examples of this kind of culture are most usually found in highly competitive, 'high-tech' industries such as those associated with computing. But there are also many examples within the care sector where managers have been able to convince staff that every new 'problem service user' presents an opportunity for the staff to learn new skills and demonstrate their competency.

Effective communication is seen to be the single most important factor in minimizing the discomfort associated with change. Managers need to explain the impending change programme fully and openly and to establish systems for receiving feedback from everyone affected. There are two critical outcomes of this process: a general acknowledgement that the changes are necessary and a shared vision of the desired result. People affected by the change process must also feel assured that sufficient resources have been identified to allow for successful implementation (Thompson 1995). Many changes have failed because the 'change agent' underestimated the time or money that would be needed to implement the change successfully.

Key factors for success

- The first thing to be changed should be something where success is certain.
- Each change proposed should have an identified 'project leader' and appropriate resources allocated to it.
- Knowledge about the action, the process and the outcome should be shared with all those affected in good time.
- Efforts should be made to develop a culture that has a 'bias for action', that is a culture that is willing to experiment and one that will tolerate and learn from mistakes.
- Throughout the change process the organization must stay 'close to the customer' and take account of users' views.

Regardless of how effectively the changes have been implemented some people will still have negative feelings. They may have resented the changes from the start and they may feel demotivated and deskilled. It is essential to identify this group of people and assist them to cope with the new situation. A re-emphasis of 'what is in it for them' and an offer of appropriate training may be useful but often the situation is resolved by giving the aggrieved employees an opportunity to express their anger and disappointment (Stoner and Hartman 1997).

Need for regular review

All organizations should have a process of regularly reviewing their services in terms of effectiveness, efficiency, and financial performance. The review, which should also 'scan the horizon' for external influences, should inform all of the activity within the service. For example, an annual training schedule for care staff should be based partially on the evidence of 'skill gaps' gleaned from the previous year and partially on assumptions made about the type of people who will be using the service in the coming year. It should also take account of the training offered by competitor organizations. In addition to this annual review there may be occasions when more frequent investigation is required. For example, there has been a recent revival in interest in the provision of respite and rehabilitative services but little detail has emerged about what purchasers are looking for and how they wish to purchase it. As more is disclosed about this 'newly' identified need there will more urgency for providers to review their situation and decide whether the proposals present an appropriate opportunity for their business.

Risks associated with development

There are obvious risks to an organization if it cannot flex and change to meet the evolving needs of its customers. There is also a danger that an organization can get so caught up in a programme of change that it loses sight of the need to manage day-to-day operations, and as a result the quality of the service declines. There is an even more widespread hazard for those organizations that implement development programmes but do not take sufficient account of the wishes, feelings and aspirations of the workforce and end up with a disaffected staff group. The organizations that fall into this trap are often hierarchical and bureaucratic and frequently rely on systems of control and compliance that are inappropriate and only demotivate the staff group further. Sometimes the disaffection comes from a lack of belief in the change being proposed and sometimes from a belief that the developments are only a temporary whim of senior managers.

Sustaining the improvement

All organizations seeking long-term success need to develop the ability to:

- continuously search for new opportunities *and* develop the ability to respond to them;
- gather information about the competition *and* develop the ability to cope with/counter it;
- appreciate that continuous improvement and innovation gives a competitive edge *and* that employees need to be empowered in order to act quickly.

These three attributes are central to all service development, but they will only be achievable where organizations recognize the importance of their workforce in rejuvenation (Bartlett and Ghoshal 1995). Bartlett and Ghoshal argue that organizations need to instil the characteristics of discipline, support and trust in place of control and constraint. Employees who are self-disciplined, who readily give and receive support and who trust the organization are more able to respond positively to change and to focus on future possibilities. The application of this type of approach in a dementia care setting is demonstrated in Case Study 16.1.

In this case study, the benefits for the organization result from staff feeling more accountable and from the organization learning to trust the staff group. By doing this it is possible to create a work environment that stimulates the staff group to be more motivated, more creative and more entrepreneurial.

Case study 16.1   Involving staff in the change process

A large residential home of 60 places for people with dementia is run on very traditional lines with a management team made up of manager, deputy and three senior care staff. The rate of staff sickness and absenteeism is high and there is considerable use of agency staff, the costs of which are threatening the viability of the business. The staff often comment that the resident group is getting more difficult to care for and there is a high level of reported accidents and incidents. A new residential home has opened in the area in the last few months and there has been a sharp decline in the number of referrals being received.

The owner appreciates that something must be done and a decision is made to operate the home on a small group living basis. The building is altered to provide five units of 12. Alongside these structural changes the management team is restructured to give five team leaders reporting directly to the manager. Each team leader is responsible for the service provided on a unit and has a dedicated staff team. Each unit team creates its own roster and arranges its own cover. Care staff supervision is now provided by the team leader and one to one supervision now alternates with unit meetings.

As the new way of working beds in, a number of things emerge:

- There is less absenteeism; staff feel more responsible about letting close colleagues down. There is a substantial saving on the costs of cover. Senior staff spend much less time ringing around looking for cover; they use the time working with care staff, ensuring a high quality of care is delivered.
- The roster is compiled without argument; the staff negotiate 'time off' with each other.
- The small units make it easier for staff to see each resident as an individual. They start compiling 'life histories' on each resident.
- Relatives visiting the home report an improvement in the quality of the service; they see the same staff looking after their family member and an increase in the consistency of care practices.
- Staff are 'managing' challenging behaviour more appropriately; they are more familiar with 'their' residents and more aware of the signs that someone is getting anxious or distressed. The level of psychotropic medication used in the home decreases and residents appear more alert. There is a decrease in the number of reported accidents and incidents and an improvement in the management of continence.
- The manager is not called upon so frequently to manage crises and has more time to review policies and processes and make them 'dementia aware'. The manager also has time to research and introduce new approaches to dementia care.
- Staff feel more responsible for 'their' unit and the amount of damage to the decoration and fabric of the building and equipment has decreased. Money saved on redecoration and replacement of broken equipment is spent on sending some staff on dementia care courses.
- There is a degree of competition between the units; as a result the units become much less institutional. The individual talents of staff are better identified and as a result the number of potential activities and outings available to residents rises.
- The staff have increased pride in the service and talk about the positive changes that have been achieved in the home to their neighbours in their local community. As a result, the number of enquiries for placements and for job vacancies increases and the home has a waiting list of potential residents and potential staff.
- The staff become concerned about the people on the waiting list and their carers. They offer to establish a carers' support group.
- The carers' group is popular and well attended; the staff involved learn a great deal from the relatives. Over a period of time they expresses concern over the lack of services to support carers as they wait for residential places to become available. They suggest to the home's proprietor that a day care service is established in an adjacent empty property . . . [the process of change and development continues].

FURTHER READING

Hall, D. and Bennett, D. (2000) *The Hallmarks of a Successful Business*. Chalford: Hall Marks.

Hanson, P. and Lubin, B. (1995) *Answers to Questions Most Frequently Asked About Organisational Development*. London: Sage.

Horovitz, J. (1999) *Seven Secrets of Service Strategy*. Harlow: Prentice Hall.

Smale, G.G. (1996) *Mapping Change and Innovation*. London: HMSO.

SYLVIA COX

Developing quality in services

17

KEY POINTS

- Quality as a concept is difficult to define. It can be understood as a dynamic system of values, objectives, standards, measurement and review.
- The challenges posed in responding to the needs of people with dementia affect the way that quality is implemented. The establishment of explicit values is an integrating concept.
- The various quality approaches, systems, tools and techniques can be judged against criteria that are relevant to a person-centred approach to dementia care.
- Research and practice confirm that there is no one approach or system that can incorporate all aspects of a quality improvement programme for people with dementia.
- Quality programmes need to be tailored to the particular stage of development and objectives of the organization; the involvement of people with dementia and other stakeholders, particularly front-line staff, is an essential component.

INTRODUCTION

This chapter draws on the research literature as well as the author's experience of a range of quality development initiatives in dementia services. It provides an overview of key quality issues and approaches and discusses the lessons for dementia services.

Services for people with dementia are provided within a melting pot of informal care (family friends, neighbours, and friends) and formal care (statutory, not-for-profit and market sectors). People with dementia are cared for in a variety of living environments. The care setting can have a major impact on their quality of life and care (see Chapter 12). Nowadays fewer people are cared for in hospital on a long-term basis but the quality of provision for people with dementia admitted for acute hospital care is a particular concern (Audit Commission 2000).

It is generally agreed that every organization needs to have the means of ensuring the quality of its service delivery. Given the range of services used by people with dementia, the starting point of this chapter is the common concerns of the various service sectors as they respond to the person's needs.

CHALLENGES FOR QUALITY IN DEMENTIA CARE

The challenges for improving quality in dementia services relate to issues discussed throughout this book. These challenges can be summarized as follows:

- Dementia is a condition that affects the person's whole life; quality services must address this.
- Dementia is almost always progressive; variability and unpredictability are therefore key factors in planning and delivering services.
- Dementia is often associated with attitudes of stigma, negativism and hopelessness; these attitudes must be overcome.
- The community, health, housing and social services involved in dementia care are mainly mainstream, not specialist, services; this has implications for the levels of expertise in dementia care.
- Accessing appropriate services can be problematic for people with dementia and their carers; this needs to be improved.
- Communication with people with dementia can be difficult; services need to find better ways of hearing the views of people with dementia.
- People with dementia are often marginalized in western society, and people from different cultural and ethnic backgrounds may be further marginalized; this must be addressed.
- People with dementia often require assistance with personal care and intimate care; it is difficult to monitor the quality of such care.
- Dementia services operate at the interface between health and social care; they have traditionally taken different approaches to improving quality.

THE NATURE OF QUALITY

Quality is a word that is used frequently, often indiscriminately, and yet it remains an elusive term to capture and almost paradoxical to explain (Kelly and Warr 1992; Gaster 1995). The often quoted definition of quality is 'degree of excellence, relative nature or kind or character' (*Concise Oxford Dictionary*).

The notion of quality attracts approval exactly because it can be defined in a number of ways depending on the purpose and perspective of the person (Nocon and Qureshi 1996). Definitions range between detailed conformance to very specific standards and a very wide, almost metaphysical, or abstract, concept (Pirsig 1974; James 1992).

Some writers suggest that quality is an 'integrating concept' which enables people to get on with the job 'grounded in the hardnosed detail of everyday life' (James 1992: 46). Yet values are also of fundamental importance to the whole framework of quality processes. Beresford *et al.* (1997: 72) argue that 'Definitions of quality, of course, are based on and emerge from values, whether these are explicit or implicit.'

Different definitions of quality may encompass elements that are irreconcilable, suggesting that an agreed definition may depend on the balance of power among the stakeholders (Nocon and Qureshi 1996). The issue of power is crucial when considering the needs of vulnerable groups in society, especially older people and those with cognitive and communication difficulties.

In the field of health and social services it is not always helpful to equate quality with excellence. The notion of continual improvement is a more productive way forward. This is especially so for dementia care where the art of the possible is continually changing but where constraints of resource are ever present (Marshall and Cox 1998).

Gaster (1995: 34) suggests that definitions of quality fall into three broad categories:

- those that define various quality dimensions, for example structure, process and outcomes;
- those focusing on process, especially gaps between the expectations of users and their experience of the service; and
- those that take a negotiating stance, with more emphasis on meeting agreed needs of consumers.

It is important to realize that the quality of a service in terms of its organizational effectiveness may have little impact on the nature and shape of the quality of life of users. Quality of life depends on many other factors. However, by addressing the challenges posed by dementia we can begin to define and develop the dimensions of services that are more likely to support and encourage the provision of high-quality opportunities and experiences.

Across health and social care provision the quality of personal relationships is crucial to the quality of the service. Hardy and Wistow (1997) identify a range of other complex factors that impact on service quality, including:

- contract specifications;
- ensuring that the consumer controls the service;
- specifying and measuring outcomes such as dignity and quality of life;
- providing personal, often intimate, care;
- providing services 'behind closed doors';
- employing front-line staff who are often unqualified and untrained, thus with no professional code of conduct.

Across the UK and in Europe there has been increasing emphasis on quality concerns (Moriarty and Webb 2000). Good quality care is seen to be non-standardized and tailored to the needs of the individual (Tester 1999). There is no doubt that issues of cost, efficiency and effectiveness affect quality. The relationships between these factors are complex and much of the emphasis, especially in policies relating to older people, has focused on cost containment (Tester 1999).

Some people argue that a definition of quality should not include the components of economy and efficiency since policies designed to improve value for money may not improve quality if the test of quality is meeting individual needs (Gaster 1995). However, increasingly the notion of quality is underpinned by the notion of 'best value' and reviews by the **Accounts Commission** (1999) and **Audit Commission** (2000) in the UK have included quality and cost. Best value is the required process for all local councils in the UK. It evaluates the delivery of services to clear standards and councils must 'challenge, compare, consult, and compete' (Filkin 1997). It has important implications for the way quality in services is perceived and managed.

Interests in quality

Any service organization has a range of people with an interest in how the service is delivered. These include users or customers, relatives, professionals, managers, purchasers, commissioners, regulators, the wider community and others.

There has been an increasing emphasis on putting the user at the centre of services in both independent and public services. Thus the British Quality Foundation (an independent, not-for-profit membership organization for industry and business) identifies customer satisfaction, employee satisfaction and impact on society as being important for all types of private, public and voluntary non-profit-sector organizations, large and small.

A person-centred approach to care has been advocated for people with dementia (Kitwood and Bredin 1992b) for some years. However, it is only recently that the person with dementia has come to be seen as a citizen who has intrinsic rights and who should not be excluded or marginalized within society.

QUALITY AS A SYSTEM

In order to understand the way quality processes are implemented within organizations it is helpful to have a model. Figure 17.1, based on Gaster (1995: 6), shows a quality system with different stages and components and which is cyclical in nature. All these stages in the cycle are influenced and informed by a range of stakeholders: person with dementia as citizen, front-line staff, family carers, managers, commissioners, regulators and others. Gaster suggests that this model or framework may be used as an aid to thinking and an aid to action.

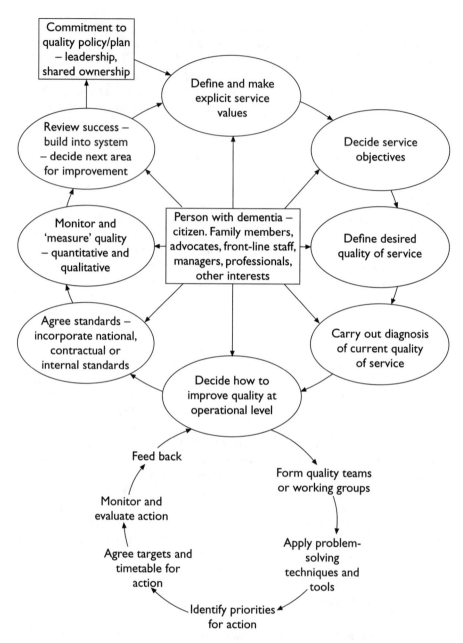

Figure 17.1 A model for developing service quality in dementia care
Source: Adapted from Gaster (1995: 6)

In order to improve the quality of services there has to be: good people management and a climate which listens and learns, encourages innovation and creativity, does not punish mistakes inappropriately or pursue so-called quality objectives for cost-saving or job-cutting ends. Building such a culture requires:

- valuing and empowering staff;
- leadership and support;
- working in problem-solving teams which include service users wherever possible;
- providing a culture that listens, learns and acts.

Values

Values are the foundation of the whole quality debate since they affect how quality is defined, interpreted and implemented (Towell 1988; Gaster 1995; Evers 1997). The model of service quality (Figure 17.1) shows how service values relate to strategic objectives and processes of quality development and improvement.

There are a number of value-based approaches to quality which can be useful and relevant in dementia services organizations (for example King's Fund Centre 1986; HMSO 1989). Within service organizations, there may be a wide gap between stated values and those that inform everyday activity. There may also be tensions between professional, managerial, personal and political values (Gaster 1995).

It is very difficult for people with dementia to assert their preferred type of service within an organization which sees them as passive recipients of service with no hope of improvement (Bamford and Bruce 2000).

Cox et al. (1998) identify five core values for dementia care services:

- maximizing personal control;
- enabling choice;
- respecting dignity;
- preserving continuity (linking past, present and future for the person in the provision of services, living environment and care processes);
- promoting equity.

Values are translated into action in a particular service by informing the objectives, the nature of the service and the way quality is measured and evaluated. Values can help those involved decide what is important so that priorities can be negotiated and prioritized.

Netten (1993), in a comparison of different residential care regimes, reports that outcomes for users related closely to the extent to which staff were, and felt themselves to be, valued. She came to the conclusion that the precise nature of the institution's caring and therapeutic philosophy seemed of less importance than the fact that there was one, and that the staff felt committed to it.

Table 17.1 Some key service outcomes for people with dementia

Process outcomes	Quality of life outcomes
• Having a say in services	• Opportunities for social contact and companionship
• Being valued	• Access to activity and stimulation
• Having one's own unique needs recognized and acted on	• Living in a clean and comfortable environment
• A positive relationship with staff	• Feeling safe and secure
• Being able to relate to other users of the service	• Maintaining a sense of personal identity
	• Maximizing a sense of personal control

Source: Summarized from Mozley *et al.* (1999) and Bamford and Bruce (2000)

Outcomes

There has been much more emphasis recently on the relationship between values, process outcomes and better valued outcomes for individuals (Nocon and Qureshi 1996; Bamford and Bruce 2000).

Research by Qureshi *et al.* (1998) suggests that identifying social care outcomes is essential if services are to improve. Due to the complex interaction of organizational and management systems underpinning health and social care services and the lack of any universal measurement instrument, they suggest that it is essential to look at both **process outcomes** and quality of life outcomes. Research on frameworks for domiciliary care (Henwood *et al.* 1998) and outcomes of community care for people with dementia and their carers (Bamford and Bruce 2000) also emphasizes process and outcome indicators. Both of these research programmes included people with dementia in defining the process and quality of life outcomes. Mozley *et al.* (2000) highlight the lack of any gold standard for judging quality in their study of the outcomes of residential and nursing home care for residents (Mozley *et al.* 1999). Interestingly, both the research on community care outcomes and the research on care home outcomes emphasizes that having something interesting, pleasurable and useful is one of the key desired outcomes. Key process outcomes and quality of life outcomes are summarized in Table 17.1.

QUALITY – APPROACHES, SYSTEMS, AWARDS AND TOOLS

A quality plan or policy may be very simple or very sophisticated but it basically spells out how the organization will approach and develop quality in its service, taking into account the particular needs of its users and other stakeholder interests. The organization cannot assume that what works for the person without dementia will also work for the person with dementia.

Quality demands answers to questions about what the organization believes it is trying to do, where it is going, how it sees its users and its staff. Quality is not a simple add-on; it begs fundamental questions about the culture of the organization and how it achieves its goals.

There is a wide range of quality approaches and systems in use including 'off the shelf', customized and in-house versions. Some have been transferred from the private sector, often from manufacturing services. It is difficult to choose any one that is most appropriate for a particular organization and to ensure that the approach or system can incorporate the most important aspects of quality for people with dementia. A number of quality approaches are presented briefly below.

Quality control

This approach first developed in manufacturing industries. It mainly sees quality as a problem; it is essentially about detecting human error and seeking to produce conformance to a specification. In a service context this usually involves conformance to a uniform set of standards that have been predetermined. As long as the specification is explicit and detailed enough, inspection can be carried out by experts or lay people. However, specifying services for people with dementia can be complex and too much specification may lead to standardization at the expense of variation and flexibility.

Quality assurance

Quality assurance is usually defined as 'building in quality' through identifying key points that can be checked with agreed standards across a system. The underlying philosophy of prevention differentiates it from other approaches. It lends itself to external verification such as BSEN Information Systems ISO 9000 (see Table 17.2). While it provides a systematic approach it can become too procedure-driven if care is not taken to involve other stakeholders especially users, carers and advocates.

A more positive approach is achieved if it is developed internally and incorporates the following (Gaster 1995):

- analysing the service process;
- identifying procedures consistent with the service value framework;
- providing appropriate staff training;
- promoting tools for self-evaluation.

'Quality assurance' is sometimes used loosely as a general term for all quality initiatives.

Total Quality Management (TQM)

This is one of the most widely known approaches to quality improvement. It is much broader than quality assurance although it may include quality assurance as part of its approach. The focus is on creating a quality culture that energetically pursues a proactive approach to quality development. There are several types of TQM. TQM has the following features (Pollitt 1997):

- a corporate perspective (that is, emphasizing the organization as one entity, the sum of its parts rather than a collection of different departments or functions);
- specific quality goals within an organization-wide plan;
- generates commitment and enthusiasm throughout the whole organization;
- cuts across departmental and disciplinary boundaries;
- substantial investment in training – especially in the early stages;
- an ongoing process of continual improvement not one-off standard setting;
- avoids mistakes rather than correcting them once they have happened;
- may be top-down and not involve all stakeholders.

Customer care

Customer care programmes are open to different interpretations and modes of implementation. They emphasize the immediate impressions made on a service user by a service. However, it may be a positive development if it can be seen as part of a wider quality programme, including the valuing of front-line staff as well as the service user (Gaster 1995).

Setting standards

Quality is often seen as the setting and meeting of standards. These may be generated externally or internally. Those developed internally, and developed 'bottom up' rather than 'top down', are more likely to be meaningful and more likely to be implemented. Burton and Kellaway (1998) provide a useful account of this type of process within a learning disability service. However, there is debate about the capacity for standards to provide protection for vulnerable people and Nocon and Qureshi (1996: 21) suggest that 'outcome specifications are preferable to service standards because the former will be less likely to inhibit flexibility and variety of approach'.

There appears to be increasing acceptance in the UK that the enforcement of minimum standards will not in itself drive out poor practice. There are suggestions that a culture of continual improvement and the careful use of complaints, whistleblowing and advocacy is the key to ensuring that standards do not fall below acceptable levels.

Dementia-specific standards have been developed in Australia (Ministerial Task Force on Dementia Services in Victoria 1997). This model aimed to encourage best practice and provide a tool for self-monitoring and service improvement. The Alzheimer's Society in conjunction with the Royal College of Nursing (Ray 1999) are in the process of developing standards for care homes.

Inspection

Studies in America and the UK have pointed to the limitations of using an inspection process to identify serious abuse and improve practice. This chimes with findings from investigations of major accidents in organizations (Reason 1997). In the field of residential care, research points to the unreliability and inconsistency of inspectors' judgements (Gibbs and Sinclair 1992). In the UK the process of inspection for residential and domiciliary care is being changed. Parallel working groups in Scotland, England and Wales are developing care standards to underpin new legislation.

Organizational audit

This refers to a cyclical process of organizational activity that involves a systematic review of practice, identification of possible improvements, implementation of these improvements and a process of further review. Audit investigates if the right thing is being done and does not necessarily involve outcome measurement. Audit within services (that is micro-level audit) often refers to the appraisal of records, for example medical audit or clinical audit in hospitals. Sometimes there is little relationship between the standards of the records and the care provided and outcomes for clients/patients. Case Study 17.1 (p. 272) provides a useful example of linking audit with an observational tool.

Performance management

Health and social services have used a number of techniques to monitor performance in commissioning and providing services. These include data collection set against set **performance indicators, thematic reviews,** and evaluative studies and surveys that make comparisons between services.

Peer review

There are different approaches to **peer review** but they usually involve the assessment of an individual or group of individuals by a group of fellow professionals, often senior or very experienced members of the profession. However, there is a continuum of approaches ranging from those that are holistic, supportive and non-judgmental to approaches that are more constrained by specific standards.

Clinical governance

This is likely to impact increasingly on quality approaches in the health services and their partner agencies in the UK. It emphasizes the importance of quality of care being at the centre of the NHS and greater accountability among professionals for clinical performance.

The approach includes:

- utilization of evidence-based practice;
- clinical audit;
- significant event analysis;
- exploitation of the educational value of complaints; a key aspect is patient and user involvement.

Benchmarking

This involves systematically comparing, evaluating and learning from good role models irrespective of the sector and geographical location. The aim is to gain insight and knowledge that can be used to bring about effective improvements in one's own activities. This term is now used rather loosely within the UK public sector; it is more difficult to assess the extent to which it has been put into practice. Riseborough (1998), discussing **benchmarking** in housing associations in the UK, notes that it does not usually involve consumers and other stakeholders.

Dementia Care Mapping (DCM)

A more detailed review of Dementia Care Mapping (DCM) is included here since it is probably the most widely used dementia-specific quality approach in the UK.

DCM was developed by Kitwood and Bredin (1992b) in the late 1980s. Since then it has been through a series of revisions. Their assumption is that relative well-being of the person with dementia is equated with good quality care. The approach was developed at a time when the idea of consumer-led services, especially for people with dementia, had barely been considered (Innes et al. 2000). It is one of a number of observational tools (Selai and Trimble 1999).

DCM is designed for use with people in a group care setting. It involves the 'mapper' participating but also observing at least five people with dementia for a minimum of six hours. Mappers note aspects of behaviour, well- and ill-being, personal detractions and positive events during each five-minute period. They also make a judgement about the appropriate behaviour code and well- and ill-being value for each person observed.

There is a qualification framework; from basic user status, which entitles people to carry out mapping in their own care setting, through to advanced trainer status, which entitles people to train others in DCM.

If carried out by trained people the approach appears to have the potential to:

- evaluate the quality of care in a group setting – a report analysing the data is fed back to staff identifying areas of improvement and suggestions for care planning;
- contribute to the development of care practice – an action plan;
- identify staff development needs;
- focus on a particular person if there are concerns;
- monitor developments over time.

There have been a number of reports about the usefulness of DCM as an observation method (Barnett 1995b; Brooker 1995) and as a research and development tool within an action research project (Lintern *et al.* 2000). However, there are some suggestions that used in the wrong way it can demotivate staff, alienate them and create anxiety (Buckland 1996). Mapping is conducted in the public areas of a care setting but there are some concerns that poorer quality care may take place in private areas such as bedrooms, bathrooms and toilets (Lee-Treweek 1994). This may not show up in mapping. It seems that DCM works best when there are already good management structures, positive support and where it is a part of an overall approach to improving quality (Buckland 1996; Lintern *et al.* 2000).

DCM affirms the person-centred approach to care. However, there is a curious lack in the DCM method of the involvement of the person with dementia or the family carer. Feedback to staff is emphasized but feedback to residents and to family carers and advocates is not. DCM could also result in blaming front-line staff for lack of engagement when they have neither the time, training, skills nor support to understand and respond to the needs of people with dementia.

There is clearly a place for DCM in the range of quality tools. However, it is not a substitute for consulting and involving people with dementia directly wherever possible. It should not be relied on as the only method of monitoring quality.

More quality tools for improving the quality of care are being developed and produced, for example lifestyle and care planning tools for front-line staff. It is likely that these will proliferate with the expansion of new technology approaches. A range of quality systems and awards are summarized in Table 17.2.

CHOOSING QUALITY APPROACHES

Organizations have to determine how quality approaches are to be pursued in a way that is congruent with the business they are in, their values, and the appropriateness for their users and for other stakeholders. Organizations, large or small, public or private, can expend a large amount of staff, time and financial resources on quality systems and still not ensure that the quality of life experienced by every user is as good as it could be. On the other hand

Table 17.2 Quality systems and awards

BSEN ISO 9000

This is consistent with a quality assurance approach. It refers to a series of international standards of quality. An organization seeks registration for processes or systems. There have been criticisms of the system relating to the lack of emphasis on user satisfaction; the bureaucratic approach that does not involve or motivate staff; and costs (Gaster 1995). Registration with the British Quality Institute means that the organization's system conforms to this standard.

Investors in People (IiP)

IiP is accessed via Local Enterprise Companies in Scotland and Learning and Skills Councils (formerly Training and Enterprise Councils) in England and Wales. It assesses how well an organization manages the training and development needs of staff. The resulting accreditation is said to ensure that the staff practice within an organization meets and maintains expected standards by a process of continuous improvement. IiP can be applied to the whole organization or a part of it.

Business Excellence Model

This is a continuous improvement system that can result in the UK Quality Award for Business Excellence by the British Quality Foundation. There is a self-assessment process – ASSESS – which is available in written or software format. It is said to provide an improvement framework to manage initiatives such as IiP, Charter Mark and ISO 9000.

SERVQUAL

This is a type of TQM but sees service quality problems as 'gaps' in the performance of the organizations. The biggest gap is often that between what consumers expect and what they actually experience in terms of service. SERVQUAL has been used to measure patient satisfaction with health services.

Inside Quality Assurance (IQA)

This developed out of the 'Caring in Homes Initiative' funded by the Department of Health. It is essentially a self-assessment system but now can involve accreditation by an external verifier.

Charter mark

Award of a charter mark gives public recognition that an organization provides services that meet specified written standards. The standards focus on the involvement and experience of consumers. Examples include the Patient's Charter and the Citizen's Charter.

QUARZ

A quality assurance system published by the Sainsbury Centre for Mental Health. It provides a number of schedules covering a range of processes.

Integrated Care Pathway (ICP)

Originated in North America it determines locally agreed multidisciplinary practice based on guidelines and evidence where possible, for a specific client group. The ICP forms part of the clinical record, documents care given and enables the evaluation of outcomes for continuous quality improvement.

---

there are many market and consumer demands placed on services and they have to develop a quality strategy that enables them to achieve their priorities. This includes the necessity of meeting statutory requirements (for example, national standards, health and safety); contract compliance standards; the requirements of running an effective organization; and the requirements of enhancing the quality of life and care of service users and staff.

For non-specialist organizations, one strategy is to identify the common aspects of quality improvement for a range of service users, ensuring that services used by people with dementia are 'dementia friendly' and that safeguards are built in for involving and communicating with people with dementia and their family carers. For larger organizations it may be necessary to use more than one quality approach. For instance, having clear written policies and procedures in a range of areas may be essential and it may make sense for verification/accreditation to be pursued. For a small voluntary agency on the other hand, written procedures may be kept to a minimum but systems still need to ensure that key information such as data on complaints is monitored.

The criteria that might be used for selecting a quality system or tool are set out in Table 17.3.

Table 17.3   Suggested criteria for selecting a quality system/tool

- Is the purpose of the system/tool improving the quality of life of users, demonstrating added value in the market, or satisfying contract compliance?
- Is the system/tool people-centred or technically orientated? There is a place for a focus on both aspects.
- What are the methods for involving users – people with dementia, relatives and supporters, wider community?
- Is the quality system consistent with the service's value base?
- Does it facilitate a positive approach to risk?
- Is the approach consistent with the wider social purpose/context, for example equity in relation to black and ethnic minority issues or equal opportunities?
- Does it have a continuous learning approach?
- What are the expectations and methods for involving staff at all levels (management, supervisory, front-line, and support services)? Is it 'top-down' or 'bottom-up'?
- If relevant, does it mesh with 'best value' approaches?
- Is it based on continual improvement rather than pursuing an impossible ideal or mere conformance to standards?
- Is it affordable? One of the key variables is staff time.
- What are the timescales involved for initial completion and longer term planning? There are advantages in early feedback.
- Does the quality system integrate with other organizational processes, for example contract compliance, inspection, identifying staff development and training needs, business planning?
- Does the quality system enable the service to identify what it does well and what needs to be improved and how?

Given the range of services that people with dementia use there is unlikely to be one type of programme, approach or specific system which will meet all the needs of an organization. The important thing is that the different strands of quality development should be working together, not at loggerheads.

If we consider again the challenges highlighted at the beginning of the chapter it is not surprising that most organizations providing services for people with dementia are struggling to find quality approaches that are workable and affordable and meet even some of these criteria.

Of course, a prerequisite of quality dementia care is that organizations understand dementia and are positive about what can be achieved. There are many pressures and constraints on organizations, not least changing fashions and new policy directions. Linking quality approaches may be one way of moving quality forward (Riseborough 1998). This might involve, for example, linking external user-based evaluations of service quality with TQM self-assessment and accreditation approaches. There are already some examples of more integrated approaches (Lintern *et al.* 2000). However, these often depend on external facilitation, which may not be available or may be too expensive for an organization to bring in. Using independent advocates may become an essential part of an integrated quality approach since there are often power imbalances between people who are cared for and people who are caregivers.

LESSONS FOR DEVELOPING QUALITY IN SERVICES

The case studies describe different approaches to improving quality in three different service settings: acute care, nursing home care and day care. They highlight the importance of leadership and clarity of purpose, the development of a learning culture and the need for policies and procedures. These factors are similar to the factors that are identified as being important in more general organizational development (see Chapter 16).

An evaluative research project by Lintern *et al.* (2000) confirms the complexity and challenges of developing quality dementia care in care homes. They make

---

Case study 17.1   Improving quality in acute hospital care for people with dementia

Commitment to change
A hospital audit included a standard on 'maximizing the well-being and quality of life for people with dementia'. A review of a sample of patient pathways through the service identified repeated moves and inconsistency in approach. This often resulted in challenging behaviour from the patient, complaints from other patients and their relatives, and expressed concerns from staff, particularly about risk. There was some evidence of repeated admissions, delayed discharges and inappropriate moves to assessment and long-stay psychogeriatric wards. Dementia care mapping was used to evaluate the care provided in the assessment ward.

Consensus on values and objectives

The values of continuity, equity, personal control, dignity and choice are underpinning the developments. A quality group was set up consisting of managers, nursing assistants, relatives, occupational therapist and advocacy worker. There were two external facilitators. Various methods were used to explore what was happening, including direct observation at different times of the day and night; audit of care plans; and discussions with relatives and patients (those with dementia and those without) exploring likes and dislikes, concerns and specific incidents. Reports of critical incidents were reviewed, and key factors identified. An audit of occupational therapy input on wards confirmed that people being discharged were prioritized. This often excluded people with dementia who were assumed to be moving on to a care home or long-stay ward or requiring more specialist rehabilitation.

Action plan priorities

Three areas were identified for improvement:

- A user-friendly care profile was developed that could be used on admission and accompany the person wherever he/she went. The relatives and person with dementia were to be involved in this along with the named nurse and key associate nurse or key worker.
- The system was examined to see if moves between wards could be reduced. If a move was unavoidable, a link nurse or associate nurse would provide continuity to staff in the new ward by reinforcing messages from the care profile. Relatives were supported by the link nurse to understand the importance of continuity. For those without visitors a contact was made with the advocacy/befriending services.
- Care pathways continue to be audited to see if there are any changes in the pattern. These changes are linked to a training programme for staff and a support system for nursing assistants.

Results

The process created a better understanding of the needs of people with dementia and the roles of staff. It has:

- unlocked commitment and enthusiasm particularly of the nursing assistants;
- opened up a dialogue with relatives, the advocacy service and voluntary organizations to explore volunteer involvement in the wards in an appropriate way – not taking over existing staff roles;
- improved targeting of resources, ensuring that people do not stay in hospital longer than they need to and that there are no avoidable moves;
- given responsibility to nursing assistants for activities;
- linked training with individual support and supervision;
- impacted on the wider system – future work is examining the interface between the acute sector, the community mental health team and the early discharge team.

The use of the care profile is the main priority in 'building in quality'. This is seen as tangible evidence that the values are being put into practice. Relatives, patients where possible and staff are to provide feedback on its effectiveness and use in care processes.

Case study 17.2   Improving quality in a nursing home

The purpose-built nursing home is designed on dementia principles (see Chapter 12). It consists of four 12-bedded units: two units for older people with mental health problems and two units for people of all ages with dementia.

The home had received accreditation with ISO 9000 series but there were concerns from management that the particular needs of residents were not being addressed within the systems and procedures in the home. Some criticisms had been made by the local authority purchasers of care and by the Registration and Inspection team.

Commitment to change

The new home manager was committed to improving the quality of care but found it difficult to know where to start. Some nursing staff found it difficult to believe that people with dementia could be more involved in improving quality in the home and there was some resentment that the dementia units were better staffed than the frail elderly units. Care assistants were technically co-key workers but in practice the care planning and implementation process was controlled by the nurse managers in the units.

Reviewing the performance

A method was needed to identify the areas in which the home was doing reasonably well and those in which it needed to do additional work. There were reservations about the available systems. A self-assessment review system based on the quality elements of the Business Excellence Model (British Quality Foundation) was piloted within the home.

Action plan priorities

The review process highlighted areas of good practice but also four major areas for improvement:

• care planning process;
• involvement of residents – particularly those with dementia or other communication difficulties;
• limited range of enjoyable and stimulating activities;
• food and meal times concerns.

While the review was underway a critical incident occurred which questioned existing procedures in relation to safety within the home. An analysis of this incident confirmed that the system verified by ISO had not sufficiently taken into account the needs of people with dementia. (It is important to note that an internal review may not identify system issues or predict serious incidents. A separate process needs to be undertaken to ensure that appropriate systems are in place.)

Values and objectives

The review process involved setting up various self-assessment teams involving all stakeholders. Involvement of residents with dementia is a challenge. However, innovative ways are being developed by key workers and advocacy workers, to reach out to residents so that their voice can be fed back into the process. There has been spin-off with relatives who now have their own regular meetings and a route to communicate with managers of the home and individual key workers.

Results

The action plan arising from the review highlighted priorities for immediate action.

An external consultant is facilitating work with front-line staff and nurse managers to understand the objectives of the care planning process and introduce a user-friendly care plan and a resident profile which involves care assistants, relatives and residents in a more integrated way. The relinquishing of some control by nurse managers to care staff has resulted in more individualized approaches to people's quality of life within the home.

The process has also fed into a clarification of roles and responsibilities, which assists in the management of the safety issues.

The priorities for learning and the development of appropriate training are now much clearer. This will focus on person-centred approaches, activities and coaching in the care planning process.

Residents, relatives, purchasers, regulators and staff at all levels now feel that they are working together to tackle the issues and that improvements can be made. Communication systems and feedback are more effective and new ideas are being generated.

---

the point that improvements took several years to implement even though the care home was intended to be 'person-centred' from the start and had excellent environmental facilities. The research examines the process of translating changes in staff attitudes and behaviour into improved well-being for the residents. The researchers identify the need for 'determination and will at a management and organisational level to overcome barriers to individualised person centred care' (Lintern *et al.* 2000: 7). This work is useful because it confirms that:

- training alone did not lead to improved outcomes for residents;
- improved attitudes and skills shown by staff may not result in good outcomes for residents if there are organizational obstacles to positive change;
- timing of feedback to staff is essential to maximize effectiveness;
- measures of staff competence such as the Dementia Care Practitioner Assessment (DCPA) may assist in the evaluation of staff training at an early stage rather than reliance on DCM, which depends on residents' functional ability and health.

Work by Beck *et al.* (1999) in North America also confirms the central role of front-line staff and the barriers to improving quality. They suggest that quality nursing home care is more likely to happen when 'the nursing home culture and organisational milieu are part of a "shared governance" environment where all the partners in nursing homes have a voice and value CNAs' [Certified Nursing Assistants] central role in residential care' (p. 209).

The three case studies provided reinforce the messages from this research. They suggest that there needs to be:

- an understanding of, and priority for, the outcomes valued by users;
- commitment and determination at a management/organizational level to overcome barriers to individualized person-centred care;

Case study 17.3   Day opportunities for younger people with dementia

---

The day service operates within a small centre three days a week and on a Saturday morning it provides a drop-in service. An outreach service provides day activities at home or in the community, linked with respite and support for family carers.

Commitment and values

This voluntary service was firmly committed to a person-centred planning approach (Sanderson et al. 1997). It provided a carefully thought-out induction programme for staff combined with a supervision and support system provided by the manager. Standards had been set by the central management of the voluntary organization for the day care centre activities. But there were concerns about demonstrating quality in the outreach service because of its varied and individualized nature.

An external evaluation took place. This explored stakeholders' expectations of the service and the impact of the service especially on service users and their family carers. At the same time Dementia Care Mapping took place in the day care centre. The careful records monitoring the activity of the service and the diary-type notes kept by the outreach workers and the manager assisted the evaluation process.

Relatives were encouraged to feed back concerns through the manager, the outreach workers and the day centre staff. Careful liaison also took place with the social work care manager who was involved in purchasing and monitoring the care package.

Valued outcomes

People valued the continuity of the service, with provision by people who were trusted and knew the person with dementia and the family circumstances. Also highly valued was the ability for the user and carer to control the intensity of the service. The main shortcoming was that, on occasions, access to a higher level of home support or respite to get the family through a crisis was unavailable.

Results

The information available from the Dementia Care Mapping at the centre and the diary information from the outreach workers facilitated a comparison between the two approaches and facilitated two-way learning. The centre staff have become more aware of available resources in the community. The involvement of care managers in the quality improvement process has alerted them to greater opportunities to integrate and link different services. For instance, a local care home is to provide a small respite unit specifically for people in the younger age groups and admissions will be organized through the day support service.

Work is starting on developing care standards for the outreach service using the framework developed by the Nuffield Institute (Henwood et al. 1998). As a result of the review, additional hours are to be purchased by the local authority, which will also allow an assistant coordinator post to deputize for the manager.

- good communication between care staff to plan and implement care sensitively – this requires effective and user-friendly care planning and lifestyle planning tools;
- good two-way communication between management and front-line staff in order to reinforce a person-centred approach through continuous feedback on performance;
- good support and supervision arrangements for staff – especially for front-line staff;
- involvement and communication with other stakeholders, especially people with dementia themselves.

These lessons must be set against the reality of the experience of those who struggle to implement person-centred care on a day-to-day basis (Packer 2000). This reality includes research findings which show that less than 50 per cent of care and nursing assistants have received training in basic care skills and very few have received training to help them understand dementia and its behavioural and psychological implications (Mozley *et al.* 2000).

There is a real danger that the 'rhetoric' of person-centred care is introduced but not real changes to basic values and practice (Smale *et al.* 1993; Packer 2000). A combination of approaches is needed, operating in different ways and at different levels to promote positive risk, protect vulnerable people and improve the quality of life and care. A key test is the level of involvement of people with dementia at all stages of the development of quality within a service.

FURTHER READING

Burton, M. and Kellaway, M. (eds) (1998) *Developing and Managing High Quality Services for People With Learning Disabilities*. Aldershot: Ashgate Publishing Ltd. Gives clear guidance on the process of developing and improving services.

Cox, S., Anderson, I., Dick, S. and Elgar, J. (1998) *The Person, the Community and Dementia: Developing a Value Framework*. Stirling: Dementia Services Development Centre. Looks at how values inform the process of understanding dementia and negotiating the provision of care and support.

Ellis, R. and Whittington, D. (1993) *Quality Assurance in Health Care: A Handbook*. London: Edward Arnold. An overview of quality assurance guidance on techniques and systems.

Evers, A., Haverinen, R., Leichsenring, K. and Wistow, G. (eds) (1997) *Developing Quality in Personal Social Services: Concepts, Cases and Comments*. Aldershot: Ashgate Publishing Ltd. An overview of developments in different European countries.

Gaster, L. (1995) *Quality in Public Services: Managers' Choices*. Buckingham: Open University Press. Provides a useful conceptual and practical framework for understanding and developing quality in public services.

Nocon, A. and Qureshi, H. (1996) *Outcomes of Community Care for Users and Carers: A Social Services Perspective*. Buckingham: Open University Press. A useful overview of the literature on quality and social care outcomes.

18

JAN KILLEEN

Involving people with dementia and their carers in developing services

KEY POINTS

- People with dementia have a right to be involved in decisions and developments which affect their lives.
- Many people with dementia are prepared and able to communicate their immediate and anticipated needs for services.
- We need a variety of approaches to involving people with dementia in the development of services.
- Effective involvement of people with dementia in service development requires dedicated staff time, expertise and appropriate funding.
- Carers of people with dementia must have opportunities to be involved in service developments in their own right.

INTRODUCTION

This chapter looks at ways of involving people with dementia and their carers in developing the services that affect their lives. In so doing it makes a distinction between people with dementia and carers, who have different voices and different needs. The chapter examines the policy context for the development of service user participation and considers why the involvement of people with dementia, and to a lesser extent their carers, has been so slow. It sets out different types of involvement in service development for people with dementia and their carers and examines the different methods available to engage people with differing circumstances and characteristics. Carers are regarded as beneficiaries of services and also as partners with service agencies in providing care. They are also often the best advocates for people with dementia who have severe difficulty in communicating their views.

THE POLICY CONTEXT

The principle of public participation in planning local services has been recognized as a democratic right for the past 30 years, but it has only gained real momentum in the past ten years. Commitment to the development of meaningful local participation strategies, which include people with disabilities and others marginalized because of poverty, age, gender or ethnicity, has generally been slow and poorly resourced in the UK. Approaches to involvement in the late 1960s and 1970s varied widely. At one end of the spectrum were community development initiatives, which aimed to empower communities to be involved in local decision making. At the other end of the spectrum were consultations on local authorities' 'structure plans' (encompassing transport, housing and public amenities) through one-off public meetings and meetings with 'special needs groups'. Initially the latter were typically approached negatively by staff who assumed that service users would not have the interest or ability to express their views. This of course proved to be wrong and service users identified a whole range of environmental and other public service issues that concerned them.

A radical shift towards **consumerism** was demonstrated in the 1990s in the field of health and social care, exemplified by the NHS and Community Care Act (1990) and the Department of Health's (1992) *Health of the Nation*. These policy documents state quite clearly that people providing services have a duty to consult fully with users and carers in the drawing up and monitoring of community care plans. More recently the government's policy report *Our Healthier Nation* (DoH 1998b) and the White Paper *The New NHS* (DoH 1997c) stress the importance of patient-centred care and the involvement of the public in planning local services. This has been reinforced in the *NHS Plan* (DoH 2000).

The Carers' (Recognition and Services) Act 1995 and the subsequent *National Carers' Strategy* (DoH 1999a) endorse the right of carers to a separate assessment of their own needs. Proposed new legislation will entitle carers to services in their own right. This further strengthens the need for services to involve carers in shaping the developments that will be of direct benefit to them, while at the same time consulting directly with people with disabilities.

The development of independent advocacy has gradually gained strength since the 1970s although it has not received statutory backing, despite attempts to give people with disabilities a right to representation within the Disabled Persons (Services, Consultation and Representation) Act 1986. However, the importance of access to independent advocacy has been recognized in a plethora of central government health and community care guidance documents (for example Home Office and DoH 2000). Access to advocacy is also encouraged by the government's Better Government for Older People initiative and *Social Inclusion Strategy* (Scottish Office 1999). Advocacy services have been most highly developed in the mental health and learning disability fields, but access to advocacy for people with dementia remains a problem in most areas. In Scotland, the health department has issued guidance to health boards and their planning partners on the development of independent advocacy schemes in their areas. These services have to be in place by December 2001. However, the services will be generic and authorities may have to be persuaded that specialist input for people with dementia and for carers is necessary (Killeen 1996).

While the consumer movement has gained in strength and momentum, the involvement of people with dementia is far from an established norm. Public consultation exercises on health and community care issues are predominantly targeted to local and national organizations representing the interests of people with dementia and their carers. Only a few initiatives have directly involved people with dementia. It is useful to look at why this has been the case in order to identify barriers that can be removed.

THE SERVICE CONTEXT

Barriers to change

The barriers to involving people with dementia in developing services to meet their needs include: ill-informed attitudes about the abilities of people with dementia to express valid opinions; lack of knowledge and training; lack of dedicated dementia service planning groups; poor multi-agency joint working; inadequate provision of specialist dementia care services; little research into service effectiveness from the perspective of people with dementia and their carers; lack of dedicated resources to involve people with dementia in planning and developing local services. Examples of good practice are beginning to emerge but progress is very variable across the UK.

Attitudes

A culture of **paternalism**, particularly in relation to people with dementia, has predominated within the health and social care professions until recent years. This is seen, for example, in medical attitudes to telling people their diagnosis. The tendency towards paternalism also persists within social care and appears to be primarily influenced by the issue of responsibility and risk. A paternalistic approach may place independence and choice in jeopardy and shift the focus of attention away from the rights of the individual.

However, these attitudes are balanced by a growing appreciation that early psychosocial interventions are worthwhile (Mittleman and Ferris 1996; Brodaty *et al.* 1997; Moniz-Cook and Woods 1997). Multidisciplinary diagnostic, assessment and support services, which provide pre- and post-diagnostic coun-selling, emotional support, rehabilitation and carer training, are well placed to empower people with dementia. This can enable people with dementia not only to make plans for their own lives, but also to have their say about the types of service that they would find useful immediately and in the future.

The movement for change

There has been a growing groundswell of understanding about the nature of dementia and how negative attitudes and behaviour in the community have served to disempower people with dementia. Campaigning by organizations such as Scottish Action on Dementia (now Alzheimer Scotland-Action on Dementia) and the Alzheimer's Disease Society (now Alzheimer's Society) in the mid-1980s and the work of the Dementia Services Development Centre movement which began in the late 1980s has contributed to the change. This has promoted a social model of care and created an appreciation of the need for 'person-centred' services that reflect the views and wishes of the individual.

Over that period we have learnt how the environment and the way in which we communicate disempowers people with dementia and what we need to do to remove the barriers we have constructed. We have learnt that people in the advanced stages of dementia have the ability to communicate what they think and feel (for further discussion see Chapters 5 and 9).

Understanding the balance of power

What can we learn from other fields about effective user involvement in de-mentia care planning and development? A major lesson concerns the balance of power. In the past those with the resources have set the agenda and how it is managed. Service users and carers have been expected to fit into fairly bureaucratic planning structures in which they have felt disempowered and from which they have received little or no information about how their views have influenced developments. As service users and carer groups have become more organized they have begun to set the agenda and terms for negotiating rather than simply responding to invitations from providers.

As Barnes and Wistow (1992a) observe, this indicates a wider shift in thinking about relationships between those who provide and those who receive services. They look at the potential implications of the shift in professional–client rela-tionships, not only for those previously excluded from decision making, but also for those who feel that their professional competence is being scrutinized. Barnes and Wistow stress the importance of professional–client relationships being regarded as creative rather than confrontational and the need for new sets of skills and new ways of working. They emphasize that the benefits of this new type of relationship need to be realized at a system level so that there can be generalized learning for effective partnerships between users and providers.

An example of a strategic approach to changing attitudes and promoting better understanding and communication between service users, carers and professionals in the mental health field is a project called Allies for Change. This project has focused on joint training for users, carers and professionals. In this project cognitive impairment is not a significant factor and any similar venture to involve people with dementia would require close attention to methods of communication and use of language.

But more than this is needed to shift the balance of power. A fundamental shift is required which would make resources available to enable people with dementia to learn how to use the unique knowledge that they have to inform policy makers, planners and providers. People with dementia, particularly those in the early stages, will have the capacity, with support, to set the agenda and the terms on which they will meet service providers. The expectation that people with dementia, or their carers, will fit into established patterns and ways of proceeding is not realistic.

EFFECTIVE INVOLVEMENT

What is meant by effective involvement? For the person with dementia and their carer it may mean that their views have been sought, listened to and acted upon. For planners it may mean that over 100 people turned up to a public meeting or filled in questionnaires. For both groups it may mean the establishment of an ongoing relationship with a two-way system of feedback about plans and service developments.

Involvement versus consultation

One-off consultation meetings, questionnaires or focus groups are limited forms of involvement from which participants may or may not receive feedback on the impact of their views. It could be argued that such consultation exercises do not constitute 'involvement', which requires a commitment of time and resources by providers to find more meaningful and ongoing ways of learning from service users and carers about the quality and types of services most appropriate to their needs.

Dick and Cunningham (2000) define effective involvement as a process, and not as one-off events, although such events can be part of the process. Their study looks at the involvement of people with learning disabilities in supported accommodation. Dick and Cunningham argue that the concept of involvement as a process is particularly important where people have not been accustomed to making decisions and where life experiences, including experiences of care, have discouraged involvement. They describe the process of becoming involved as 'a cumulative one, where the experience of influencing a decision in one area may lead to greater self-determination in others and new opportunities to express opinions may lead to greater confidence to do so in other situations' (p. 27).

From the start of any programme of user/carer involvement, a clear understanding of objectives and shared expectations is essential. This requires time to be taken to provide information for users and carers and to involve them in the process of planning any consultation exercise. While people with dementia will have had a lifetime of making decisions, the disease process and service responses leave many feeling deskilled and lacking in confidence. In designing any programme to facilitate the involvement of service users and carers it is important to be clear about who is to be involved and why, then to work out with them what resources they need to aid full participation.

The five core components for effective user involvement identified by Dick and Cunningham (2000) are applicable to people with dementia. These are:

- having the information needed in order to become involved;
- knowing what the options and choices are;
- feeling free to express views and wishes;
- being listened to and understood and having views respected and heard;
- being able to influence what happens and make decisions that matter.

Objectives for involvement

The objectives for involving service users may be categorized in terms of the contribution they can make to:

- developing services which are more sensitive to the needs of users by working with service commissioners;
- identifying gaps in services for strategic and locality planning purposes;
- assessing quality of service and the development of good practice;
- evaluating a specific service;
- developing new services;
- empowering users both in respect of control over services they receive (including a potential role in management) and their own lives more generally.

Only a few studies have evaluated the involvement of service users and carers. Barnes and Wistow (1992a) identified the following benefits from their evaluation of service user and carer participation in community care planning in Birmingham: the recognition and valuing of individual worth; collective expression of solidarity; improved information and expertise; some service improvements. They also found significant developments in the relationships between users and providers with regard to sharing information, a sense of working together and mutual trust. It is important to recognize these 'process' outcomes which contribute to sustaining user involvement in service development.

Representation

It is worth mentioning the issue of '**representation**' which Barnes and Wistow (1992b) address in their study. They identified two major difficulties which representation presents for planners: the practicalities of making contact with people normally excluded from the decision-making process, and the weight to be placed on the views of people who have not been nominated to speak on behalf of a larger group. These concerns need not be a problem if there is clarity about objectives. For example, in a carer consultation programme, service providers and carers themselves may be concerned about the carers' status as 'representatives'. This concern may centre on different concepts. It may be concern about whether the carers represent the characteristics of a larger population of carers in terms of a set of agreed characteristics. There is no requirement of 'accountability' within this concept. It may, however, be related to accountability and whether the carers are able to represent the views of others. This would require a mechanism for referring back to a wider network of carers (discussed later in relation to carers' groups and panels). The approach taken to addressing the 'representation' issue will depend on the nature and objectives of the involvement programme.

ENABLING SERVICE USERS AND CARERS TO PARTICIPATE EFFECTIVELY

Access

Factors including culture, geography, gender, age and socio-economic circumstances of potential participants should be taken into account in designing a programme for involving any group of people with dementia and their carers. The development of such a programme would be best informed by input from local organizations directly involved with the service user and carer groups to be targeted.

A review by Thornton and Tozer (1994) of different initiatives for involving older people showed that many operated in isolation from other similar projects so there was no shared learning about the most effective ways of working. Approaches to involvement often appeared to be adopted without first exploring the preferences of the service users to be 'involved'. Thornton and Tozer also found that options for involvement were usually limited to a single approach, for example through regular consultation with a forum for older people thus excluding the views of people who were housebound. It is also unusual for initiatives to evaluate their impact or acceptability to participants. More sensitivity to service user requirements will be achieved where users themselves are involved in planning how they can contribute.

Information and skills development

People with dementia and their carers, like other user groups, need accessible information about community care services and about planning mechanisms; they also need the opportunity to develop skills so that they can participate effectively. Involvement is subjective – we need to know when carers and people with dementia 'feel' involved and what helps nurture this feeling of involvement.

Practical help

It is important that people with dementia, at whatever stage, feel competent to contribute meaningfully. Some attention will need to be given to the sort of practical help they might need and would feel acceptable. It would be essential to discuss this with them. It might be anticipated that memory aids such as small tape recorders, invaluable to most professionals, would be equally useful to service users to record and play back their views and to record meetings. Appropriately designed visual aids may also be helpful.

INVOLVING PEOPLE WITH DEMENTIA IN SERVICE DEVELOPMENT

To improve the quality of life for people with dementia it is essential to accept that they have a voice, to facilitate it and hear it.

Service providers may involve people with dementia as a means to achieving a variety of service objectives. Depending upon their objectives they will have to use a range of methods and techniques if they are to involve people with dementia effectively. These objectives, methods and techniques are summarized in Table 18.1.

Examples of services involving people with dementia are as yet limited. Peer groups of people with dementia and their carers who initially met together for social activities and companionship have been known to turn to campaigning. One such group invited local politicians to meet to talk about the need for services for people in the early and later stages of the illness. They involved the media and achieved good coverage in the local press. Staff supporting such groups need to be alert to the potential for such activity.

The majority of older community care users, either carers or people with dementia, are not members of a social club or self-help group, but comparatively little attention has been given to extending opportunities for involvement to these individuals in their own homes. Contact with service providers in the home is both a source of information and an opportunity for making views known. Indeed, it has been suggested that older people think that their views have been heard if they express them to service providers. There are few formal mechanisms for aggregating users' views via direct care providers in the statutory sector and the lack of recognition of the role of information provision in this context is a particular concern.

Some voluntary organizations providing home support services report that they rely on their home support staff to feed back the views of the older people they visit. In this way organizations are able to gain the views

Table 18.1 Involving people with dementia in service development

Service development objectives	Methods and techniques
Identify gaps in services for strategic plan/locality plan	Meetings with service user support groups and panels, on their own ground, using semi-structured interviews/questionnaires, use of tape recorder, visual aids
Identify priorities for development for strategic plan/locality plan	Semi-structured discussion with individuals, small groups, peer groups Use of visual aids
Improve responsiveness of current services	Conversational; semi-structured questionnaires. Use of visual aids
Improve hands-on quality of care	Feedback from individual service user via the service delivery system; input to training sessions
Monitor services and quality e.g. inspection	Membership of inspection team by persons with dementia with the use of the 'buddy' system; carer membership of team Feedback on service from individuals and groups, for example, residents' committee
Identify what type of service and delivery best supports the quality of life for people with dementia from their perspective and from the perspective of carers	Peer group project
Involvement in service management	Formation of formal organization managed by carers; representation on management by people with dementia

of those who are very unlikely to participate in any formal consultation process. Provider organizations may do this on a formal basis, for example using a semi-structured questionnaire with the older person every six months.

An initiative in Preston (Dabbs 1999) piloted a method of gaining the views of people with dementia with the objective of informing the future strategy and development of service provision. Unstructured tape-recorded interviews were held on a one-to-one basis. The interviews explored factors affecting social, emotional, physical and financial well-being. They were conducted at a time and place chosen by each person interviewed. The study identified specific recommendations for services, including the importance of companionship, choice of activity and basic health care. Dabbs concludes that the pilot stimulated interest and commitment by commissioners and service providers to develop more appropriate and effective services for people with dementia in Preston, not least by consulting them on a regular basis.

The involvement of people with dementia in inspection teams is a largely unexplored area. However, there is considerable potential for individuals or small groups of people with dementia to be engaged in visits to services to observe and comment on quality of care.

A new Glasgow-based project, 'Involving People with Dementia in Service Development', will use a range of methods to engage and sustain the interest of people with dementia in the development of local services. While there have been a number of one-off surveys to gain the views of people with dementia about services, there has been little work to support their involvement over a period of time. This innovative three-year project will work with several small groups of people with dementia in ways which are responsive to their concerns and using a variety of means of communicating their views to policy makers, planners and providers, including the use of video. It is hoped that those taking part in the project will actively encourage other people with dementia to become involved. Initial recruitment will be through memory clinics and projects for people in the early stages of dementia.

Involving people with dementia – some lessons from research

There is a new focus on the involvement of people with dementia in research related to the development of service provision (Cottrell and Schultz 1993; Keady 1996; Downs 1997; Woods 1997; Keady and Gilliard 1999). A growing number of small-scale research projects (for example Sperlinger and McAuslane 1993; Dabbs 1999; Keady and Gilliard 1999; Stalker *et al.* 1999a) have been conducted which provide evidence that people with dementia, at all stages of the illness, are capable of expressing their views about services. They also show that people with dementia have something important to say to those responsible for the quality and provision of services. For example, a recent study (Stalker *et al.* 1999a) involving people with learning difficulties and dementia showed that they were able to express clear preferences. On the basis of this small in-depth study researchers concluded

> that those involved needed to become more aware of this fact and more responsive to individual choices; that it may be helpful for professionals and carers to review their own behaviour and attitudes and how these may restrict the choices available to people.
>
> (Stalker *et al.* 1999a: 27)

Stalker *et al.* (1999b) have reviewed research that aimed to gain the perspective of the person with dementia. Their findings are instructive in relation to gaining the involvement of people with dementia in service development. For example, it has generally been assumed that methods for involving people with learning disabilities can be emulated for people with dementia but this assumption is challenged. Stalker *et al.* (1999b) draw comparisons between the methods that work for people with learning disabilities and those that work for people with dementia. They conclude that the significant difference is that people with dementia have skills, knowledge and experiences which are in the process of being diminished because of the disease process and because of the social constructs placed on people with dementia. People with dementia were once 'empowered' but are in the process of being 'disempowered' – unlike people with learning disabilities whose experience of life is hopefully being built up and their confidence encouraged. The key point is made that different methods and approaches are required for each group to take into account their different life experiences (although approaches need to be individualized in any case to take account of the person's cultural and educational background, and individual life experience).

Involving people in the early stages of dementia

Researchers have used a range of methods including small group discussions, informal conversations, and structured and semi-structured interviews to obtain the views of people in the early stages of dementia. Some examples are described below.

Group interviews with people with dementia about service use have been conducted by Bamford (1998) who argues in favour of this method as a non-threatening approach to getting information. The growing number of support groups for people with dementia may provide a ready-made focus for service planners who could explore with members how they might contribute to service developments. While closed groups may be perceived as elitist for other client groups, they are necessary for people with dementia to provide continuity, to build on the memory of what went before and on the understanding of how people in the group best communicate.

Murphy (1998) describes an evaluation of a drop-in centre for people with dementia which relied on conversations with them to elicit their views of services. Sperlinger and McAuslane (1993) used in-depth interviews in their pilot study of the views of service users with dementia in a London borough. They interviewed six people who were in the early stages of dementia and found four of the six had issues and concerns to which they wished to draw attention. Although many aspects of care were discussed it was the social aspects that were of greatest concern to the service users. They conclude that 'our experience suggests that generally people using these services have plenty to say . . . it is clear from the pilot study that it is possible to consult with some users of the dementia services in a meaningful way' (p. 4).

A study by Phair (1990) also describes the use of interviews with people using services at a centre. Phair showed that both the mentally alert and the mentally frail centre members were able to give their perceptions of the unit. She went on to stress the importance of gaining the views of those who were mentally confused because their perceptions were different from those of their carers and those providing the service.

Involving people with advanced dementia

Goldsmith (1996) interviewed a number of people with severe dementia. He concluded that it is possible to communicate with some of the people some of the time. The first challenge is to discover ways in which more people might be enabled to communicate more of the time. The second challenge is to act on what is communicated. The first challenge is more important because it is one of attitude – it involves believing that communication is possible to a much later stage than had hitherto been thought. It is then important to devise services to meet the expressed needs of the people with dementia. This may mean occasionally adjusting services that were designed to meet the needs of people with dementia as perceived by other people. Hearing the views of people with dementia in the later stages can be a difficult and taxing job that requires time and resources.

To elicit the views of those in an advanced stage of dementia, Kitwood (1997c) proposed a seven-point strategy that includes:

- careful listening to what people say in some kind of interview or group;
- attending carefully to what they say in the course of the day;
- consulting people who have undergone an illness with dementia-like features;
- learning from observing their behaviour and reactions.

The conventional approach to conducting semi-structured interviews may need to be adapted in working with people with dementia. As Kitwood (1997c) suggests, it may be more appropriate to follow the person's lead rather than impose a structure on the conversation. Killick's (1994) work in long-stay environments provides an example of such an approach.

In conducting interviews with people with dementia, the following should be borne in mind:

- Questions in and of themselves can be threatening to someone with cognitive impairment.
- People with cognitive impairments function best in familiar surroundings.
- People with cognitive impairments can most easily comment on their immediate surroundings.
- People with cognitive impairments may need the aid of stimulus materials to discuss abstractions (cf. Bamford 1998).
- Family carers and staff may feel they need to be present, and this may influence the response.

INVOLVING CARERS IN SERVICE DEVELOPMENT

Carer involvement in developing services varies widely. It may mean membership of voluntary organizations that consult on local and national service development issues. It may mean closer involvement through input to purchasing, policy and planning processes established by local statutory authorities. Carers may have input to existing services through membership of advisory groups, management committees or through regular feedback and evaluations undertaken by services. Carers may have input to training for professional staff and to the evaluation of carer training. A number of approaches to carer involvement are discussed below.

Panels

Carer panels differ from support groups in that their objective is to influence local service developments. The panel approach involves recruiting a limited number of carers who meet regularly and set their own agenda. Groups are usually supported by paid workers. An example of this type of approach is described in Case Study 18.1.

Case study 18.1   A carer panel: Glasgow carers as capacity builders

This well-established panel, supported by Alzheimer Scotland – Action on Dementia, has been in operation for some years and has representatives on the main community care planning forums. Some individual members have gained bursaries from the City's millennium citizen participation programme and have been able to use that to the advantage of the whole group. The panel consults with other carers through a network of carer support groups and other community groups with shared interests. It also has an input to professional training programmes. Two members of the panel are members of Registration and Inspection teams. The panel has been a victim of its own success in terms of demands made upon it and the group has sought expert advice on how to manage its workload and involve more carers.

Case study 18.2   A carer panel – improving effectiveness

The carer panel in the Scottish Borders was keen to explore how it could be more effective in representing the views of carers to statutory bodies in the area. A full day session, attended by 15 carers, ended with the formation of an Action Plan. It was agreed to make a report of the points raised to inform local authority planners and also to invite local planners to meet with the panel to discuss the report. The panel requested involvement in drawing up the dementia service section of the new three-year community care plan and the Mental Health Framework plan. Consultation meetings have since been held with officials on these plans.

The project clearly demonstrated that carers of people with dementia are able to make a unique contribution to planning and improving services. However, a key lesson was that for such participation to be sustained, the support of a paid worker is essential.

Case study 18.3   Meeting carers' information and training needs

The Local Advocacy and Training Project in Scotland received funding for two years to increase the knowledge, skills and confidence of carers in campaigning and making effective representations to local authorities, health authorities and other agencies to improve services. The methodology was two pronged: the provision of training workshops for carers and the production of accessible information and briefings on community care and campaigning issues for use by carers of people with dementia across Scotland.

The workshops recognized the fact that people learn best from the starting points that relate to their own experiences. Training needs and community care issues were identified by participants at preliminary meetings. While there was much common ground, programmes were modified to relate to specific local issues raised by carers. Workshop planning meetings revealed that carers knew very little about community care and their rights under legislation, so this was the starting point.

A range of educational techniques were used including short formal presentations, working in small groups and the use of case examples of how others have worked successfully to influence services. Carers developed a detailed checklist designed to ease the task of analysing community care plans so that they could respond to consultation exercises. The checklist, *Whose Plan Is It Anyway? Getting Involved in Community Care Planning: A Guide for Carers and Carer Groups*, has been evaluated by other carers who have found it to be a very useful tool.

Meeting the information and training needs of carers

Training and information have been identified above as key ingredients for effective participation but there is no blueprint for how this might best be delivered. Case Study 18.2 provides an example of one approach that has proved successful.

Telephone conferencing

Telephone conferencing with carers has been a rewarding experience in some remote rural areas and where carers find it difficult to leave the house. It not only helps to reduce the sense of isolation many such carers feel, but provides concrete information and ideas about how needs can be met in the face of geographical barriers.

Carers as service providers

Service provision can be carer-led. The Dementia Care Initiative (DCI) is the name of a charitable organization managed by a board of trustees, all of whom are carers or ex-carers. They employ a coordinator and 120 staff who provide 200 care packages to people with dementia in their own homes and run six independent living houses. DCI grew from a carers' support group which started in 1987. Twelve members of this group became advisers to a pilot care management project set up in 1992 as a partnership project between health and social services. The service found it very difficult to meet the needs identified by carers and the carers themselves decided that, at the end of the pilot period, they would like to take over the organization and management of the service. Twelve carers became trustees in 1993 and the Dementia Care Initiative became recognized as a charity in 1994. The criterion for Trust membership is that the person must be a carer or an ex-carer.

CONCLUSION: ISSUES FOR IMPLEMENTATION

The importance of gaining the views of people with dementia has been highlighted by recent research into staff and carers' perceptions of the views of people with dementia (Phair 1990; Barnett 1996). These studies found that staff and carers' perceptions rarely reflected those expressed by people with dementia themselves. As a consequence, many of the aspects of services that were significant to people with dementia went completely unrecognized. This means that efforts made by staff and carers to improve the services would often be in vain, misdirected or irrelevant to people with dementia themselves. Consequently as Jacques and Jackson (2000) explain:

> both relatives and staff need constant reminders that the person with dementia can express choice, can be involved in decisions and generally can be an active participant in their own life. They need to be reminded that participation can bring enormous satisfaction to someone who fears that her [sic] competence is failing. They need to be reminded that rational disagreement is perfectly possible.
>
> (Jacques and Jackson 2000: 298)

Training

All those aiming to involve people with dementia need to improve their ability to communicate and listen if they are to ensure that the preferences of people with dementia are heard (for example Stokes and Goudie 1990; Goldsmith 1996). For further discussion about communication with people with dementia see Chapter 9.

We note above that the training and information needs of carers and people with dementia need to be recognized and met so that they can participate effectively. However, training or awareness raising is also essential for policy makers, planners and providers. They need to understand about the benefits of involving people with dementia and their carers in service developments affecting their care, not only to improve the quality of their lives, but also in terms of the provision of cost-effective services.

Recompense

There is a general expectation by statutory authorities that service users and carers will contribute their time freely and willingly; and mostly they do. However, consideration should be given not only to the payment of expenses but also to payment for the time spent in taking part. This will not always be appropriate. But where there is an individual engaged in a planning group working alongside paid professionals, it would be appropriate to pay a fee. This would overcome the sense that carers and users sometimes feel that they are taken for granted and that their contribution is undervalued compared with the views of the professionals.

Monitoring user and carer involvement

A Scottish initiative, described in Case Study 18.3, produced materials to enable carer panels/groups to monitor the involvement of carers of people with dementia within the community care planning process. Key questions identified were:

- Have separate planning arrangements been made for services for people with dementia and their carers?
- What representation of carers of people with dementia is there within the planning structure?
- How are people with dementia included in the consultation exercises?
- Are venues and times of day suitable for carers?
- Are alternative care arrangements offered so more carers can participate, including those who cannot attend meetings?
- Is adequate time allowed for participation?
- Is there a mechanism for providing feedback to participants?

Basic principles

The philosophy of normalization has been influential particularly in learning disability services (Wolfensberger 1972). It emphasizes the rights of people with disabilities and others with special needs to live ordinary lives. In the context of normalization philosophy, involvement in decision making about how to live one's life is seen as a right to be exercised by people with disabilities no less than their non-disabled counterparts. In line with this philosophy, this chapter concludes with a reminder of the key principles that should underpin the involvement of people with dementia and their carers in developing services:

- People with dementia and their carers have the same right as anyone else of access to public services.
- People with dementia and their carers have a right to services which are appropriate to their individual needs.

- People with dementia and their carers have the same right as anyone else to be consulted about services that directly affect the quality of their lives.

FURTHER READING

Ahlquist, L. (1997) *Empowerment in Action: Practising Empowerment*. Edinburgh: Age Concern Scotland, the Poverty Alliance and Greater Glasgow Health Board.

Allan, K. (2001) *Communication and Consultation: Exploring Ways for Staff to Involve People with Dementia in Developing Services*. Bristol: Policy Press.

Cheston, R., Bender, M. and Byatt, S. (2000) Involving people who have dementia in the evaluation of services: a review, *Journal of Mental Health*, 9(5): 471–9.

Jacques A. and Jackson G. (2000) *Understanding Dementia*, 3rd edn. Edinburgh: Churchill Livingstone.

Welsh Consumer Council (1990) *Putting People First. Consumer Consultation and Community Care*. Cardiff: Welsh Consumer Council.

19

CAROLINE CANTLEY AND GILBERT SMITH

Research, policy and practice in dementia care

KEY POINTS

- Research in dementia care should draw upon the full range of experimental, quantitative and qualitative methodologies.
- It is important to understand that research is only one of the many influences in the processes of policy development and implementation.
- We should aim for the development of dementia services to be soundly based in knowledge and research.

INTRODUCTION

This chapter is about policy implementation in dementia care and particularly the role of research in influencing policy and practice. The key point to the chapter is this. Practitioners (and indeed informal carers as well) frequently, and quite naturally, assume that what they do makes a difference. Their actions would indeed make little sense without that assumption. Nevertheless, a substantial amount of social science research has made it clear that a great deal of individual action has comparatively little effect in comparison with the impact of factors such as gender, age, family structure, socio-economics, politics and organizational constraints. At the very least it is essential to understand the way in which such factors shape the social environment in which individual practice takes place. The 'individual versus social' debate in science has generated much intellectual, and on occasions political, heat. But any insistence in the study of dementia care that we can find a valid knowledge-based approach to good practice solely by studying the social and policy context or solely by focusing on individual skills and actions would seriously oversimplify a complex debate.

So the question we shall explore is this. For individuals seeking to provide high-quality services in the fields of dementia care how may research contribute to the policy processes that provide the context in which they work? The question breaks down into several parts, particularly when we remember that the discussion in this chapter is directed towards the interests of practitioners themselves.

First, we shall consider the nature and types of research that are relevant to dementia care. In discussing these different methodologies we shall note the different basic assumptions and ideological frameworks upon which they are founded. Second, we examine current claims that are made of 'evidence-based' practice. Third, we will examine the role of research – however conducted – in the policy development and implementation process; for it would be simplistic indeed to assume that the process is entirely rational. In important ways it involves the exercise of influence and control by a range of interest groups. Finally, we shall take stock of this discussion in pointing to some of the issues that must be addressed if research in dementia care is to have a positive impact on service delivery.

RESEARCH DESIGN AND METHODOLOGY

It is beyond the scope of this chapter to provide a comprehensive overview of research design and methodological issues in dementia care. This section more simply examines some of the strengths and limitations of some key research designs and data collection methods as they might be applied to studies in dementia care.

Quantitative and experimental research

Much discussion about research in dementia care is predicated on the idea that investigations should be 'scientific'. This notion of 'scientific' research is generally taken to mean a particular class of investigation that resembles that which is found in the physical sciences. Here there is a clear formulation of the hypothesis, a notion of the **dependent and independent variable** and an ability to control a whole range of other variables such that the impact of factors in which the investigator has a particular interest can be isolated and understood. Such investigations are somehow (it is not always very clear just how or why) viewed as stereotypically (and by implication ideally) 'true science'.

For many researchers studying, for example, the efficacy of anti-dementia drugs, or the effectiveness of a therapeutic intervention in dementia care, the **experimental** model of research described above, in the form of the clinical trial, is regarded as the 'gold standard' of scientific investigation. Such researchers often take the view that any other kind of investigation lacks the rigour

Case study 19.1   An experimental research design in dementia care

McNamara and Kempenaar (1998) report plans for an experimental design to assess the effects of the use of sensory stimulation by therapists and carers of people with dementia living in the community. The study aims to include 26 clients in the experimental group and 26 in the control group which will receive no intervention. The study involves assessing the clients and carers at weeks 1 and 6 to establish baseline measures. The baseline includes measures of the client's cognitive and affective state and measures of the carer's level of well-being. A therapist will then undertake sensory work with each client in the experimental group over a period of eight weeks. Following this, clients and carers will be reassessed again using the baseline scales. The therapist will then teach the carers how to implement the sensory intervention. The carers will be asked to undertake the sensory intervention for 12 weeks after which there will be a further assessment of client and carer using the baseline scales.

necessary for definitive conclusions. They regard other kinds of investigation as either precursors to or deficient forms of the ideal scientific design. This stance is often described as the 'medical model' of research.

This 'medical model' of research is appropriate to the kinds of study we have mentioned above. Many examples of research that have used this type of methodology are reported in Chapter 10 and an example of this type of study is described in Case Study 19.1.

However, when applied more generally to service-related research, the medical model of research contains within it some very important errors and misunderstandings and is by no means the only way of establishing a sound knowledge base. It is therefore crucial that practitioners are aware of the fact that a rich variety of methodologies is available in the medical and social sciences and that the majority have something to offer practitioners as they seek to improve their practice.

It is also important to note at this point that debates about 'real science' and experimental design are often implicitly tied up with the notion that powerful research must involve high levels of quantification – or, at its crudest, that if you cannot count it, it is not worth knowing about. Research which does not assign precise numbers to variables may thus well be dismissed as elementary, imprecise, lacking rigour or even as 'merely social science'. The issue is important in the context of this book since such arguments – or prejudices (for often that is what they really are) – may lead practitioners to think that research should not be taken seriously unless it includes large numbers and statistical tests. Of course quantification *is* important in some areas of research; for example in establishing the prevalence of different types of dementia in a population or comparing the extent to which different groups of service users and carers make use of different types of services. Quantification should not however be an end in itself.

Adherence to the view that quantification should be a goal of research derives from a failure to be clear about the underlying status and nature of the social and medical phenomena with which we are concerned. It may sound simple but nevertheless it is important to stress that quantification is appropriate, first, only at the level at which the phenomena being measured can be quantified and, second, only if it serves the purpose for which the research is being conducted. Frequently in social life measurement is only justified at a nominal or ordinal level. At the nominal level, for example, numbers may be used to identify bedrooms in a home. But it makes no sense to say that room 2 plus room 4 is equal to room 6. At the ordinal level relatives may, for example, be able to place particular residential homes in order of preference without it being sensible to presume that the differences between one preference and another can be quantified so as to give any meaning to a total preference score. Inappropriate use of quantification not only constitutes poor science but can also obscure potentially valuable insights that could be gained from a more qualitative research approach.

One of the key challenges in dementia care research is to develop more appropriate outcome measures (Downs 1997). Nocon and Qureshi (1996: 149), in summarizing what is required for community care outcomes more generally, provide sound advice for dementia care researchers:

- The existence of different stakeholders should be explicitly recognized and incorporated into the work.
- The views of service users and their carers are of key importance.
- Professional expertise and research-based knowledge are both useful in constructing measures.
- An understanding of the context in which measures are to be implemented has an important bearing on their likely usefulness.

Limitations of the experimental model of research

The experimental model of research can be powerful in assessing cause and effect relationships between variables when the wider environment has no impact or can be controlled. However, this model of research cannot be transposed simply from the traditional concerns of medical research to wider service-related research. The reasons for this are several.

First, adherence to the medical model leads to research that is insensitive to the complexities of social life. In most social settings the full range of variables that potentially have some effect on the situation are so many and so complicated that the notion that any attempt could be made to control them in any systematic way is absurd. Even if it was technically possible to construct experimental or quasi-experimental tests (and in some particular contexts it is) there are a whole host of moral and political difficulties in actually achieving this in the real world. There is also the difficulty of change over time. Most social settings are not at all stable. So the complexities of the great plurality of variables are magnified substantially by the fact that the object of study and the environment in which those objects are located are themselves constantly variable.

There have been attempts to apply experimental designs which are sensitive to these issues. The danger, however, is that since the difficulties are so great the experimental approach frequently ends up forcing the object of study into the design rather than adapting the design to the social world in all its variety. Too often simplifying assumptions are made not because they are justified but because the design of the study would not be possible without them. That, unfortunately, is the wrong way round. Methodologies must adapt to the real world. Researchers cannot expect the real world to fit into their research design just because they would otherwise be presented with problems that they would find insurmountable.

Second, the view that research can only be 'scientific' if it is experimental neglects the importance of understanding the *processes* of social life. Even if we are able to establish reliably that a particular intervention is accompanied by particular consequences – for example that a particular design of residential accommodation appears to reduce the levels of stress of elderly residents – this is of only limited value to the practitioner if it is not understood *why* that occurs. Straightforward correlations, even if links can be drawn in a causal way (and that is really very difficult indeed), do not tell practitioners how and why the factors are associated with each other. Yet it is the 'how' and 'why' which are so important if research findings are to be of practical use in informing care strategies. Without that understanding practitioners would be operating in the dark, simply applying stimuli in a mechanical manner without being able to grasp why it was that what they were doing was of benefit. Such a stance would be unacceptable to most professionals as well as ineffective and potentially quite dangerous. Even the most rigorous experimental work thus needs to be complemented at the very least with research that describes the processes linking cause and effect.

So it is important to be aware of the limitations of what some would claim to be the gold standard of the experimental method or the clinical trial, but it is equally important to be aware of the power of such research designs where they can be justifiably employed. It is also important not to get locked into some dogmatic methodological position (not unknown in academia) which precludes the fruitful adaptation of a methodological design to the problem in hand.

Qualitative research

Methods

It is well beyond the scope of this chapter to give a full account of all qualitative methods of data collection but a brief overview is feasible. These methods fall into five main groups. They involve talking to people (interviews of various kinds and focus groups); watching and recording behaviour (observation); joining in activities (participation); reading and analysing written material (documentary analysis); and picking up on a whole range of signs and indications without disturbing the situation that is being researched (unobtrusive measures). Examples of research using qualitative methods in dementia care include studies that use:

- interviews to explore the experience of dementia from the perspectives of people with dementia and their carers;
- non-participant observation to describe daily life for people with dementia in different care settings;
- participant observation to describe aspects of care provision;
- focus groups with people with dementia to explore their views about services and how they would like to see services developed.

It is important to stress that data derived from this range of qualitative methods are not inferior to more quantified materials. They are different. Both qualitative and quantitative data can be precise or imprecise, accurate or inaccurate, meaningful or meaningless, revealing or confusing and based on legitimate or illegitimate methodological techniques. It is especially important not to fall into the trap of assuming that just because a high degree of skill in statistical technique is not required in conducting good qualitative research, it does not require high levels of research expertise at all. It does. It is also true that some of the skills of interviewing, observing, describing and analyzing documentary material have much in common with many of the skills of professional practice and may thus come more easily to those not experienced in research. However, the interaction between independent researchers and their research respondents is in important respects different from that between practitioners and their colleagues or service users. Having said that, there are some forms of reflective practitioner research in which the traditional boundaries between the roles of researcher and practitioner are blurred (see Chapter 6 for further discussion).

Research design in context

Qualitative research approaches are well suited to the circumstances in which research is often commissioned. (For we should never forget that research is an expensive business and generally needs a particular agency to provide funds in its support. It does not just happen in an ivory tower quite insulated from the political realities of resource allocation.) What often happens is this. A new programme, treatment or policy is introduced for some political or professional reason. A new kind of dementia care unit is established, perhaps, or a home attempts to introduce a new person-centred care planning approach, or professional responsibilities are altered in setting up a new community dementia care team. Policy makers and managers then require research to assess the change and report on the success or otherwise of the new measure. The demand for research is particularly likely if the new service is more expensive than the previous practice. (If the new measure has saved money, policy makers generally do not want to know if it has been successful or not. They would rather simply claim greater efficiency in a state of ignorance unencumbered by research evidence.) The policy makers or managers then commission researchers to conduct a study to evaluate the initiative and report on the lessons learned.

On the face of it the commissioning of evaluative research on new services is sensible. However, if we think about the comments that we have made so far in this chapter, there are usually some difficulties about the design of this research. Typically the evaluation is launched so late that it is impossible to collect data on what was happening before the change was introduced. Lots of other changes are also taking place at the same time so it is hard to determine the impact of one particular factor. Neither are the innovations themselves generally stable. Novel practices and services evolve as they are introduced. In these circumstances an evaluation following the experimental model of research is not feasible. However, a variety of study designs are nevertheless possible. We consider two approaches below: case studies and action research.

Case study research

Many lessons for practice and policy have been learned from single case studies of services. Here a detailed account of the service intervention is assembled from the perspectives of those involved. This **ethnography** often spans a considerable period of time. On the basis of the ethnography, judgements are made about the progress of the initiative and the effect that it has had. There is a degree of subjectivity involved in such judgements. But all data, not just qualitative data, are in some ways subjective; the experimental researcher, for example, makes judgements about the choice of relevant variables and how they will be measured. The important factor in qualitative research is that subjectivity in data collection and analysis is dealt with explicitly as an integral aspect of the research design.

Qualitative case studies can produce a detailed and informative account of a service that is not otherwise available. Conclusions about the service can then be reached in a variety of ways. For example, a study of a residential home might include looking at the impact of a new management style on the life of the home. Interviews with staff might confirm that this new management style includes greater emphasis on staff spending time in meaningful interaction with residents with dementia. Observation of the life of the home could then help us to understand how staff put this new approach into practice. But it might also alert us to other changes in the life of the home. For example, qualitative observations might show that changes in staff interactions with residents were associated with changes in the way staff interact with each other and perhaps also changes in the way residents with dementia interact with each other.

As mentioned above, the case study approach is also important in service evaluation. A number of approaches to evaluation using qualitative research methodologies have been described (Murphy *et al.* 1998). Smith and Cantley

---

Case study 19.2   A multiple case study research design in dementia care

---

The evaluation of the Mental Health Foundation's Dementia Advice and Support Service uses a multiple case study design to assess the operation of a number of pilot services nationally. In each location the pilot services offer people with dementia, and their carers, befriending, advice and help in accessing existing services; other services are also offered in some pilot sites to fit local needs and circumstances. The evaluation of the Mental Health Foundation's scheme involves a case study in each location. The data collection in each location is mainly qualitative and involves interviews, focus groups, telephone interviews and records analysis. There is also some quantitative data collection, for example on numbers of referrals to and from the pilot services. The case study approach ensures that the research captures the variety of experiences in the different pilot sites, but the research also looks across the case studies to learn the wider lessons of the scheme as a whole.

(1985) make the case for 'pluralistic evaluation' which involves assessing the success of a service on the range of criteria that are variously identified and pursued by different interest groups. Smith and Cantley (1985) have demonstrated the application of pluralistic evaluation in the context of a detailed case study of a day hospital for older people with mental health problems.

We can also learn from research that involves multiple case studies. An example of this type of research in dementia care is described in Case Study 19.2. And finally we should note that while case studies very often involve mainly qualitative data collection methods, they may also use quantitative methods, either alone or in combination with qualitative approaches. For fuller discussion of case study research see Yin (1994).

In an important sense the case study approach systematizes the way in which we learn from innovation as a regular part of professional life. But we need not be apologetic about that. Nor need this method of accruing knowledge about service development be regarded as any the less 'scientific' in consequence.

Action research

Another qualitative research approach of particular value in the context of service development is 'action' research. The term is often used in a rather casual and imprecise way simply to refer to research which is taking place in a rapidly changing environment and in which the researchers try to track this change usually by employing a range of qualitative methods. At its most rigorous, however, there is more to action research than this.

Although there are a variety of models of action research (see Hart and Bond 1995), action research essentially involves studies that do not insist on drawing a clear distinction between the 'action' providing the service and the 'research' examining the service. Rather, the research designs seek to capitalize

---

Case study 19.3   An action research project in dementia care

A social services department commissioned a two-year action research project to develop care planning in two residential homes for older people. The researcher used a variety of data collection methods (interviews, focus groups, observations and records analysis) to develop a picture of care planning in the broader context of the life of the home. This picture was shared with staff and managers and was used to inform the development work. The researcher worked with staff to develop and test out a range of approaches to improving care planning. This included life story work, 24-hour diaries, activity diaries, interviews with family members, staff discussions about individual residents, and review of existing care planning documentation. The impact of the various developments was assessed, again using a variety of data collection methods, and the findings shared with staff and managers as part of the continuous action research process of enquiry, intervention and review.

---

upon a set of practical, methodological and political factors that from the point of view of researchers seeking to mimic the experimental method would be a severe embarrassment. Unlike experimental studies that seek to maintain as much control and stability as possible over the independent variables, the methodology of action research seeks to achieve almost the direct opposite. Action research does not seek to avoid the researchers contaminating, or having an impact on, the service that is being studied. Nor do the researchers refrain from expressing views and making judgemental statements until the conclusion of the project. Rather, the key point about action research is that it is seen as a continuous learning process – for both the research and the action. Initial findings are not just fed back. They are *tested*. For the 'action', practice is modified to see if new ways of doing things are more effective than the old in the light of research findings. For the 'research', there is the chance to see, by putting the implications of understanding into practice, whether or not understanding is correct. In this way, it is hoped, knowledge is advanced and practice is improved. The development of research and its implementation in policy and practice are thus closely entwined. (We shall return to this later in the chapter.) Case Study 19.3 provides an example of action research in dementia care.

It will be apparent from this description of action research that not only is the process of the research very different from that of the experiment or the clinical trial, but also that the types of data that are collected are likely (but not absolutely necessarily) to be very different. An exploration of the processes of change and a descriptive understanding of practice regimes or the effects of a particular policy can seldom be captured in measurement techniques rooted in high levels of quantification. In order to convey meaning and understanding, data that reflect qualitative as well as the quantitative aspects of the phenomena under review will be required.

EVIDENCE-BASED PRACTICE

In the field of health and social care the concept of 'evidence-based practice' is relatively novel. In these fields the authority of the professions has long been at least a partial substitute for science, with the result that many practices have been of dubious value and a significant proportion have undoubtedly done more harm than good. Why some professions should enjoy such authority while others (such as engineers) do not is a question for the history and sociology of the professions that is beyond the scope of this chapter. The point of note here is that recently from within the field of medicine there has developed a 'movement' (far and away the best term for describing briefly what is happening) devoted to advancing the cause of evidence-based practice. The essence of the approach is that when the patient says, in effect, 'Why should I accept that advice?', the legitimate reply should be not, 'Because I say so' but, 'Because that is the conclusion that we draw from the evidence.'

The most widely accepted definition of evidence-based medicine (EBM) comes from Sackett et al. (1997: 2): 'The practice of evidence-based medicine means integrating individual clinical expertise with the best available external evidence from systematic research.' The authors argue that it is the responsibility of the profession therefore to identify information needs, track down the best evidence, appraise this evidence, apply the results and evaluate performance.

Such an approach moves a long way towards the idea that professional practice should be science-based. The concept of external evidence from systematic research is a powerful one. Important features of the scientific model are apparent here with clear importance placed upon the rationality of a process which links evidence to good practice. And there is also the assumption here that science (research) will make a difference. Like many theories of the advancement of knowledge, underlying the approach is the implicit view that the growth of western scientific knowledge will make a difference to practice and service delivery and that this change process is inevitably beneficial.

Yet, despite these powerful arguments, evidence-based practice is proving to be difficult to achieve. There is a growing literature on how to encourage greater implementation of EB practice (see for example, Oxman et al. 1995; Kitson et al. 1998; Wye and McClenahan 2000). We can suggest a number of factors that contribute to the problems of achieving evidence-based practice, particularly as they affect dementia care.

First, the approach taken to persuading practitioners of the merits of EB practice and teaching them how to implement it, is somewhat individualistic. It substantially neglects the social and policy context in which practice takes place. We noted in Chapter 15, for example, how the different professions in dementia care are underpinned by different knowledge bases. These knowledge bases will inevitably impact on the way the professions respond to evidence-based practice. As Fitzgerald et al. (1999) point out: 'Perceptions of evidence vary by specialty, by profession and by individual . . . There is no one accepted view of "evidence"; individuals and groups strongly defend their versions of reality' (p. 204).

Second, the scientific model of evidence-based practice can only succeed when there is clear evidence to inform professional decision making. But it is apparent throughout this book that in many areas of dementia care definitive evidence is not currently available (cf. Briggs and Askham 1999).

Third, evidence-based practice assumes that, even if our knowledge is currently inadequate, science will eventually provide the answers to the questions that face practitioners in their everyday dealings with service users and carers. But in areas like dementia care this fails to take account of the way in which many crucial decisions in practice involve difficult value judgements. This is highlighted in Chapter 6 in discussing the development of an evidence-based approach to managing continence in people with dementia.

Fourth, there are risks that over-simplistic application of an evidence-based approach will have the effect of deskilling practitioners. Thus, for example, we see how the Cochrane review (Spector *et al.* 1999b) demonstrates the lack of evidence to support the effectiveness of reminiscence therapy and highlights the need for further research. But that is not the same thing as saying that this therapeutic approach has no value. Practitioners need to consider evidence in broad context and make practice decisions accordingly.

Fifth, evidence-based practice sits uneasily alongside professional dominance. The introduction of 'evidence' potentially reduces this dominance since professional judgement can now be challenged on the basis of data and conclusions to which professionals, clients and other professionals alike have access. Thus in medicine, where the introduction of EB practice has been most developed, we see much debate about the role of 'clinical expertise' and whether professionals should retain the right of final decision over patient treatment, particularly if their views run counter to the best available evidence.

Sixth, many social scientists would argue that the whole notion of science-based professional practice is massively over-rationalistic in that it neglects the complex set of policy and social variables that are a part of the context in which clients are provided with support and services. In the remaining part of this chapter we shall therefore turn, as we have previously indicated, to consider the impact of the policy implementation process and the power of a range of different groups within this process.

RESEARCH AND THE POLICY PROCESS

As we indicated at the start of this chapter it is always important to remember that dementia services are provided within a policy and organizational context. There are national and local policies. There are the resources that is takes to provide a service. There is the setting within which the service is sited. There are the human resources: the recruitment, training, supervision, regulation and authorization of staff. For many services there is also a basis of legislation, sometimes quite complex. There are, too, for example, the rules and other factors governing the interaction between agencies within and across different service sectors.

Chapter 14 outlines recent themes in the development of policy relevant to the care of people with dementia and their carers. In this chapter we are more concerned to highlight the process through which that policy is formed and implemented. For, again, rationalist accounts have dominated sections of the literature. But there are weaknesses in such accounts of which it is important to be aware if practitioners are to understand the way in which the links between research, policy and the practices of care are shaped.

Typically a rationalist account of policy making runs like this. Issues of public concern are raised in a variety of ways: through the press, by pressure groups, by professional associations and so on. Suggestions are put forward in the form of policy statements to solve these problems. If necessary there is a political process leading to legislation. The new policy is then implemented and under the best of circumstances also evaluated. On the basis of the evaluation, improvements can be made either in the methods of implementation or perhaps in some features of the policy itself if it is found to be particularly weak. This is essentially a 'top-down' model of the translation of policy into practice. In the light of the recent emphasis on evidence-based policy making and service provision, a rational model presumes that significant research results would be brought to bear on the process, particularly at the stage of formulating the problem and evaluating the effectiveness of the implemented measures.

Many practitioners, through reflecting on their experiences of being part of the policy process, will be aware of some of the weaknesses of a purely rational model as a way of understanding policy development and implementation.

First, in spite of the emphasis on the importance of a knowledge-based service, such an ideal is seldom realized. The use of research to inform policy debates, to inform policy formulation and legislation, and to inform implementation and service delivery, is seldom as systematic as the rational model implies. Often the research is not available. Where it has been conducted it may not have been systematically reviewed and presented in such a way as to make it usable. Or it may simply be ignored by those whose interests are not served by paying attention to it. Or it may form one consideration in a complex process alongside other factors such as experience, political pressures and political judgements. Or its conduct may be used as a delaying tactic or as a means of enhancing status through academic associations (cf. Weiss 1986).

Second, as we noted above and in Chapter 15, interest group (sometimes called stakeholder) activity is a significant component of all aspects of organizational life and service provision. Some professional groups are more powerful than others for a whole host of reasons. Different groups are able to wield very different levels of economic power. Different groups have varying political significance. These and other differences have long been recognized in the political science literature as being of major importance.

Third, a rational account of policy making has an important weakness in that it pays insufficient attention to the ambiguities of policy and the different meanings that can be assigned to a particular policy objective. Most social organizations have multiple, conflicting and changing goals. Students of organizations have long been aware of that (see Chapter 15). The same is true of social policies. For example the policy objective of, say, improving the care of older people with dementia will clearly be interpreted very differently depending upon the particular approach that is taken to a definition of what constitutes high-quality care. Even a quite specific objective, like opening a new day hospital for older people with mental health problems, can be interpreted very differently by the different groups involved in the initiative (Smith and Cantley 1985). Thus what the policy is intended to achieve becomes a matter of interpretation and practitioners may well find themselves a part of this defining process during the course of their work.

One alternative to the rational model of the policy process is the incremental model which views policy making and implementation much more as a process of trial and error in which progress is made in small stages rather than in accord with some grand policy plan. This model takes greater account of 'bottom-up' influences on policy and of the ongoing processes of negotiation through policy development and implementation. Hill (1997) provides an overview of theoretical perspectives on the policy process and Harrison (1996) explores the implications of different 'top-down' and 'bottom-up' assumptions for the implementation of research and development findings.

Thus, as we have sought to examine some of the relationships between policy, research and the practice of dementia care, the variable power positions of different groups of professionals, service users, carers, politicians and researchers, among others, have repeatedly featured as significant.

CONCLUSION: ISSUES IN RESEARCH IN DEMENTIA CARE

This chapter has described different research methodologies and commented on basic assumptions and ideologies that underpin them. We have examined the way in which research is but one component in a complex policy process. We conclude with five observations.

First, we note that research in dementia care raises some complex ethical issues, particularly in relation to the ability of people with dementia to give informed consent to participating in research. These ethical issues are discussed in Chapter 13.

Second, the different research approaches described in this chapter tend to sit more or less comfortably with different theoretical disciplines and hence also, to a large extent, with different professions. This has important implications for research in dementia care which we would argue, by its nature, should increasingly involve working across disciplinary, professional and agency boundaries.

Third, there are differences between service sectors in dementia care in the extent to which they have a culture of using and doing research. This is related to different levels of access to research findings, research funding, research expertise and research training. Again these differences have implications for research that involves work across sector boundaries.

Fourth, we draw attention to the ways in which different research designs and methodologies may be more or less appropriate for research which has different purposes. These purposes can be thought of as ranging along a continuum from 'curiosity-driven' academic research at one end to applied research commissioned by service organizations at the other end. It is important that dementia care research, no matter where it sits along this continuum, is high-quality research. But this must involve the notion of 'fitness for purpose'. Thus as Booth (1988) argues:

> Good policy research must aim to be useful, understandable, relevant, timely and practical. Technical adequacy alone does not ensure usefulness; usefulness cannot be taken for granted. It has to be planned for and built into the design of studies as an essential aspect of their methodology.
>
> (Booth 1988: 251)

Finally, we have commented on arguments in favour of evidence-based practice. We have expressed caution about adopting too narrow an approach. But this caution should not detract from the challenge of ensuring that decisions about service provision have a sound basis in knowledge and research.

FURTHER READING

Abbott, P. and Sapsford, R. (1998) *Research Methods for Nurses and the Caring Professions*, 2nd edn. Buckingham: Open University Press. For an introduction to using and doing research.

Baker, M.R. and Kirk, S. (1998) *Research and Development for the NHS: Evidence, Evaluation and Effectiveness*, 2nd edn. Abingdon: Radcliffe Medical Press. For discussion of a range of research and development issues in health care.

Bond, J. and Corner, L. (2001) Researching dementia: are there unique methodological challenges for health services research?, *Ageing and Society*, 21: 95–116.

Ham, C. and Hill, M. (1993) *The Policy Process in the Modern Capitalist State*, 2nd edn. London: Harvester Wheatsheaf. For an introduction to policy development and implementation.

CAROLINE CANTLEY

Conclusion: the future development of dementia care

DEMENTIA AS A SOCIAL PROBLEM

Dementia is a significant social problem. The processes by which issues become identified and treated as social problems rather than as private troubles are complex (see for example Manning 1985). Gubrium (1986) has described the social construction of the problem of Alzheimer's disease in the United States. Although it is beyond the scope of this conclusion to provide a detailed analysis of the processes by which dementia has become a social problem, we can identify a number of contributory and interrelated factors. These factors include:

- growth in the number of people with dementia;
- the 'structured dependency' of older people in our society;
- fears that families are becoming less willing and able to provide care;
- the emergence of carers as a social and research issue (and with this, the recognition of the particular problems of carers of people with dementia);
- the emergence and growth of pressure groups such as Alzheimer's Society focusing on dementia;
- the prospect of solutions to the problem in the form of biomedical 'golden bullets' and new approaches to care;
- growth in academic interest as dementia increasingly becomes a fertile field of research for biomedical and social science;
- the promotion of new approaches to care through initiatives such as Dementia Services Development Centres;
- growing professional interest as specialist knowledge is identified and offers a source of professional expertise and status;
- higher media profile related to new treatments and potential cures;
- higher media profile from celebrities 'going public' about having dementia;

- the commercial interests of drug companies in establishing the need for new treatments;
- growing public awareness as a result of the above and as more people have personal contact with someone with dementia;
- increased attention in national policy discussions as attention is focused on the 'knock-on' effects of dementia on health services more generally, for example through people with dementia 'blocking' acute beds;
- fears about the resource implications of providing new treatments and long-term care.

Our views of the nature of the problem of dementia care and solutions to that problem are by no means static. Changes in the wider social and service contexts of dementia care will have a big impact. We can seldom accurately predict the extent or timing of change; but we can anticipate broadly the types of changes that will be significant. These changes include:

- demographic changes that will affect not only the proportion of older people in our society but also, more specifically, the numbers of people with dementia from minority ethnic communities and from other groups with special needs;
- social changes in family patterns, employment patterns, and social and geographical mobility that will affect people who have dementia and those who provide care;
- changing expectations of people with dementia and their carers as population cohorts with different life experiences age;
- advances in diagnostic techniques and in drug treatments;
- advances in genetics that may provide options for prevention as well as new forms of treatment;
- advances in information technology that will increase public access to specialist knowledge and change the practice of health and social care professionals;
- advances in technology that will make 'smart' environments more sophisticated and more widely available;
- changes in the organizations that deliver dementia care, especially growth in the influence of primary care and new arrangements for integrated provision of health and social care;
- changes in the configuration of the professions in response to growing demands for working across traditional boundaries;
- the impact of the recent Human Rights Act legislation and other reforms in legislation covering the way we deal with mental incapacity (for example DoH 2000b);
- economic changes, with varying levels of growth and prosperity affecting how we individually and as a society respond to meeting the care needs of people with dementia.

In looking to the future, we need to take account of the long-term effects of current policies and ways of doing things. Evandrou (1998) argues that in developing social policies for older people we need an approach that combines two things: planning across different areas such as income support, housing, health and social care; and planning that takes account of the impact of policies over the individual's lifetime. Current employment and pension policies, for example, will shape the experience of older people, including those with dementia, for many decades to come. We need, therefore, to begin now to think about the foundations we are laying for care of people with dementia well into the future.

CONCEPTUAL FRAMEWORKS

This book has shown how a very wide range of conceptual frameworks is relevant to understanding dementia and to developing dementia care. These frameworks include: biomedicine, psychology, sociology, philosophy and theology, practice development theory, ethics, social policy, organization and management theory, research and the perspectives of people with dementia and their carers. Other frameworks for thinking about dementia, for example law and epidemiology, have been mentioned although detailed discussion has been beyond the scope of this book. We can, however, identify three additional frameworks with significant growing influence in dementia care: anthropology, economics and the arts. They should not pass without comment, even if only briefly.

We know relatively little about how dementia is experienced and understood in cultural context, particularly in non-Western cultures (Ineichen 1998). Pollit (1996) argues that anthropological perspectives and cross-cultural research have an important contribution to make. For western societies this type of research can increase awareness of the cultural content of our assumptions about old age and the disorders of old age. It can also help us to view critically our approaches to treatment and care by allowing us to see them reflected back from a different cultural perspective.

The economics of dementia care is reviewed by Wimo *et al.* (1998). Understanding the costs of dementia is complex. There are considerable personal costs as well as financial costs to the state, and to individuals and their families (Bosanquet *et al.* 1998; Knapp and Wigglesworth 1998). Increasingly policy makers want decisions about service provision to be informed by cost data. Knapp and Wigglesworth (1998) point to a number of areas in which economic research might inform dementia service planning, particularly since there is evidence of links between costs and cognitive function in both community and institutional settings. So, for example, they suggest that economic evaluation can contribute to assessing the impact of the new anti-dementia drugs or to establishing the most appropriate care settings for people with dementia who need multiple care inputs. But as Knapp and Wigglesworth stress, it is important to look at costs across the full range of services and informal provision and to act to ensure that costs are not simply shifted from one part of a system to another. Additionally, they are cautious about taking too narrow a view of costs:

Focusing simply on the *costs* of community-based care is not enough, for the outcomes achieved from these costs must also be taken into account ... there could be a strong case for *increasing* expenditure on a particular dementia patient or group of patients if the benefits in terms of health status and quality of life are substantial.

(Knapp and Wigglesworth 1998: 241)

From a very different stance, the arts can contribute to dementia care in a variety of ways (see for example Pickles 1997; Batson 1998; Perrin 1998; Hill 1999; Killick and Allan 1999; Allan and Killick 2000). We have visual, literary, dramatic and documentary representations of the experience of dementia and of caring for people with dementia. We have different types of art therapy being used with people with dementia (for example music, painting and dance). We have the use of the arts as a means of giving people with dementia opportunities for self-expression and more generally for enhancing the quality of their lives; for example through involvement in painting, dance, sculpture and music. Individual practitioners who have particular artistic interests and skills are currently the main promoters of the use of the arts. There is clearly scope for innovative research to enhance our understanding of how the arts might be used more widely to improve dementia care.

RESEARCH

From the discussions in this book we can identify a range of broad themes for future research in dementia care. Biomedical and clinical research is important but needs to be accompanied by extensive programmes of research on:

- the experiences of people with dementia and their carers: particularly looking at diversity in experiences, quality of life, what people want from services and how they experience services;
- maintaining and improving the individual potential of people with dementia and carers: particularly learning more about which therapies, activities and support strategies work, for whom and in what circumstances;
- quality of care practice: including the perspectives of care staff, the nature of best practice and how to achieve good quality in a range of service settings;
- service organization and delivery: evaluating different service models, learning about how best to change organizational culture and how to work across professions and organizations to achieve a 'whole systems perspective';
- social policies and their impact on dementia care: we need to know more not just about the impact of health and social care policies but also wider policies on income support, housing, employment, leisure and so on.

Perhaps the most important point, however, is that there is a need to build stronger links between researchers, practitioners and managers in order to ensure the relevance of research to practice and to facilitate better uptake of research findings. Developing these links requires an understanding of the policy and organizational context of research in dementia care.

THE SERVICE CONTEXT

This book demonstrates the complexity and fluidity of the professional, or-ganizational and policy environments of dementia care. We see, for example, how professional frameworks of knowledge cut across disciplinary frameworks in a variety of ways, sometimes facilitating integration of ideas and sometimes reinforcing conceptual barriers. We are alerted to the diversity in organizations that provide dementia care, and to how the multiple and sometimes conflicting interests within them create incentives, pressures and constraints that affect development work. We also see how different approaches can be used to bring about change in services; for example, through practice development, organ-izational development, quality management and the involvement of service users and carers.

Overall this book shows that if change is to be successful, practitioners and managers need to work in a variety of ways, with different groups of people, at different levels and in different organizational and policy contexts. In its complexity dementia services development is no different from development in other service areas; and we can therefore learn from experience elsewhere.

SERVICE DEVELOPMENT

'Service development' means different things in different contexts. Hawley and Hudson (1996) suggest that it is helpful to think of four main types of activity: researching problems and piloting solutions; replicating successful pilot schemes; promoting wider uptake of successful initiatives; and imple-menting universally programmes that have a proven value.

If we use Hawley and Hudson's (1996) ideas in dementia service develop-ment, it is clear that we need a variety of activities of different kinds. So, for example, there are many areas in dementia care where we do not yet know what the solution should be; for these we need research and opportunities to test out different options and ways of working. There are other areas of pro-vision in which there have been successful pilot schemes; these often need to be tried out in different contexts to see if the benefits are transferable. There are some areas of work where we know what constitutes good practice and the development issue is how to ensure that this good practice is more widely applied.

Different development challenges require the involvement of different groups of people and the use of different development methods. Success in this activ-ity will depend on an understanding of the people, organizations and policy context of the work. For as Hawley and Hudson (1996: 23) point out: 'A mechanistic approach to service development is neither possible, nor desir-able, nor credible. In practice, the world of policy and service development is complex and messy'.

Yet too often work on developing dementia care has been based implicitly on the assumption that we are dealing with a problem that is straightforward and easily understood. Originally the conception of the problem was of a medical disease where increasing numbers of people affected could be dealt with either by finding a 'cure' or, in the absence of a cure, by simply providing more of the same, or at least similar, care services. The 'new culture of dementia care' opened the debate and highlighted the fact that the problem was not as straight-forward as first thought. Nevertheless, the focus was still very much on indi-viduals and the 'malignant social psychology' that surrounds them. In this book, we have employed a very wide range of conceptual frameworks to understand-ing the issues involved in developing dementia care. In doing this we have shown that these issues are not nearly as simple as we might first have thought. For if we take seriously the very varied ideas presented in this book, we can see how dementia services development is intertwined with a whole raft of academic, policy, organizational, professional and ethical debates. If we are to find the most effective solutions to the problems that we face in developing dementia care, we need to acknowledge and address this complexity.

In dealing with this complexity, we would do well to heed the distinction that Clarke and Stewart (2000) make between 'wicked' and 'tame' problems. Tame problems are problems that are easily defined and for which solutions are readily available. Wicked problems are intractable and complex, and re-quire us to develop new ways of thinking and working. Clarke and Stewart (2000) suggest that while some problems fall into one or other of these cate-gories, many sit along a continuum between the two. If dementia services development is, as we have argued, more of a 'wicked problem' than we have generally assumed, then we need to adapt our problem-solving approaches accordingly.

There are a number of approaches to dealing with 'wicked problems'. First, we need to develop different ways of understanding and thinking; ways that are more holistic, that make connections, that accept different perspectives and that accept uncertainties. Second, we need to develop different ways of working and involving people; ways of working across organizational bound-aries, unconventional ways of doing things and ways of involving a wide range of people who are otherwise excluded. Third, we need constantly to be open to learning; this will involve experimentation, reflection and diversity.

By opening up our thinking about the development of dementia care in this way we can identify a number of lessons for the future. The first lesson is the importance of moving on from the current position in which practitioners and academics from different backgrounds often present their different concep-tions of dementia care as alternative, if not competing, approaches. We see this in debates, explicit or implicit, about the relative importance of the biomedical as compared with the social psychological, the individual as compared with the broader social or organizational, values and feelings as compared with knowledge and skill and so on. It will be much more productive in future for us to accept different perspectives and to look for ways in which we can make connections and develop more holistic conceptualizations of dementia care.

The second lesson is that we should increasingly be thinking and working across boundaries in dementia services development. This means challenging conventional boundaries as well as working across the familiar boundaries between health and social care. It also means paying attention to the boundaries that exist within organizations between different levels of service provision, service management and policy making. And we need to involve a broader range of people; crucially this will mean greater involvement of people with dementia themselves. It will also mean identifying and involving people whose particular expertise may not yet be contributing to dementia services development.

The third lesson about being open to learning means that we need to be prepared to experiment in dementia care and not to reject ideas because they do not fit our preconceptions about what is appropriate. We also need to be prepared to think critically about what is useful and valuable.

This book has shown that we have an enormous resource of ideas and knowledge that we can use to inform service development in dementia care. It has also discussed ethical and value issues in dementia care. We need to be aware that as different ideas about dementia care are applied in different organizational and policy contexts so different value stances are, implicitly or explicitly, supported or undermined in the process.

The diversity and complexity of dementia care that we have described in this book offer few certainties to the practitioner, manager or policy maker. But if we are to develop dementia care as fully and effectively as possibly we need to grapple with that complexity and diversity; this is what makes dementia care such a challenging and exciting field for both practice and research.

Glossary

'7S analysis': management tool for assessing an organization's performance in the areas of strategy, structure, systems, style, shared values, skills and staff.

Accountability: the duty to explain decisions and actions taken on behalf of others.

Accounts Commission: see Audit Commission.

Action research: a strategy for research that combines the development of knowledge and action to improve practice in a continuous and interactive learning process.

Advanced Directive: (also known as advance statement and living wills) – a formal communication made in advance, generally indicating a person's wishes regarding treatment (its extent, form and location) or care. Good practice will respect these and they are increasingly used within mental health services.

Advocacy: speaking up for someone or for a group of people, particularly to defend their rights or promote their interests.

Ageism: the negative stereotyping of individuals on the basis of age.

Agnosia: inability to recognize familiar objects.

Altruism: doing good without regard to personal benefit. Some doubt that altruism exists – motives always have some degree of self-interest. Others believe that humans can be altruistic.

Alzheimer's disease (AD): the most common cause of dementia with characteristic pathological changes in the brain (senile plaques and neurofibrillary tangles). Memory disorder is the most striking feature but symptoms are typically progressive and involve more global aspects of the individual's functioning.

Anti-dementia drugs: medication to improve cognitive function, mainly used in Alzheimer's disease.

Appointeeship: the appointment of a person, by the authority of the Secretary of State for Social Security, to make claims and receive payments on behalf of a claimant who is unable to manage his or her own affairs.

Assessment: the systematic, initial and ongoing process of establishing information about an individual for the purposes of planning services for them or determining their eligibility for services.

Assistive technology: any device or system that enables an individual to perform tasks that they would otherwise be unable to do, to perform tasks more easily or to perform tasks more safely.

Attachment theory: theory on the function and consequences of long-lasting emotional ties between two humans, in particular infant and mother.

Audit: a cyclical process that involves a systematic review, identification of possible improvements, implementation of these improvements and a process of further review. Clinical audit applies this process to clinical practice; organizational audit applies it to organizations or organizational units.

Audit Commission: for England and Wales ensures the proper stewardship of public finances by helping public services achieve economy, efficiency and effectiveness. The Accounts Commission is a similar body in Scotland.

Autonomy: the principle of 'self-rule' which champions the right of people to choose and follow individual courses of action. The ability to reason and the possession of mental capacity are sometimes seen as prerequisites for autonomy. Autonomy can be threatened by the actions of others and some argue that autonomy is usually qualified by context and human interdependence.

Benchmarking: involves systematically comparing, evaluating and learning from good role models.

Beneficence: ethical principle of doing good.

Best interest(s): principle for making decisions or choices on behalf of others in accordance with what is believed to be best for him or her. Best interests offers a framework for decision making that sets the individual's interests at the centre, not those of the decision maker.

'Best value': required process for all local councils in the UK. It evaluates the delivery of services to clear standards and councils must 'challenge, compare, consult, and compete'.

Biography: the representation of individual experience in the form of a descriptive product of retrospective and prospective reflection.

Biomedical: the application of biological sciences in medicine.

Boarding out: providing care for an individual in someone else's home, sometimes called fostering in child care.

Brain stem: area of the brain involved in regulation of basic biological functions.

Bright-light therapy: exposure to bright light usually for one hour in the morning in order to restore normal circadian rhythm.

Burden (carers): carers' subjective views on those aspects of caring that they see as difficult.

Bureaucracy: an organization that is characterized by a hierarchical structure and rule-governed culture.

Care management: the process of assessing, planning, determining and maintaining effective delivery and review of care services for an individual. Used to describe both the general process of organizational management and the management of individual care plans. It is distinct from case management in social work and 'integrated care management' in health care.

Care manager: a person responsible for community care assessments and the allocation, coordination and management of resources in individual care packages. Often a social work role but sometimes undertaken by other professions. Sometimes used more loosely to refer to the line management or supervisory function in care provision.

Care plan: the formal written record detailing an individual's package of care.

Care planning: those stages of care management concerned with assessing need, planning care and implementing the care plan.

Care Programme Approach (CPA): a health service-led framework for managing the care of people with mental health problems in the community.

CarenapD: an assessment tool for use with people in community or day care settings.

Carer panels: an ongoing group of carers whose specific purpose is to influence service development.

'Carers as experts' model: a model for professionals working with carers based on developing a shared understanding so those interactions more fully reflect a partnership and empowerment approach.

Carers' assessment of difficulties index (CADI): based on the transactional model of stress; an individual profile of stressful events compiled for each carer.

Carers' assessment of managing index (CAMI): tool that assesses the coping strategies and tactics used by carers.

Carers' assessment of satisfactions index (CASI): 30-item assessment tool based on the transactional model of stress.

Cerebellum: area of the brain involved in balance, posture and movement.

Cerebral cortex: collective term for the four major regions (lobes) of the brain: temporal, frontal, parietal and occipital.

Cerebrovascular: related to the blood vessels of the brain.

Challenging behaviour: behaviour by the person with dementia which is a challenge to those providing care to understand and to help, for example, aggression, withdrawn behaviour, and repetitive behaviour.

Cochrane review: refers to an approach to systematic review of evidence of effectiveness.

Cognitive behavioural: the psychological approach based on the relationship between cognitions (thoughts), mood, behaviour and physiological factors.

Cognitive therapy: therapy based on the theories linking cognitions, emotions, behaviour and physiological factors. The therapy provides the client with strategies to challenge and replace negative thought patterns and modify behaviour.

Commissioning (of services): the process of meeting the duty placed upon statutory agencies to ensure that services are available to meet the assessed needs of an area or population.

Community: a social group or class having common interests.

Confusion/Acute confusion: inability to think clearly and coherently. Acute confusion is of sudden onset and usually has an underlying cause, for example, physical illness.

Consent (informed): an agreement to a course of action made on the basis of full information and knowledge of risks and their likelihood. Duress or undue influence would negate consent, as it would not have been willingly provided. A person should have a broad understanding of the issues involved and an ability to make a decision.

Consumerism: viewing the users of services in the same way as 'consumers' of other goods/services.

Controlled trials: a research design that has at least two sample groups and that seeks to measure and attribute change in the groups to a purposeful intervention.

Coping strategies/tactics: efforts employed to deal with potentially stressful or threatening situations.

Creutzfeldt-Jacob disease (CJD): a rare and rapidly progressing dementia caused by a brain protein called prion protein. Prion disease may be inherited or transmitted through infected material. 'New variant' CJD appears to be linked with prion disease in cattle (**BSE**).

CT (Computerised Tomography): a method of brain imaging which uses conventional X-rays to produce a three-dimensional picture of the brain. CT scans are most useful to show brain atrophy (shrinkage) or brain abnormalities such as stroke or tumour.

Culture: distinctive social institutions, norms, manners, attitudes and ways of thinking which are passed from one generation to another; the tradition of formal and informal rules shared by a particular group of people.

Culture (organizational): the totality of the values, attitudes, customs, beliefs, knowledge, ways of thinking and ways of doing things that exist in an organization.

Customers: people who buy goods and services – in this context may also include service users for whom a third party makes the payment.

Delirium: acute confusion due to an underlying physical cause.

Delusions: fixed false beliefs not shaken by logical argument.

Demand: the level of expressed desire or need for particular services or products.

Dementia Care Mapping (DCM): an observational evaluation tool to assess the well-being of individuals with dementia in formal dementia care settings. Usually used for the purpose of improving well-being.

Dementia with Lewy bodies (DLB): recently recognized form of dementia due to brain lesions called Lewy bodies. It is characterized by fluctuation in attention level, the presence of visual hallucinations and parkinsonism.

Dependent variables: see experimental research.

Deviance/deviant: a shift away from the normal and valued attributes of the social group.

Differential diagnosis: the process of listing the possible causes of a patient's symptoms and presentation.

Disability: limitation in the performance of an activity resulting from an impairment (see below).

Disablism: the negative stereotyping of individuals on the basis of disability.

Down's syndrome: a congenital (genetic) abnormality leading to mental retardation, short stature and a typical physical appearance previously known as Mongolism. The genetic abnormality is on chromosome 21, the same chromosome that carries an abnormal gene (APP gene) in some rare cases of early onset familial Alzheimer's disease.

Dysarthria: difficulty with articulation of words.

Dysphasia: abnormalities of language skills.

Dyspraxia: abnormalities in visuospatial and practical abilities.

Early onset dementia: usually used to refer to dementia in people aged under 65 years.

ECG (Electrocardiogram): an electrical record of the heart's activity.

Effectiveness: the ability to create a desired outcome. The ability of an organization to meet the demands of individuals and groups involved and affected by it. 'Doing the right things'.

Efficiency: managing resources to maximize the return. 'Doing things right'.

Empowerment: in the context of community care refers to the process by which power is gained, developed, facilitated or given. Enpowerment is about people's ability to control their own lives and act as autonomous individuals.

Enduring Power of Attorney: a legal power under the Enduring Power of Attorney Act 1985 which allows a person to make arrangements in advance for the management of his/her financial affairs, which will come into place if he/she subsequently loses mental capacity. The power has to be registered with the Court of Protection. Separate arrangements operate in Scotland.

Engagement: interaction between individuals or between an individual and some aspect of their environment.

Epidemiological: related to patterns of disease in populations.

Ethnocentric: focused on a majority ethnic group.

Ethnography: research-based description of a social setting or way of life, usually based on qualitative data.

Ethnomethodology: the idea that social order is achieved through our taken-for-granted assumptions about everyday life and through the way we typify objects, events or experiences.

Evidence: information used to prove/disprove an issue. Contemporary use often refers solely to research based information.

Evidence-based practice: a process of systematically finding, appraising and using research evidence as a basis for making decisions about practice.

Existential: referring to questions and answers touching on the meaning of existence.

Experimental research: studies in which the aim is to standardize a situation so that the researcher can manipulate some variables (the independent variables) and measure the effect of this on other variables (the dependent variables).

Feminism: theoretical critique of gender stratification in society in which social relations between men and women are dominated by men and women are oppressed by men.

Frontal lobe dementia (FLD): sometimes referred to as fronto-temporal dementia. A less common form of dementia in which neurones are lost from the frontal lobes or from parts of the temporal lobes of the brain. About 50 per cent of cases have so called Pick's bodies (abnormal structures in the neurones). The frontal type is characterized by personality change; in other variants there is early loss of language and visual skills. Tends to be more common in younger people.

Frontal lobes: region of the brain influencing speech, personality, decision making, complex behaviour and judgement.

Functional (ability): the ability to perform everyday tasks.

Gender: whereas sex refers to biological differences between men and women, gender concerns the psychological, social and cultural differences between males and females.

Generalizability: ability of research findings to be applied to a wider group of people or situations than those in the original study.

Gerontology: the science and study of ageing.

Hallucinations: a false perception occurring in the absence of an external stimulus. Most commonly experienced as seeing things or hearing noises when there is nothing there.

Hippocampus: area of the brain involved in memory function especially new learning.

Humanistic: taking a perspective on life and ethics which makes human interests of paramount importance.

Huntington's disease (HD): an inherited form of dementia, associated with abnormal movements (chorea) of trunk and limbs.

Hypertension: abnormally high blood pressure.

Identity (personal): the story of a person's life as seen from the inside.

Ideology: a system of independent ideas held by a social group or society which reflects, rationalizes and defends its particular social, moral, religious, political or economic institutional interests or commitments.

Ill-being: an emotional state of inner distress and low self-esteem characterized by observable behavioural signs.

Impairment: anatomical, psychological or physiological loss or abnormality.

Incapacity: a term, used generally in legal and medical contexts, reflecting language used in mental health legislation. The Law Commission has recommended that a new legal definition of incapacity should be adopted including the ability to make a decision on the matter in question or inability to communicate a decision (1997).

Independent sector: includes both private and voluntary sector welfare organizations.

Independent variables: see experimental research.

Insight: a meaningful understanding of a particular process, typically illness.

Institutionalization: processes in a formal care setting where the needs of the individual are subjugated to the needs of those running the institution with the result of dehumanizing those in care.

Intervention: efforts to change or alter an existing situation for the better.

Justice: the ideal of justice may be explained in administrative terms through fair legal systems and processes, be based on need or deserving characteristics, on notions of fairness, on human rights (such as the right to life and liberty) and equality of citizenship. Justice is a complex yet intuitive and compelling force.

Knowledge bases/knowledges: different ways of understanding a situation or process by drawing on a variety of philosophical positions.

Labelling: refers to a social process by which individuals or groups classify the social behaviour of other individuals.

Lesions: disease-related damage.

Life history: the presentation of the facts of an individual's life.

Malignant social psychology: a term coined by Tom Kitwood to describe the cumulative effect of ways of interacting with the person with dementia that are damaging to them and do not promote well-being.

Managerialism: the application of commercial sector management practices in health and welfare organizations.

Maslovian: after AH Maslow who developed a model of the hierarchy of human needs which has a baseline of the satisfying of basic physical and physiological need and culminates in higher order issues such as the achievement of self-actualization

Medicalization: defining behaviour as a medical problem and mandating the medical profession to find some form of treatment for it.

Memory clinic: an outpatients clinic to which people with a range of memory problems are referred for investigation, diagnosis, assessment and some forms of treatment.

Methodology: the theoretical basis of research designs.

Mid-brain: area of the brain involved in regulation of basic biological functions.

Mini-mental state examination (MMSE): a test of cognitive impairment.

Mixed economy of care: care provided in combination by different service sectors – public, private, voluntary and informal.

MRI: a method of brain imaging (magnetic resonance imaging) which uses a very high strength magnetic field. Produces very high quality three-dimensional pictures of the brain which are superior to CT scans. Most useful for seeing very small abnormalities in the brain, particularly in the white matter.

Multi-infarct dementia (MID): term used to describe dementia resulting from multiple small strokes.

Multiple sclerosis: a neurological disease associated with degeneration of white matter in the brain. Characterized clinically by speech and swallowing difficulties, impaired vision and muscle weakness. Can be associated with a dementia syndrome involving the frontal lobes.

Mutation: relatively stable, and heritable, change in genetic material.

Neuro. . . : related to the nervous system, including the brain.

Neurofibrillary tangles: abnormal structures within brain cells, composed of an abnormal protein called tau.

Neuroleptic: a class of drugs used to control psychotic symptoms, particularly hallucinations and delusions. These drugs, which are most effective in schizophrenia, are frequently given to patients with dementia to treat psychosis, reduce agitation and aggression, and control other unwanted behaviours. They may be associated with undesirable side effects, particularly in dementia with Lewy bodies.

Neurones: nerve cells.

Neurotransmitters: chemicals involved in nerve cell communication.

New culture of dementia care: culture based on respect for the uniqueness of the individual; it respects the emotional and psychological needs of individuals and recognizes that we exist in relationships and have attachment needs.

New Right: a pro-market and anti-state political stance particularly associated with the Thatcher governments.

Non-malficence: ethical principle of doing no harm.

Normalization: a set of ideas promoting the rights and social value of disabled people which emphasizes dignity, social inclusion and the value of an ordinary life. Much used within learning disability services as a philosophy for practice, it is also applicable to other groups.

Normative: normative data refers to the information collected from a range of measures for a large group of people of a similar age, educational status, cultural and ethnic background. This then provides an indication of whether individual scores can be considered to be within the range of what is considered 'normal' for this group.

Norms: norms are prescriptions serving as common guidelines for social action.

Objectivity: independence of perception from an individual's conceptualizations.

Occipital lobes: region of the brain concerned with processing visual stimuli.

Occupation: to be involved in life, to use one's abilities.

Old culture of dementia care: care culture which denies the human emotional and psychological needs of those in care. Care is primarily physical and plays down a need for attachment.

Operational definition (of behaviour): a precise definition of the essential details of the behaviour and a description of the characteristics of the behaviour.

Outcomes: impact, effect, or consequence of care, services or policies.

Outcomes (better valued): the type of impact or effect which is valued, i.e. matters most to the user or carer rather than the professional or service provider.

Outcomes (process): impact or effect on a service user or carer of the way that services are put together and delivered.

Palliative care: care before death that is concerned with relief of symptoms rather than cure.

Paradigm: a scientific paradigm refers to the shared agreement or shared assumptions of a community of scientists.

Parietal lobes: region of the brain involved in perception of the individual self, perception of the outside world and execution of tasks involving complex movements.

Parkinson's disease: neurological disease leading to disorder of movement characterized by slowness to initiate movement, muscle rigidity and resting tremor.

Pastoral care: help and advice in regard to personal and ethical issues given by a minister of religion or other counsellor.

Paternalism: describes an institutionalized culture or attitude whereby those with authority assume a superior knowledge of what is in the 'best interests' of another person.

Peer review: involves the assessment of an individual or group of individuals by a group of fellow professionals.

Performance indicators: specific data which monitors/measures the performance of an organization/service. Performance indicators should measure rather than just describe and should relate to service user outcomes where possible.

Person-centred: a value base that is focused on the worth of all human beings and appreciates their uniqueness regardless of illness, age or disability.

Personal detraction: refers to brief examples of negative interaction with a person with dementia which may undermine self-esteem and well-being.

Personality: the motivations, attitudes and behaviour that characterize an individual.

Personhood: a term developed by Tom Kitwood to describe the essence of the whole person. The term is often used in relation to discussions of ways of preserving and maintaining well-being in the person with dementia by recognizing them as an individual with the same rights and needs as all members of the human race.

PEST analysis: management tool for assessing the impact on an organization of four aspects of the external environment (Political and legal; Economic; Social and cultural; and Technological).

Phenomenology: is about perceiving the world as objects or events which are, in essential respects, common – the same for others as they are for ourselves.

Philosophical: concerning the ultimate nature of existence, reality, knowledge and goodness.

Pick's disease: see frontal lobe dementia.

Pluralism: theoretical perspectives which see power as being spread across different groups and decision making as the outcome of negotiation and competition between these groups.

Political economy: theoretical perspective that emphasizes the importance of social structures rather than individual characteristics for the understanding of human behaviour.

Postmodernism: theoretical perspective critical of modernism and the ideas of the Enlightenment, which rejects the notion of human rationality and the presence of absolute truth.

Pre-morbid: prior to the onset of disease.

Prevalence: measure of proportion of people in a population affected by a particular condition.

Primary care: health services that can be directly accessed by the service user. Often used to refer to general medical practices and their linked community health services.

Primary carer: the family member or friend who provides most of the care for an individual.

Principlism: approach to health care ethics involving the application of ethical principles with a view to resolving or clarifying practical questions.

Process: an organized series of events or activities which are put together to achieve the delivery of a service.

Professionalization: process by which an occupational group claims professional status by establishing that they have an expert knowledge base, autonomous practice and control over an area of work.

Protocol: statement of the steps to be taken in a process of care or treatment.

Psychodynamic: the psychological approach based on theories concerning the interaction of conscious and unconscious elements in the mind.

Psychotherapy: a global term to describe therapeutic approaches based on psychological theories and methods derived from them.

Psychotic: severe psychiatric illness typically manifest as delusions and hallucinations.

Psychotropics: drugs which have effects upon mental function.

Qualitative (research): research that uses a variety of non-numeric data and is principally concerned with understanding how and why something happens.

Quality (in services): can be understood as a dynamic system of values, objectives, standards, measurement and review.

Quality assurance: sometimes used loosely as a general term for all quality initiatives. More specifically it is defined as 'building in quality' through identifying key points which can be checked with agreed standards across a system.

Quality control: involves detecting human error and seeking to produce conformance to a specification.

Quality of life: overall physical, mental and social well-being.

Quantitative (research): research that uses numerical data.

Racism: the false attribution of psychological and social characteristics on the basis of a person's race.

Randomized controlled research: research that randomly allocates individuals to a treatment or no treatment option – often the person is unaware which group they are in. This helps to control for placebo effects and the rate at which the improvements would have been seen by chance.

Rationality: the belief that all phenomena have natural causes.

Reality Orientation: therapeutic approach that aims to reprovide information that people have lost through neurological impairment, primarily to orientate the person to place, time and person.

Receivership: the appointment of a person by a court to administer the property of a bankrupt or mentally incompetent person, or property which is the subject of litigation.

Reciprocity: mutual cooperation and exchange.

Reductionist: a characteristic of scientific theories in which complex data and phenomena are reduced to a simple explanation.

Re-engineering (business or process): a comprehensive approach to examining and re-designing all of the processes involved in a business.

Reflective practice: a process that encourages people to learn from their practice experiences.

Reflexivity: a process of turning back on oneself and understanding the influence we as individuals have on events.

Rehabilitation: to return an individual to a previously higher level of functioning.

Religious: practising a faith in a God or gods, encompassing prayer, ritual and particular way of life.

Reminiscence therapy: involves the sharing of memories often evoked through the use of stimulating material.

Representation: where an individual or delegation is nominated by a defined group to put forward the views of that group to public authorities or others.

Respite care: short-stay care, usually residential care, designed to give a family carer a break.

Rights (Human Rights): the idea that being human equates with fundamental rights is culturally, politically and historically relevant. These are often disputed but the growing adoption of codes and laws (such as the Human Rights Act) provides a legal framework which is open to personal redress.

Risk: usually defined as the probability of an adverse effect; but can be conceptualized as a property of knowledge.

Rogerian: after Carl Rogers, the founder of an influential school of person-centred counselling

Role: the part played by an individual and the associated patterns of behaviour.

Secondary (care): health services that are accessed by referral from a medical practitioner or other professional.

Secondary carer: someone who supports the main or primary carer, for example a child who supports a parent, who is in turn looking after a person with dementia.

Secular: dealing with life in disregard for or outside the context of religious considerations.

Self/Selves: self refers to an enduring personal identity, based on our sense of the uniqueness of our lived experience. Selves refers to the various representations of our identity, based on our understanding of what is socially or culturally acceptable to others.

Self-determination: refers to personal autonomy or exercise of free will. The principle of self determination is highly valued and is based on respect. For those with limited capacity, respect may also mean it is possible to bring other judgements into the delivery of care.

Senile plaques: abnormal structures, composed largely of a protein (beta-amyloid), which engulf neighbouring brain cells and their connecting fibres. Characteristic feature of Alzheimer's disease.

Sick role: describes the expectations that people in society have about people who are sick and defines the rights and duties of people who are sick.

Significant others: partners and other close relatives and friends who are important to us.

Single case research design: research where baseline recordings are taken over a long enough period to be contrasted with a treatment effect on a single individual; the individual acts as his or her own control.

Snoezelen: multi-sensory stimulation in the form of music, projected images, bubble-tubes, aromatherapy, fibre-optic sprays and so on, set up in a specific room.

Social constructionist: theoretical perspective which treats as problematic taken-for-granted facts and issues. Facts are created through social interaction and people's interpretations of these. Therefore there exist multiple realities.

Social control: the maintenance of order and stability through a combination of compliance, coercion and commitment to social values.

Social environment: encompasses people, social interactions and relationships for example surrounding a person with dementia.

Social psychology: the study of the influence of the direct environment and the interactions of people within that environment. Theoretical approaches have been developed to consider the effects that these have on the psychological state of the individuals and of society as a whole.

Socio-economic class: refers here to a hierarchy of occupational categories used by the Registrar General to classify the population into groups with broadly similar social and economic characteristics.

Spiritual: concerned with higher levels of meaning and value in life, usually associated with belief in a power or force beyond the material world.

Stakeholders: all those who have an interest in a service – this includes front-line care staff, users, carers, professionals and so on.

Standards: a defined level of efficiency/value/quality in a service.

Statistically significant: refers to research findings which have been subjected to a statistical test to ensure that any improvement seen would not have arisen by chance alone.

Stigma: refers to a social attribute which is discrediting for an individual or group.

Strategy: the means by which an organization plans and achieves its objectives and purpose.

Street level bureaucracy: term used by Lipsky to refer to the way front-line staff in welfare bureaucracies process clients and make life manageable for themselves.

Stress (carers): the potentially detrimental effects of caregiving upon well-being.

Structural functionalism: sociological perspective based on the key assumption that all our social behaviour is the result of the organization and structure of society in which we live.

Structured dependency: sociological perspective rooted in political economy. It describes the development of a dependent status resulting from the restricted access to a wide range of resources, particularly income.

Style (organizational): the way an organization does things, its formal and informal customs, practices and beliefs.

Substituted judgement: a judgement made on behalf of someone in accordance with what is understood to be his or her preference.

Supervision (peer, group, professional): mechanism that encourages reflective practice through discussion.

Support groups: sometimes known as self-help groups. A group of people who are experiencing a similar situation who come together to share their experiences.

SWOT analysis: management tool for assessing an organization's strengths, weaknesses, opportunities and threats.

Symbolic interactionism: theoretical perspective that emphasizes understanding the individual by attempting to look at the world from the perspective of the other and appreciating how the world looks to them.

Systematic review: strategy to evaluate all research on a specified topic area and produce recommendations based on this meta-analysis.

Systemic therapy: therapy based on the conceptualization of a problem in terms of the relationships between members of the 'system' which may be a family, an organization or a system of care. The therapist seeks to work with the members of the system to identify dysfunctions and potential areas for change.

Systems: refers to the way things are done in an organization – it includes procedures, processes and policies. Systems theory is a theoretical perspective for understanding organizations.

Tau: abnormal protein involved in the production of the neurofibrillary tangles that are characteristic of Alzheimer's disease.

Teamwork (open): 'open' teamwork is a term used by Payne to describe an approach to multiprofessional working that combines traditional teamworking with networking.

Temporal lobes: region of the brain that regulates memory and mood.

Thematic reviews: a critical examination (internal or external) of the aims, objectives, methods and outcomes of an organization/service by focusing on one specific aspect, function or theme.

Theology: the study of God and religion, including God's relationship with man.

Total institution: term used by Goffman to describe a closed institution and the characteristics of the social world that develops within it.

Total quality management (TQM): involves creating a quality culture which energetically and proactively pursues quality development.

Transactional model of stress: approach based on the belief that potentially stressful events are 'appraised' by an individual and consequently what one person finds difficult may not be a problem for another.

User involvement: service user participation, both formal and informal, in a range of activities, over time, to influence service planning and development.

Utilitarianism: approach that seeks to maximize the benefits for the greatest number in society and to permit individual liberty of action unless it harms others.

Valid/validity: refers to whether research data give a true picture of what is being studied, for example whether what is being measured is a true reflection of the outcome of therapy.

Validation therapy: works to understand and to authenticate the emotional state of the person with dementia.

Value for money (VFM): getting the best service/product for a specified amount of money. It may not necessarily equate to the 'cheapest'. The government's emphasis on VFM has now been replaced by 'Best Value' initiatives.

Values: underlying philosophy/mindset that implicitly or explicitly underpins the mind/behaviour/action of an individual or organization.

Vascular dementia (VaD): dementia due to stroke disease or impaired blood flow in the brain. Onset often sudden and symptoms may be focused on a specific area of functioning rather than a more global impairment. Deterioration may be stepwise.

Visual access: what you can see from a particular viewpoint.

Visuospatial: awareness of the location of objects and figures in three dimensions. Visuospatial abnormalities can be demonstrated by simple tests such as copying or drawing a simple line figure.

Well-being: an emotional state of inner peace and high self-esteem characterized by observable behavioural signs.

References

Abberley, P. (1997) The limits of the classical social theory in the analysis and transformation of disablement – (can this really be the end; to be stuck inside Mobile with Memphis Blues again?), in L. Barton and M. Oliver (eds) *Disability Studies: Past, Present and Future*. Leeds: The Disability Press.

Abbott, P. (1998) Conflict over the grey areas: district nurses and home helps providing community care, in P. Abbott and L. Meerabeau (eds) *The Sociology of the Caring Professions*, 2nd edn. London: UCL Press.

Abbott, P. and Meerabeau, L. (1998a) Professionals, professionalization and the caring professions, in P. Abbott and L. Meerabeau (eds) *The Sociology of the Caring Professions*, 2nd edn. London: UCL Press.

Abbott, P. and Meerabeau, L. (eds) (1998b) *The Sociology of the Caring Professions*, 2nd edn. London: UCL Press.

Abbott, P. and Wallace, C. (1998) Health visiting, social work, nursing and midwifery: a history, in P. Abbott and L. Meerabeau (eds) *The Sociology of the Caring Professions*, 2nd edn. London: UCL Press.

Abdalati, H. (1975) *Islam in Focus*. London: The Islamic Cultural Centre.

Abdul-Rauf, M. (1982) The aging in Islam, in F. Tiso (ed.) *Ageing: Spiritual Perspectives*. Lakeworth: Sunday Publications Inc.

Abrams, P. S., Abrams, R., Humphrey, R. and Snaith, R. (1989) *Neighbourhood Care and Social Policy*. London: HMSO.

Accounts Commission for Scotland (1999) *Care in the Balance: Evaluating the Quality and Cost of Residential and Nursing Home Care for Older People*. Edinburgh: Accounts Commission for Scotland.

Achenbaum, W.A. (1985) Societal perceptions of aging and the aged, in R.H. Binstock and E. Shanas (eds) *Handbook of Aging and the Social Sciences*. New York, NY: Van Nostrand Reinhold.

Adams, T. (1999) Developing partnership in the work of community psychiatric nurses with older people with dementia, in T. Adams and C. Clarke (eds) *Dementia Care: Developing Partnerships in Practice*. London: Baillière Tindall.

Adamson, J. (1999) Carers and dementia among African/Caribbean and South Asian families, *Generations Review*, 9(3): 12–14.

Alaszewski, A., Harrison, L. and Manthorpe, J. (eds) (1998) *Risk, Health and Welfare*. Buckingham: Open University Press.

Allan, K. (ed.) (1994) *Wandering*. Stirling: Dementia Services Development Centre.

Allan, K. (2000) Hearing the views of people with dementia. Report on a 2-year study exploring the process of consulting people with dementia on their views on services. Paper presented at the Journal of Dementia Care Conference, Bournemouth, 17–18 May.

Allan, K. and Killick, J. (2000) Undiminished possibility: the arts in dementia care, *Journal of Dementia Care*, 8(3): 16–18.

Allen, H. and Baldwin, B. (1995) The referral, investigation and diagnosis of presenile dementia: two services compared, *International Journal of Geriatric Psychiatry*, 10(3): 185–90.

Allen, N.H.P., Gordon, S., Hope, T. and Burns, A. (1996) Manchester and Oxford Universities Scale for Psychopathological Assessment of Dementia (MOUSEPAD), *British Journal of Psychiatry*, 169: 293–307.

Allinson, K. (1997) *Adult Placements for People with Dementia: An Alternative to Residential Care*. Stirling: Dementia Services Development Centre.

Almond, B. (2000) Commodifying animals: ethical issues in genetic engineering of animals, *Health, Risk and Society*, 2(1): 95–106.

Alzheimer's Disease Society (1994) *Home Alone: Living Alone with Dementia*. London: Alzheimer's Disease Society.

Alzheimer's Disease Society (1995a) *Dementia in the Community: Management Strategies for General Practice*. London: Alzheimer's Disease Society.

Alzheimer's Disease Society (1995b) *Right from the Start: Primary Health Care and Dementia*. London: Alzheimer's Disease Society.

Alzheimer's Disease Society (1996) *Younger People With Dementia: A Review and Strategy*. London: Alzheimer's Disease Society.

Alzheimer's Disease Society (1997) *No Accounting For Health. Health Commissioning For Dementia*. London: Alzheimer's Disease Society.

Alzheimer Scotland Action on Dementia (1996) *Putting Quality First: The Need to Improve Long-stay Care for People with Dementia*. Edinburgh: Alzheimer Scotland Action on Dementia.

Alzheimer's Society (2000) Help for gay carers, *Alzheimer's Society Newsletter*, April: 6.

Anderson, I. and Brownlie, J. (1997) A neglected problem: minority ethnic elders with dementia, in A. Bowes and D. Sim (eds) *Perspectives on Welfare: The Experiences of Minority Ethnic Groups in Scotland*. Aldershot: Ashgate Publishing.

Anderson, D. and Philpott, R. (1991) The changing pattern of referrals for psychogeriatric consultation in the general hospital: an eight-year study, *International Journal of Geriatric Psychiatry*, 6: 801–7.

Aneshensel, C.S., Pearlin, L.I. and Schuler, R.H. (1993) Stress, role captivity, and the cessation of caregiving, *Journal of Health and Social Behavior*, 34 (March): 54–70.

Aneshensel, C.S., Pearlin, L.I., Mullan, J.T., Zarit, S.H. and Whitlatch, C.J. (1995) *Profiles in Caregiving: The Unexpected Career*. London and San Diego, CA: Academic Press.

Arber, S. and Ginn, J. (1991) *Gender and Later Life: A Sociological Analysis of Resources and Constraints*. London: Sage.

Archbold, P.G., Stewart, B.J., Greenlick, M.R. and Harvath, T.A. (1992) The clinical assessment of mutuality and preparedness in family caregivers of frail older people, in S.G. Funk, E.M.T. Tornquist, S.T. Champagne and R.A. Wiese (eds) *Key Aspects of Elder Care: Managing Falls, Incontinence and Cognitive Impairment.* New York, NY: Springer.

Archibald, C. (1990) *Activities 1.* Stirling: Dementia Services Development Centre.

Archibald, C. (1993) *Activities 2.* Stirling: Dementia Services Development Centre.

Archibald, C. (1994) *Sexuality and Dementia: A Guide.* Stirling: Dementia Services Development Centre.

Archibald, C. and Murphy, C. (1995) *Not Them and Us, Simply Us: Activities Training Pack.* Stirling: Dementia Services Development Centre.

Archibald, C. and Murphy, C. (eds) (1999) *Activities and People with Dementia: Involving Family Carers.* Stirling: Dementia Services Development Centre.

Ashburner, L. and Birch, K. (1999) Professional control issues between medicine and nursing in primary care, in A.L. Mark and S. Dopson (eds) *Organisational Behaviour in Health Care.* Basingstoke and London: Macmillan.

Ashida, S. (2000) The effect of reminiscence music therapy sessions on changes in depressive symptoms in elderly persons with dementia, *Journal of Music Therapy,* 37: 170–82.

Askham, J. (1995) Making sense of dementia: carers' perceptions, *Ageing and Society,* 15: 103–14.

Askham, J. (1998) Supporting caregivers of older people: an overview of problems and priorities. Paper presented at the World Congress of Gerontology, Adelaide, August 1997.

Askham, J., Henshaw, L. and Tarpey, M. (1995) *Social and Health Authority Services for People from Black and Minority Ethnic Communities.* London: HMSO.

Askham, J. and Thompson, C. (1990) *Dementia and Home Care: A Research Report on a Home Care Scheme for Dementia Sufferers.* London: Age Concern.

Atkin, K. (1998) Ageing in a multi-racial Britain: demography, policy and practice, in M. Bernard and J. Phillips (eds) *The Social Policy of Old Age.* London: Centre for Policy on Ageing.

Atkinson, P. (1988) Discourse, descriptions and diagnoses: reproducing normal medicine, in M. Lock and D. Gordon (eds) *Biomedicine Examined.* London: Kleuwer Academic Publishers.

Audit Commission (1986) *Making a Reality of Community Care.* London: HMSO.

Audit Commission (1997) *The Coming of Age.* London: Audit Commission.

Audit Commission (1998) *Home Alone. The Role of Housing in Community Care.* London: Audit Commission.

Audit Commission (2000) *Forget Me Not. Mental Health Services for Older People.* London: Audit Commission.

Backman, L. (1992) Memory training and memory improvement in Alzheimer's disease: rules and exceptions, *Acta Neurologia Scandinavica,* Supplement 139: 84–9.

Baker, R., Dowling, Z., Wareing, L.A., Dawson, J. and Assey, J. (1997) Snoezelen: its long-term and short-term effects on older people with dementia, *British Journal of Occupational Therapy,* 60(5): 213–18.

Bakhtin, M. ([1929] 1984) *Problems of Dostoevsky's Poetics,* edited and translated by C. Emerson. Minneapolis, MN: Minneapolis University Press.

Balloch, S., Andrew, T., Ginn, J. and McLean, J. (1995) *Working in the Social Services.* London: National Institute for Social Work.

Baltes, P.B. (1997) On the incomplete architecture of human ontogeny. Selection, optimization, and compensation as foundation of developmental theory, *American Psychologist*, 52(4): 366–80.

Bamford, C. (1998) Consulting older people with dementia, *Cash Care*, Spring: 2.

Bamford, C. and Bruce, E. (2000) Defining the outcomes of community care: the perspectives of older people with dementia and their carers, *Ageing and Society*, 20: 543–70.

Banks, P. (1999) *Carer Support: Time for a Change of Direction*. London: King's Fund.

Baragwanath, A. (1997) Bounce and balance: a team approach to risk management for people with dementia living at home, in M. Marshall (ed.) *State of the Art in Dementia Care*. London: Centre for Policy on Ageing.

Barber, R. (1997) A survey of services for younger people with dementia, *International Journal of Geriatric Psychiatry*, 12(9): 951–4.

Barker, P. and Pinkney, L. (1992) *Snoezelen: A Therapeutic Environment for Elderly People with Severe Confusion*. Chesterfield: Rompa Research Papers.

Barnes, D. (1997) *Older People with Mental Health Problems Living Alone: Anybody's Priority?* Wetherby: Department of Health, Social Services Inspectorate.

Barnes, M. and Wistow, G. (1992a) *Coming in from the Wilderness: Carers' Views on the Consultations and their Outcomes. Report 2 from the Research Evaluation of Birmingham's Community Special Action Project*. Leeds: Nuffield Institute for Health, University of Leeds.

Barnes, M. and Wistow, G. (1992b) Achieving a strategy for user involvement in community care, *Health and Social Care*, 2: 347–56.

Barnett, E. (1995a) Broadening our approach to spirituality, in T. Kitwood and S. Benson (eds) *The New Culture of Dementia Care*. London: Hawker Publications.

Barnett, E. (1995b) A window of insight into quality care, *Journal of Dementia Care*, 3(4): 23–6.

Barnett, E. (1996) 'I need to be me'. A thematic evaluation of a dementia care facility based on the client perspective. Unpublished PhD thesis, University of Bath.

Barnett, E. (1997) Collaboration and interdependence: care as a two-way street, in M. Marshall (ed.) *State of the Art in Dementia Care*. London: Centre for Policy on Ageing.

Baron, S., Gilloran, A. and Schad, D. (1995) Collaboration in a time of change: blocks to collaboration, *Social Sciences In Health*, 1: 195–205.

Barrance, S. (1999) Spirituality and dementia: formulating the questions for an ageing society. Paper presented at 'Tradition and Transition: Ageing into the Third Millennium', Annual Conference of the British Society of Gerontology, Bournemouth, 17–19 September.

Bartlett, C. and Ghoshal, S. (1995) Rebuilding behavioural context: turn process re-engineering into people rejuvenation, *Sloan Management Review*, Fall: 11–22.

Batson, P. (1998) Drama as therapy: bringing memories to life, *Journal of Dementia Care*, 6(4): 19–21.

Bayley, J. (1998) *Iris: A Memoir of Iris Murdoch*. London: Duckworth.

Beck, A.T. (1976) *Cognitive Therapy and the Emotional Disorders*. New York, NY: International Universities Press.

Beck, A.T., Rush, J., Shaw, B. and Emery, G. (1979) *Cognitive Therapy of Depression*. New York, NY: Guildford Press.

Beck, C., Ortigara, A., Mercer, S. and Shue, V. (1999) Enabling and empowering certified nursing assistants for quality dementia care, *International Journal of Geriatric Psychiatry*, 14(3): 197–212.

Bell, M. and Procter S. (1998) Developing nurse practitioners to develop practice: the experiences of nurses working on a Nursing Development Unit, *Journal of Nursing Management*, 6: 61–9.

Benbow, S.M., Marriott, A., Morley, M. and Walsh, S. (1993) Family therapy and dementia: review and clinical experience, *International Journal of Geriatric Psychiatry*, 8: 717–25.

Bender, M. (1999a) Support for all involved in the companions' club, *Journal of Dementia Care*, 7(1): 29–31.

Bender, M. (1999b) Adapting the counselling role for dementia care, *Journal of Dementia Care*, 7(2): 24–5.

Beresford, P., Croft, S., Evans, C. and Harding, T. (1997) Quality in personal social services: the developing role of user involvement in the UK, in A. Evers, R. Haverinen, K. Leichsenring and G. Wistow (eds) *Developing Quality in Personal Social Services*. Aldershot: Ashgate Publishing Ltd.

Berg, A., Hallberg, I.R. and Norberg, A. (1998) Nurses' reflections about dementia care, the patients, the care and themselves in their daily caregiving, *International Journal of Nursing Studies*, 35: 271–82.

Berger, P.L. and Berger, B. (1976) *Sociology: A Biographical Approach*. Harmondsworth: Penguin.

Bernlef, J. (1984) *Out of Mind*. London: Faber and Faber.

Billis, D. and Harris, M. (eds) (1996) *Voluntary Agencies: Challenges of Organisation and Management*. Basingstoke: Macmillan.

Blakemore, K. and Boneham, M. (1994) *Age, Race and Ethnicity: A Comparative Approach*. Buckingham: Open University Press.

Blau, P. (1964) *Exchange and Power in Social Life*. New York, NY: Wiley.

Blum, N.S. (1991) The management of stigma by Alzheimer family caregivers, *Journal of Contemporary Ethnography*, 20: 263–84.

Blumer, H. (1969) *Symbolic Interactionism: Perspective and Method*. Englewood Cliffs, NJ: Prentice-Hall.

Boersma, F., Eefsting, J.A., van den Brink, W. and van Tilburg, W. (1997) Care services for dementia patients: predictors for service utilization, *International Journal of Geriatric Psychiatry*, 12: 1119–26.

Bond, J. (1986) Political economy as a perspective in the analysis of old age, in Phillipson, C. and Bernard, M. (eds) *Dependency and Inter-dependency in Old Age – Theoretical Perspectives and Policy Alternatives*. London: Croom Helm.

Bond, J. (1992a) The medicalization of dementia, *Journal of Aging Studies*, 6: 397–403.

Bond, J. (1992b) The politics of caregiving: the professionalisation of informal support, *Ageing and Society*, 12: 5–21.

Bond, J. (1997) Health care reform in the UK: unrealistic or broken promises to older citizens, *Journal of Aging Studies*, 11(3): 195–210.

Bond, J. and Bond, S. (1994) *Sociology and Health Care. An Introduction for Nurses and Other Health Care Professionals*, 2nd edn. Edinburgh: Churchill Livingstone.

Booth, T. (1988) *Developing Policy Research*. Aldershot: Avebury.

Bornat, J. and Chamberlayne, P. (1999) Reminiscence in care settings: implications for training, *Education and Ageing*, 14(3): 277–96.

Bosanquet, N., May, J. and Johnson, N. (1998) *Alzheimer's Disease in the United Kingdom. Burden of Disease and Future Care*. London: Health Policy Unit, Imperial College School of Medicine.

Bowe, B. and Loveday, B. (1995) Strategies for training and organisational change, in T. Kitwood and S. Benson (eds) *The New Culture of Dementia Care*. London: Hawker Publications.

Bowen, M. (1978) *Family Therapy in Clinical Practice*. New York, NY: Jason Aronson.

Bowers, B.J. (1987) Inter-generational caregiving: adult caregivers and their ageing parents, *Advances in Nursing Science*, 9(2): 20–31.

Bowers, B.J. (1988) Family perceptions of care in a nursing home, *The Gerontologist*, 28(3): 361–7.

Bowers, L. (1997) Mental health, in D. Skidmore (ed.) *Community Care. Initial Training and Beyond*. London: Edward Arnold.

Bowie, P. and Mountain, G. (1993) Using direct observation to record the behaviour of longstay patients with dementia, *International Journal of Geriatric Psychiatry*, 8: 857–64.

Bowl, R. (1986) Social work with older people, in C. Phillipson and A. Walker (eds) *Ageing and Social Policy*. Aldershot: Gower.

Bowlby, J. (1969) *Attachment and Loss, Volume 1. Attachment*. London: The Hogarth Press.

Bowling, A. (1991) *Measuring Health: A Review of the Quality of Life Measurement Scales*. Buckingham: Open University Press.

Bradburn, N. (1969) *The Structure of Psychological Well-being*. Chicago, IL: Aldine.

Bradford Dementia Group (1997) *Evaluating Dementia Care: The DCM Method*, 7th edn. Bradford: University of Bradford.

Braithwaite, V.A. (1990) *Bound to Care*. Sydney: Allen & Unwin.

Bretherton, I. (1985) Attachment theory, retrospect and prospect, in I. Bretherton and E. Waters (eds) *Growing Points in Attachment Theory and Research, Monographs of the Society for Research in Child Development*. 50 (1–2), Serial No. 209.

Briggs, K. and Askham, J. (1999) *The Needs of People with Dementia and Those Who Care for Them. A Review of the Literature*. London: Alzheimer's Society.

Brodaty, H. and Gresham, M. (1989) Effect of a training programme to reduce stress in carers of patients with dementia, *British Medical Journal*, 299: 1375–9.

Brodaty, H., Gresham, M. and Luscombe, G. (1997) The Prince Henry Hospital Dementia Caregivers' Training Programme, *International Journal of Geriatric Psychiatry*, 12: 183–92.

Brodaty, H., Roberts, K. and Peters, K. (1994) Quasi-experimental evaluation of an educational model for dementia caregivers, *International Journal of Geriatric Psychiatry*, 9: 195–204.

Brody, E.M. (1981) 'Women in the middle' and family help to older people, *The Gerontologist*, 21: 471–80.

Brooker, D. (1995) Looking at them, looking at me. A review of observational studies into the quality of institutional care for elderly people with dementia, *Journal of Mental Health*, 4(2): 145–56.

Brooker, D.J.R. and Duce, L. (2000) Well-being and activity in dementia: a comparison of group reminiscence therapy, structured goal-directed group activity and unstructured time, *Aging and Mental Health*, 4: 356–60.

Brooker, D.J.R., Snape, M., Johnson, E., Ward, D. and Payne, M. (1997) Single case evaluation of aromatherapy and massage on disturbed behaviour in severe dementia, *British Journal of Clinical Psychology*, 36: 287–96.

Brown, G.D. (1995) Understanding barriers to basing nursing practice upon research: a communication model approach, *Journal of Advanced Nursing*, 21: 154–7.

Brown, R.W. (1986) *Social Psychology*, 2nd edn. New York, NY: The Free Press.

Brownlie, J. (1991) *A Hidden Problem? Dementia Amongst Minority Ethnic Groups*. Stirling: Dementia Services Development Centre.

Bruce, E. (1997) *Well-being and Ill-being Profile*. Bradford: Bradford Dementia Group, University of Bradford.

Bruce, E. (1998) How can we measure spiritual well-being? *Journal of Dementia Care*, May/June: 16–17.

Bruce, E. (2000) Looking after well being: a tool for evaluation, *Journal of Dementia Care*, 8(6): 25–7.

Bruner, J.S. (1986) *Actual Minds, Possible Worlds*. Cambridge, MA: Harvard University Press.

Buber, M. ([1923] 1937) *I and Thou*, translated by R. Gregor Smith. Edinburgh: Clark.

Buckland, S. (1996) Dementia Care Mapping: looking a bit deeper, *Signpost*, January: 5–7.

Bulmer, M. (1986) *Neighbours. The Work of Philip Abrams*. Cambridge: Cambridge University Press.

Burgio, L., Scilley, K., Hardin, J.M. and Hsu, C. (1996) Environmental 'white noise': an intervention for verbally agitated nursing home residents, *Journals of Gerontology Series B – Psychological Sciences and Social Sciences*, 51B: 364–73.

Burns, A. and Rabins, P. (2000) Carer burden in dementia, *International Journal of Geriatric Psychiatry*, 15 Suppl. 1: 59–13.

Burr, W.R., Klein, S.R. and associates (1994) *Re-examining Family Stress: New Theory and Research*. Thousand Oaks, CA: Sage.

Burtholt, V., Wenger, G.C. and Scott, A. (1997) Dementia, disability and contact with formal services: a comparison of cases and non-cases in rural and urban settings, *Health and Social Care in the Community*, 5(6): 384–97.

Burton, A., Chapman, A. and Myers, K. (1997) *Dementia: A Practice Guide for Social Work Staff*. Stirling: Dementia Services Development Centre.

Burton, M. and Kellaway, M. (eds) (1998) *Developing and Managing High-quality Services for People with Learning Disabilities*. Aldershot: Ashgate Publishing Ltd.

Butcher, T. (2000) The public administration model of welfare delivery, in C. Davies, L. Finlay and A. Bullman (eds) *Changing Practice in Health and Social Care*. London: Sage.

Butters, M.A., Salmon, D.P. and Butters, N. (1997) Neuropsychological assessment of dementia, in M. Storandt and G.R. VandenBos (eds) *Neuropsychological Assessment of Dementia and Depression in Older Adults: A Clinician's Guide*. Washington, DC: American Psychological Association.

Cahill, S. (1999) Caring in families: what motivates wives, daughters and daughters-in-law to provide dementia care?, *Journal of Family Studies*, 5(2): 235–47.

Cahill, S. (2000) Elderly husbands caring at home for wives diagnosed with Alzheimer's disease: are male caregivers really different?, *Australian Journal of Social Issues*, 35(1): 53–72.

Cahill, S. and Shapiro, M. (1998) 'The only one you neglect is yourself': health outcomes for carers of spouses or parents with dementia. Do wives and daughter carers differ?, *Journal of Family Studies*, 4(1): 87–101.

Caldock, K. (1996) Multidisciplinary assessment and care management, in J. Phillips and B. Penhale (eds) *Reviewing Care Management for Older People*. London: Jessica Kingsley.

Calkins, M.P. (1988) *Design for Dementia Planning: Environments for the Elderly and the Confused*. Owing Mills, MD: National Health Publishing.

Camberg, L., Woods, P. and Ooi, W.L. (1999) Evaluation of simulated presence: a personalised approach to enhance wellbeing in person with Alzheimer's disease, *Journal of the American Geriatric Society*, 47: 446–52.

Canadian Study of Health and Aging (1994) Patterns of caring for people with dementia in Canada, *Canadian Journal on Aging*, 13(4): 470–87.

Cantley, C. and Smith, M. in collaboration with Clarke, C. and Stanley, D. (2000) *An Independent Supported Living House for People with Early Onset Dementia: Evaluation of a Dementia Care Initiative Project*. Newcastle: Dementia North.

Cantley, C., Reed, J., Stanley, D. *et al.* (2000) Early onset team proves a success, *Journal of Dementia Care*, 8(4): 10–11.

Carr, J., Garton, C. and Munroe, H. (1998) *Dementia: A Practice Guide for Occupational Therapy Staff*. Stirling: Dementia Services Development Centre.

Carter, C.E. (1999) The family caring experiences of married women in dementia care, in T. Adams and C.L. Clarke (eds) *Dementia Care: Developing Partnerships in Practice*. London: Ballière Tindall.

Carter, S.E., Campbell, E.M., Sanson-Fisher, R.W., Redman, S. and Gillespie, W.J. (1997) Environmental hazards in the homes of older people, *Age and Ageing*, 23(3): 195–202.

Cartwright, J.C., Archbold, P.G., Stewart, B.J. and Limandri, B. (1994) Enrichment processes in family caregiving to frail elders, *Advances in Nursing Sciences*, 17(1): 31–43.

Cassidy, S. (1988) *Sharing the Darkness: The Spirituality of Caring*. London: Darton, Longman and Todd.

Cath, S.H. (1982) Psychoanalysis and psychoanalytic psychotherapy of the older patient, *Journal of Geriatric Psychiatry*, 15: 43–53.

Centre for Policy on Ageing (1984) *Home Life: A Code of Practice for Residential Care*. London: Centre for Policy on Ageing.

Centre for Policy on Ageing (1996) *A Better Home Life*. London: Centre for Policy on Ageing.

Chadwick, R. and Levitt, M. (1998) The ethics of community mental health care, in R. Chadwick and M. Levitt (eds) *Ethical Issues in Community Health Care*. London: Edward Arnold.

Challis, D., Carpenter, I. and Traske, K. (1996) *Assessment in Continuing Care Homes: Towards a National Standard Instrument*. Kent: Personal Social Services Research Unit, University of Kent at Canterbury.

Challis, D., von Abendorff, R., Brown, P. and Chesterman, J. (1997) Care management and dementia. An evaluation of the Lewisham Intensive Case Management Scheme, in S. Hunter (ed.) *Dementia. Challenges and New Directions*. Research Highlights in Social Work 31. London: Jessica Kingsley.

Chapman, A. (1997) Is multidisciplinary training possible? in M. Marshall (ed.) *State of the Art in Dementia Care*. London: Centre for Policy on Ageing.

Cheston, R. (1996) Stories and metaphors: talking about the past in a psychotherapy group for people with dementia, *Ageing and Society*, 16: 579–602.

Cheston, R. (1998) Psychotherapeutic work with people with dementia: a review of the literature, *British Journal of Medical Psychology*, 71: 211–31.

Cheston, R. and Bender, M. (1999) *Understanding Dementia: The Man with the Worried Eyes*. London: Jessica Kingsley.

Cheston, R. and Byatt, S. (1999) Taped memories: a source of emotional security, *Journal of Dementia Care*, 7(2): 28–30.

Cheston, R. and Jones, K. (2000) A place to work it all out together, *Journal of Dementia Care*, 8(6): 22–4.

Chinen, A.B. (1989) *In the Ever After: Fairy Tales and the Second Half of Life*. Wilmette, IL: Chiron Publications.

CHSR (Centre for Health Services Research and Department of Primary Care) (1998) *The Primary Care Management of Dementia. North of England Evidence Based Guideline Development Project*. Newcastle: University of Newcastle.

Clarke, C. and Gardner, A. (1999) Using action research to develop evidence based continence care for older people with a mental illness. Presentation at Clinical Excellence '99 Conference, Harrogate, December.

Clarke, C.L. (1995) Care of elderly people suffering from dementia and their co-resident informal carers, in B. Heyman (ed.) *Researching User Perspectives on Community Health Care*. London: Chapman and Hall.

Clarke, C.L. (1997) In sickness and in health: remembering the relationship in family caregiving for people with dementia, in M. Marshall (ed.) *The State of the Art in Dementia Care*. London: Centre for Policy on Ageing.

Clarke, C.L. (1998) *Developing Health Care Practice: A Facilitated Seminar Programme*. Newcastle upon Tyne: University of Northumbria at Newcastle.

Clarke, C.L. (1999) Dementia care partnerships: knowledge, ownership and exchange, in T. Adams and C.L. Clarke (eds) *Dementia Care: Developing Partnerships in Practice*. London: Ballière Tindall.

Clarke, C.L. and Heyman B. (1998) Risk management for people with dementia, in B. Heyman (ed.) *Risk, Health and Health Care*. London: Edward Arnold.

Clarke, M. and Stewart, J. (2000) Handling the wicked issues, in C. Davies, L. Finlay and A. Bullman (eds) *Changing Practice in Health and Social Care*. London: Sage.

Cohen, A.P. (1994) *Self Consciousness: An Alternative Anthropology of Identity*. London: Routledge.

Cohen, C.A., Gold, D.P., Shulman, K.I. and Zucchero, C.A. (1994) Positive aspects in caregiving: an overlooked variable in research, *Canadian Journal of Aging*, 13(3): 378–91.

Cohen, U. and Weisman, G.D. (1991) *Holding Onto Home: Designing Environments for People with Dementia*. Baltimore, MD: The Johns Hopkins University Press.

Coleman, P.G. (1986a) *The Ageing Process and the Role of Reminiscence*. Chichester: Wiley.

Coleman, P.G. (1986b) *Ageing and Reminiscence Processes: Social and Clinical Implications*. Chichester: Wiley.

Coleman, P.G. (1992) Fostering creative attitudes in work with elderly people: lessons from Great Britain, in N. Stevens, Th.A.M. Vis and M.F.H.G. Wimmers (eds) *Education in Gerontology in the 90's. International Perspectives and Developments*. Nijmegen, The Netherlands: University of Nijmegen.

Coleman, P.G., Ivani-Chalian, C. and Robinson, M. (1999) Self and identity in advanced old age: validation of theory through longitudinal case analysis, *Journal of Personality*, 69: 819–48.

Conrad, P. (1975) The discovery of hyperkinesis: notes on the medicalization of deviant behavior, *Social Problems*, 23(1): 12–21.

Cook, A.K., Niven, C.A. and Downs, M.G. (1999) Assessing the pain of people with cognitive impairment, *International Journal of Geriatric Psychiatry*, 14(6): 421–5.

Coppola, S. (1998) Clinical interpretation of 'Occupation and well-being in dementia: the experience of day-care staff', *American Journal of Occupational Therapy*, 5: 435–9.

Cottrell, V. and Schulz, R. (1993) The perspective of the patient with Alzheimer's disease: a neglected dimension of dementia research, *Gerontologist*, 33(2): 205–11.

Counsel and Care (undated) *The Right to Take Risks*. London: Counsel and Care.

Cousins, C. (1987) *Controlling Social Welfare. A Sociology of State Welfare Work and Organisation*. Sussex: Wheatsheaf Books.

Cox, S. (1996) Quality care for the dying person with dementia, *Journal of Dementia Care*, July/August: 19–21.

Cox, S. (1998) *Housing and Support for People with Dementia*. London: HACT (The Housing Associations Charitable Trust).

Cox, S. and Keady, J. (eds) (1999) *Younger People with Dementia: Planning, Practice, and Development*. London: Jessica Kingsley.

Cox, S. and Sheard, D. (eds) (1998) *Teams, Multidisciplinary and Interprofessional Working and Dementia*. Stirling: Dementia Services Development Centre, University of Stirling.

Cox, S., Anderson, I., Dick, S. and Elgar, J. (1998) *The Person, the Community and Dementia: Developing a Value Framework*. Stirling: Dementia Services Development Centre.

Crimmens, P. (1996) Unpublished address, Journal of Dementia Care Conference, Edinburgh.

Crump, A. (1992) Restless spirits, *Nursing Times*, 20 May: 26–28.

Csikszentmihalyi, M. (1992) *Flow: The Psychology of Happiness*. London: Rider Press.

Cumming, E. and Henry, W. (1961) *Growing Old: The Process of Disengagement*. New York, NY: Basic Books.

Dabbs, C. (1999) *Please Knock and Come in for Some Tea. The Views of People with Dementia and Improving the Quality of Life*. Preston: Preston Community Health Council.

Dalley, G. (1989) Professional ideology or organisational tribalism? The health service–social work divide, in R. Taylor and J. Ford (eds) *Social Work and Health Care. Research Highlights in Social Work 19*. London: Jessica Kingsley.

Dant, T. (1988) Dependency and old age: theoretical accounts and practical understandings, *Ageing and Society*, 8: 171–88.

Davis, A., Ellis, K. and Rummery, K. (1997) *Access to Assessment: Perspectives of Practioners, Disabled People and Carers*. Bristol: The Policy Press.

Davies, B. (1995) The reform of community and long term care of elderly persons: an international perspective, in T. Scharf and G.C. Wenger (eds) *International Perspectives on Community Care for Older People*. Aldershot: Avebury.

Davies, C. (1995) *Gender and the Professional Predicament in Nursing*. Buckingham: Open University Press.

Davis, R. (1989) *My Journey into Alzheimer's Disease*. Wheaton, Ill: Tyndale House.

Davison, N. and Reed J. (1995) One foot on the escalator: elderly people in sheltered accommodation, in B. Heyman (ed.) *Researching User Perspectives on Community Health Care*. London: Chapman and Hall.

Deakin, N. (1998) The voluntary sector, in P. Alcock, A. Erskine and M. May, *The Student's Companion to Social Policy*. Oxford: Blackwell.

Dean, H. and Khan, Z. (1998) Islam: a challenge to welfare professionalism, *Journal of Interprofessional Care*, 12(4): 399–405.

DeJong, R., Osterlund, O.W. and Roy, G.W. (1989) Measurement of quality-of-life changes in patients with Alzheimer's disease, *Clinical Therapeutics*, 11(4): 545–54.

Dening, T. (2000) Mental health services for older people: the policy perspective. Paper presented at SE Regional Conference, Oxford, 28 June.

Dening, T. and Brown, T. (2000) Dementia and the Department of Health. Perspectives from England on later life. Paper presented at North Sea Joint Meeting of Dementia Centres, Oslo, March 16.

Derrida, J. (1982) *Margins of Philosophy*. Hemel Hempstead: Harvester.

de Villiers, B. (1997) HIV-related dementia: the benefits of a small homely environment with a holistic client-centred approach, in M. Marshall (ed.) *State of the Art in Dementia Care*. London: Centre for the Policy on Ageing.

DeVries, H. and Gallagher-Thompson, D. (1993) Cognitive-behavioural therapy and the ageing caregiver, *Clinical Gerontologist*, 13: 53–7.

DHSS (1981) *Growing Older*, Cmnd. 8173. London: HMSO.

Dick, L.P., Gallagher-Thompson, D. and Thompson, D. (1996) Cognitive-behavioral therapy, in R.T. Woods (ed.) *Handbook of the Clinical Psychology of Ageing*. Chichester: Wiley.

Dick, S. and Cunningham, G. (2000) *Nothing About Me, Without Me*. Edinburgh: The Consultation and Involvement Trust Scotland.

Dimond, B. (1997) *Legal Aspects of Care in the Community*. Basingstoke: Macmillan.

Dingwall, R. (1976) *Aspects of Illness*. London: Martin Robertson.

DoH (Department of Health) (1989a) *Caring for People. Community Care in the Next Decade and Beyond*, Cm 849. London: HMSO.

DoH (Department of Health) (1989b) *Working for Patients*, Cm 555. London: HMSO.

DoH (Department of Health) (1991) *Care Management and Assessment: Summary of Practice Guidance*. London: HMSO.

DoH (Department of Health) (1992) *Health of the Nation*. London: HMSO.

DoH (Department of Health) (1995a) *Building Bridges: A Guide to Arrangements for Inter-agency Working for the Care and Protection of Severely Mentally Ill People*. London: HMSO.

DoH (Department of Health) (1995b) *NHS Responsibilities for Meeting Continuing Health Care Needs*, HSG(95)8, LAC(95)5. London: Dept of Health.

DoH (Department of Health) (1996) *Promoting Clinical Effectiveness – A Framework for Action In and Through the NHS*. London: NHS Executive.

DoH (Department of Health) (1997a) *Better Services for Vulnerable People*, EL(97) 62, CI(97) 24. London: Department of Health.

DoH (Department of Health) (1997b) *A Handbook on the Mental Health of Older People*. London: Dept. of Health.

DoH (Department of Health) (1997c) *The New NHS: Modern, Dependable*, Cm 3807. London: The Stationery Office.

DoH (Department of Health) (1998a) *Modernising Social Services. Promoting independence, Improving protection, Raising standards*, Cm 4169. London: The Stationery Office.

DoH (Department of Health) (1998b) *Our Healthier Nation*, Cm 3852. London: The Stationery Office.

DoH (Department of Health) (1998c) *Partnership in Action. (New Opportunities for Joint Working between Health and Social Services). A Discussion Document*. London: Dept. of Health.

DoH (Department of Health) (1999a) *Caring about Carers: A National Strategy for Carers*. London: Dept. of Health.

DoH (Department of Health) (1999b) *Fit for the Future? National Required Standards for Residential and Nursing Homes for Older People Consultation Document*. London: Department of Health.

DoH (Department of Health) (1999c) *No Secrets: The Protection of Vulnerable Adults. Guidance on the Development and Implementation of Multi-agency Policies and Procedures.* London: Department of Health.

DoH (Department of Health) (2000) *The NHS Plan.* London: NHS Executive, Dept. of Health.

DoH (Department of Health) (2001a) *Care Homes for Older People. National Minimum Standards.* London: HMSO.

DoH (Department of Health) (2001b) *Older People: National Framework for Older People.* London: Dept. of Health.

DoH (Department of Health) (2001c) *Valuing People: A New Strategy for Learning Disability for the 21st Century,* Cm 5086. London: The Stationery Office.

DoH, DETR (Department of Health, Department of Environment, Transport and Regions) (1999) *Better Care, Higher Standards. A Charter for Long-term Care.* London: Department of Health.

DoH/Home Office (Department of Health and the Home Office) (2000) *Reforming the Mental Health Act,* Cm 50161. London: The Stationery Office.

DoHSSI (Department of Health Social Services Inspectorate) (1993) *Inspecting for Quality. Standards for the Residential Care of Elderly People with Mental Disorders.* London: HMSO.

DoHSSI (Department of Health Social Services Inspectorate) (1996) *Assessing Older People with Dementia Living in the Community: Action Checklists.* Wetherby: Department of Health.

DoHSSI (Department of Health Social Services Inspectorate) (1997) *At Home with Dementia. Inspection of Services for Older People with Dementia in the Community.* Wetherby: Department of Health.

DoHSSI (Department of Health Social Services Inspectorate) (1998) *Care Management Study – Care Management Arrangements.* Wetherby: Department of Health.

DoHSSI (Department of Health Social Services Inspectorate) (1999) *Still Building Bridges: The Report of a National Inspection of Arrangements for the Integration of Care Programme Approach with Care Management.* London: Department of Health.

DoHSSI (Department of Health Social Services Inspectorate) and Scottish Office Social Work Services Group (1991) *Care Management and Assessment. Practitioner's Guide.* London: HMSO.

Dowd, T.T. (1991) Discovering older women's experience of urinary incontinence. *Research in Nursing and Health,* 14: 179–86.

Downs, M. (1997) Evaluating dementia services, in M. Marshall (ed.) *State of the Art in Dementia Care.* London: Centre for Policy on Ageing.

Downs, M. (2000) Dementia as a disability. Implications for practice, Paper presented at the Journal of Dementia Care Conference, Bournemouth, 17–18 May.

Downs, M.G. (1996) The role of general practice and the primary care team in dementia diagnosis and management, *International Journal of Geriatric Psychiatry,* 11(11): 937–42.

Doyal, L. (1985) Women and the National Health Service: the carers and the careless, in E. Lewin and V. Olesen (eds) *Women, Health and Healing: Toward a New Perspective.* London: Tavistock.

Doyle, C., Zapparoni, T., O'Connor, D. and Runci, S. (1997) Efficacy of psychosocial treatments for noisemaking in severe dementia, *International Psychogeriatrics,* 9: 405–22.

Dworkin, R. (1986) Autonomy and the demented self, *The Milbank Quarterly,* 64 (Suppl. 2): 4–16.

Eccles, M., Clarke, J., Livingston, M., Freemantle, N. and Mason, J. (1998) North of England evidence based guidelines development project: guideline for the primary care management of dementia, *British Medical Journal*, 317: 802–8.

Eccles, M., Clapp, Z., Grimshaw, J. *et al.* (1996) Developing valid guidelines: methodological and procedural issues from the North of England Evidence Based Guideline Development Project, *Quality in Health Care*, 5: 44–50.

Egan, G. (1994) *Working the Shadow Side. A Guide to Positive Behind-the-Scenes Management.* San Francisco, CA: Jossey-Bass.

Eisai Ltd and Pfizer Ltd (1998) *Is Someone You Care For Becoming Forgetful?* London: A112-30194-06-98, Eisai Ltd and Pfizer Ltd.

Elgar, J. and Marshall, M. (1998) *Dementia: A Practice Guide for Registration and Inspection Staff.* Stirling: Dementia Services Development Centre.

Ellen, R.T., Silveira, E. and Shah E. (1998) A comparison of mental health among minority ethnic elders and whites in East and North London, *Age and Ageing*, 27: 375–83.

Ellis, J. and Thorn, T. (2000) Sensory stimulation: where do we go from here?, *Journal of Dementia Care*, 8(1): 33–7.

Ely, M., Brayne, C., Huppert, F.A., O'Connor, D.W. and Pollitt, P.A. (1997) Cognitive impairment: a challenge for community care. A comparison of the domiciliary service receipt of cognitively impaired and equally dependent physically impaired elderly women, *Age and Ageing*, 26: 301–8.

Eraut, M. (1994) *Developing Professional Knowledge and Competence.* London: Falmer Books.

Estes, C.L. and Binney, E. (1989) The biomedicalisation of aging: dangers and dilemmas, *Gerontologist*, 29(5): 587–96.

Evandrou, M. (1998) Great expectations: social policy and the new millennium elders, in M. Bernard and J. Phillips (eds) *The Social Policy of Old Age.* London: Centre for Policy on Ageing.

Evans, J. (1995) *Feminist Theory Today. An Introduction to Second-Wave Feminism.* London: Sage.

Evers, A. (1995) The future of elderly care in Europe: limits and aspirations, in F. Scharf and G.C. Wenger (eds) *International Perspectives on Community Care for Older People.* Aldershot: Avebury.

Evers, A. (1997) Quality development – part of a changing culture of care in personal social services, in A. Evers, R. Haverinen, K. Leichsenring and G. Wistow, *Developing Quality in Personal Social Services: Concepts, Cases and Comments.* Aldershot: Ashgate Publishing.

Fairbairn, A. (1997) Insight and dementia, in M. Marshall (ed.) *State of the Art in Dementia Care.* London: Centre for Policy on Ageing.

Fairbairn, A. (2000) Alzheimer's disease and its management, *Prescriber Journal*, 40(2): 77–85.

Featherstone, M. and Hepworth, M. (1993) Images of ageing, in J. Bond, P. Coleman and S. Peace (eds) *Ageing in Society. An Introduction to Social Gerontology*, 2nd edn. London: Sage.

Feil, N. (1992) *Validation: The Feil Method*, 2nd edn. Cleveland, OH: Edward Feil Productions.

Feil, N. (1993) *The Validation Breakthrough: Simple Techniques for Communicating with People with 'Alzheimer's Type Dementia'.* Baltimore, MD: Health Professions Press.

Fellows, L.K. (1998) Competency and consent in dementia, *Journal of the American Geriatrics Society*, 46: 922–6.

Fennell, G., Phillipson, C. and Evers, H. (1988) *The Sociology of Old Age*. Milton Keynes: Open University Press.

Ferran, J., Wilson, K. and Doran, M. (1996) The early onset dementias: a study of clinical characteristics and service use, *International Journal of Geriatric Psychiatry*, 11(10): 863–9.

Filkin, G. (1997) *Best Value for the Public: Briefing and Discussion Papers*. London: Municipal Journal.

Finch, J. and Groves, D. (1983) *A Labour of Love: Women, Work and Caring*. London: Routledge and Kegan Paul.

Finnema, E.J., Drocs, R.M., Vander Kooij, C.H. *et al.* (1998) The design of a large scale experimental study into the effects of emotion-oriented care on demented elderly and professional carers in nursing homes, *Archives of Gerontology and Geriatrics*, 6: 193–200.

Fish, D. (1998) *Appreciating Practice and the Caring Professions – Refocussing Professional Development and Practitioner Research*. Oxford: Butterworth-Heinemann.

Fish, D. and Coles, C. (2000) Seeing anew: understanding professional practice as artistry, in C. Davies, L. Finlay and A. Bullman (eds) *Changing Practice in Health and Social Care*. London: Sage.

Fisher, M. (1994) Man-made care: community care and older male carers, *British Journal of Social Work*, 24(6): 659–80.

Fitting, M., Rabins, P., Lucas, M. and Eastham, J. (1986) Caregivers for dementia patients: a comparison of husbands and wives, *The Gerontologist*, 26: 248–52.

Fitzgerald, L., Ferlie, E., Wood, M. and Hawkins, C. (1999) Evidence into practice? An exploratory analysis of the interpretation of evidence, in A.L. Mark and S. Dopson (eds) *Organisational Behaviour in Health Care*. Basingstoke: Macmillan.

Fleming, R., Bowles, J., Todd, S. and Kramer, T. (1996) *Model Care Plans for Carers of People with Dementia*. Australia: The Hammond Care Group.

Flynn, N. (1990) *Public Sector Management*. London: Harvester Wheatsheaf.

Folstein, M.F., Folstein, S.E. and McHugh, P.R. (1975) 'Mini-mental state'. A practical method of grading the cognitive state of patients for the clinician, *Journal of Psychiatric Research*, 12: 189–98.

Fontana, A. and Smith, R.W. (1989) Alzheimer's disease victims: the 'unbecoming' of self and the normalization of competence, *Sociological Perspectives*, 32(1): 35–46.

Forster, M. (1989) *Have the Men Had Enough?* London: Penguin Books.

Foucault, M. (1967) *Madness and Civilization*, translated by Richard Howard. London: Tavistock.

Foucault, M. (1973) *The Birth of the Clinic*. London: Tavistock.

Franklin, B.J. (1996) New perspectives on housing and support for older people, in R. Bland (ed.) *Developing Services for Older People and Their Families. Research Highlights in Social Work 29*. London: Jessica Kingsley.

Freeman, M. (1993) *Rewriting the Self*. London: Routledge.

Freidson, E. (1975) *Profession of Medicine. A Study of the Sociology of Applied Knowledge*. New York, NY: Dodd, Mead and Co.

Freud, S. (1924) *On Psychotherapy, Collected Papers. Vol. 1*. London: Hogarth Press.

Froggatt, A. and Moffitt, L. (1997) Spiritual needs and religious practice in dementia care, in M. Marshall (ed.) *The State of the Art in Dementia Care*. London: Centre for Policy in Ageing.

Froggatt, A. and Shamy, E. (1992) *Dementia: A Christian Perspective*, Occasional Paper No. 5. London: Christian Council on Ageing.

Fuller, R. and Petch, A. (1995) *Practitioner Research: The Reflexive Social Worker.* Buckingham: Open University Press.

Fuller, R. and Tulle-Winton, E. (1996) Specialist teams – are they more effective?, in R. Bland (ed.) *Developing Services for Older People and their Families.* Research Highlights in Social Work 29. London: Jessica Kingsley.

Gallagher-Thompson, D. and Thompson, L.W. (1992) *Cognitive-Behavioural Therapy for Late-life Depression: A Treatment Manual.* Palo Alto, CA: Department of Veterans' Affairs Medical Centre.

Gallop (1986) *Omnibus Survey in Britain.* Princeton, NJ: The Gallop Organisation.

Garland, J. (1996) Working to change the organization, in R.T. Woods (ed.) *Handbook of the Clinical Psychology of Ageing.* Chichester: Wiley.

Garrat, S. and Hamilton-Smith, E. (1995) *Rethinking Dementia: An Australian Approach.* Melbourne: Ausmed.

Gaster, L. (1995) *Quality in Public Services: Managers' Choices.* Buckingham: Open University Press.

Gelsthorpe, L. (1992) Response to Martyn Hammersley's paper 'On feminist methodology', *Sociology*, 26: 213–18.

Gerkin, C.V. (1989) Pastoral care and models of aging, *Journal of Religion and Aging*, 6: 83–100.

Gibbs, I. and Sinclair, L. (1992) Consistency: a prerequisite for inspecting old people's homes, *British Journal of Social Work*, 22: 535–50.

Gibson, F. (1994) What can reminiscence contribute to people with dementia?, in J. Bornat (ed.) *Reminiscence Reviewed: Evaluations, Achievements, Perspectives.* Buckingham: Open University Press.

Giddens, A. (2000) *The Third Way: The Renewal of Social Democracy.* Cambridge: Polity Press.

Gilliard, J. (1992) A different kind of loss, *Social Work Today*, 3 Dec: 18.

Gilliard, J. (1996) Ripples of stress across the generations, *Journal of Dementia Care*, 4(4): 16–18.

Gilliard, J. and Rabins, P. (1999) Carer support, in G. Wilcock, R. Bucks and K. Rockwood (eds) *Manual for Memory Disorders Teams.* Oxford: Oxford University Press.

Gillies, B. (1995) *The Subjective Experience of Dementia. A Qualitative Analysis of Interviews with Dementia Sufferers and their Carers, and the Implications for Service Provision.* Dundee: Tayside Health Board and Tayside Region Social Work Dept.

Gilloran, A., Robertson, A., McGlew, T. and McKee, K. (1995) Improving work satisfaction amongst nursing staff and quality of care for elderly patients with dementia: some policy implications, *Ageing and Society*, 15: 375–91.

Given, B.A. and Given, C.W. (1991) Family caregivers for the elderly, in J. Fitzpatrick, R. Tauton and A. Jacox (eds) *Annual Review of Nursing Research*, Vol. 9. New York, NY: Springer.

Glaser, B.G. and Strauss, A.L. (1965) *Awareness of Dying.* Chicago, IL: Aldine.

Glendinning, C. and Coleman, A. (2000) Honeymoon year, *Community Care*, 6–12 July: 24–5.

Goffman, E. (1961) *Asylums. Essays on the Social Situation of Mental Patients and Other Inmates.* Harmondsworth: Penguin.

Goffman, E. (1968) *Stigma: Notes on the Management of Spoiled Identity.* Harmondsworth: Penguin.

Goffman, E. (1971) *The Presentation of Self in Everyday Life.* Harmondsworth: Penguin.

Gold, M.F. (1992) Restoring dignity, *Provider*, April: 17–24.

Golding, E. (1991) *Middlesex Elderly Assessment of Mental State (MEAMS)*. Bury St. Edmunds: Thames Valley Test Company.

Goldsmith, M. (1996) *Hearing the Voice of People with Dementia: Opportunities and Obstacles*. London: Jessica Kingsley.

Goldsmith, M. (1999a) Dementia: a challenge to Christian theology and pastoral care, in A. Jewell (ed.) *Spirituality and Ageing*. London: Jessica Kingsley.

Goldsmith, M. (1999b) Ethical dilemmas in dementia care, in T. Adams and C.L. Clarke (eds) *Dementia Care: Developing Partnerships in Practice*. London: Ballière Tindall.

Graham, H. (1983) Caring: a labour of love in J. Finch and D. Groves (eds) *A Labour of Love: Women, Work and Caring*. London: Routledge and Kegan Paul.

Grant, L. (1998) *Remind Me Who I Am, Again*. London: Granta.

Gresham, M. (1999) The heart of the home – but how are kitchens used?, *Journal of Dementia Care*, March/April: 20–3.

Groene II, R., Zapchenk, S., Marble, G. and Kantar, S. (1998) The effect of therapist and activity characteristics on the purposeful responses of probable Alzheimer's disease participants, *Journal of Music Therapy*, 35: 119–36.

Gubrium, J.F. (1986) *Oldtimers and Alzheimer's: The Descriptive Organization of Senility*. London: Jai Press.

Gubrium, J.F. (1987) Structuring and destructuring the course of illness: the Alzheimer's disease experience, *Sociology of Health and Illness* 9: 1–24.

Gubrium, J.F. (1989) Emotion work and emotive discourse in the Alzheimer's disease experience, *Current Perspectives on Ageing and the Life Cycle*, 3: 243–68.

Gubrium, J.F. and Lynott, R.J. (1985) Alzheimer's disease as biographical work, in W.A. Peterson and J. Quadagno (eds) *Social Bonds in Later Life*. Beverley Hills, CA: Sage Publications.

Gyatso, T. (1999) *Ancient Wisdom, Modern World: Ethics for the New Millennium*. London: Abacus.

Hamilton-Smith, E., Hooker, D. and James, M. (1992) *Granny is a Bit Strange: The Medicalisation of Dementia*. Adelaide: Royal Melbourne Institute of Technology.

Hammer, M. and Champy, J. (1993) *Re-engineering the Corporation: A Manifesto for Business Revolution*. New York, NY: Harper Collins.

Handy, C. (1993) *Understanding Organisations*, 4th edn. London: Penguin.

Hanson, P. and Lubin, B. (1995) *Answers To Questions Most Frequently Asked About Organisational Development*. London: Sage.

Harding, N. (1998) The social construction of management, in A. Symonds and A. Kelly (eds) *The Social Construction of Community Care*. Basingstoke: Macmillan.

Harding, T. (2000) The hole in the plan, *Community Care*, 3–9 August: 23.

Hardy, A. (1966) *The Divine Flame: An Essay Towards a Natural History of Religion*. London: Collins.

Hardy, B. and Wistow, G. (1997) Quality assured or quality compromised? Developing domiciliary care markets in Britain, in A. Evers, R. Haverinen, K. Leichsenring and G. Wistow (eds) *Developing Quality in Personal Social Services: Concepts, Cases and Comments*. Aldershot: Ashgate Publishing.

Haringey Housing and Social Services and Alzheimer's Society (1998) *The Needs of People with Dementia and their Carers within Three Ethnic Minority Groups in Haringey*. London: Haringey Council Printing Services.

Harrington, H. (1987) *The Improvement Process*. Milwaukee: Quality Press.

Harris, P. (1993) The misunderstood caregiver? A qualitative study of the male caregiver of Alzheimer's disease victims, *The Gerontologist*, 33(4): 551–6.

Harrison, S. (1996) Implementing the results of research and development in clinical and managerial practice, in M. Baker and S. Kirk (eds) *Research and Development for the NHS. Evidence, Evaluation and Effectiveness.* Oxford: NAHAT, Radcliffe Medical Press.

Hart, E. and Bond, M. (1995) *Action Research for Health and Social Care: A Guide to Practice.* Buckingham: Open University Press.

Harvath, T.A., Archbold, P.G., Stewart, B.J. *et al.* (1994) Establishing partnerships with family caregivers: local and cosmopolitan knowledge, *Journal of Gerontological Nursing*, 20(2): 29–35.

Harvey, R. (1998) *Young Onset Dementia: Epidemiology, Clinical Symptoms, Family Burden, Support and Outcome.* London: Imperial College of Science, Technology and Medicine.

Hasselkus, B.R. (1998) Occupation and well-being in dementia: the experience of day-care staff, *American Journal of Occupational Therapy*, 52: 423–34.

Haupt, M. (1996) Psychotherapeutic intervention in dementia, *Dementia*, 7: 207–9.

Hausman, C. (1992) Dynamic psychotherapy with elderly demented patients, in G. Jones and B.M.L. Miesen (eds) *Care Giving in Dementia.* London: Routledge.

Hawley, K. and Hudson, B. (1996) *Community Care and the Prospects for Service Development.* London: King's Fund.

Health Advisory Service (1983) *The Rising Tide. Developing Services for Mental Illness in Old Age.* Sutton, Surrey: Health Advisory Service.

Heard, D. and Lake, B. (1997) *The Challenge of Attachment for Care-giving.* London and New York, NY: Routledge.

Henwood, M. (1998) *Ignored and Invisible? Carers' Experience of the NHS.* Report of a UK research survey commissioned by Carers' National Association. London: Carers National Association.

Henwood, M., Lewis, H. and Waddington, E. (1998) *Listening to Users of Domiciliary Care Services: Developing and Monitoring Quality Standards.* Leeds: Nuffield Institute for Health.

Herbert, G. (1997) Which hat should we wear today? Recruiting and developing the ideal workforce for dementia care, in M. Marshall (ed.) *State of the Art in Dementia Care.* London: Centre for Policy on Ageing.

Hiatt, L.G. (1995) Understanding the physical environment, *Pride Institute Journal of Long Term Care*, 4(2): 12–22.

Hill, H. (1999) Dance therapy and communication in dementia, *Signpost*, 4(1): 13–14.

Hill, M. (1997) *The Policy Process in the Modern State*, 3rd edn. Hemel Hempstead: Prentice Hall/Harvester Wheatsheaf.

Hill, M. (2000) Organisation within local authorities, in M. Hill (ed.) *Local Authority Social Services. An Introduction.* Oxford: Blackwell Publishers.

Hinriden, G.A. and Niedireche, G. (1999) Dementia management strategies: adjustment of family members of older patients, *The Gerontologist*, 34: 92–102.

Hirschfield, M.J. (1981) Families living and coping with the cognitively impaired, in L.A. Copp (ed.) *Care of the Ageing.* Edinburgh: Churchill Livingstone.

Hirschfield, M.J. (1983) Home care versus institutionalisation: family caregiving and senile brain disease, *International Journal of Nursing Studies*, 20(1): 23–32.

HMSO (1988) *Community Care: An Agenda for Action*, Cm 849. London: HMSO.

HMSO (1989) *Homes Are For Living In.* London: HMSO.

Hockey, J. and James, A. (1993) *Growing Up and Growing Old. Ageing and Dependency in the Life Course.* London: Sage.

Hodkinson, M. (1973) Mental impairment in the elderly, *Journal of the Royal College of Physicians*, 7: 305–17.

Hofman, A., Rocca, W.A., Brayne, C. *et al.* (1991) The prevalence of dementia in Europe: a collaborative study of 1980–1990 findings, *International Journal of Epidemiology*, 20: 736–48.

Holden, U.P. and Woods, R.T. (1995) *Positive Approaches to Dementia Care*, 3rd edn. Edinburgh: Churchill Livingstone.

Holland, T. (1997) The risk of dementia in people with Down's syndrome, in S. Hunter (ed.) *Dementia. Challenges and New Directions*. Research Highlights in Social Work 31. London: Jessica Kingsley.

Home Office and DoH (2000) *No Secrets; Guidance on Developing and Implementing Multi-agency Policies and Procedures to Protect Vulnerable Adults from Abuse*. London: Dept. of Health.

Hope, K.W. (1996) Caring for older people with dementia: is there a case for the use of multisensory environments?, *Reviews in Clinical Gerontology*, 6: 169–75.

Howse, K. (1999) *Religion, Spirituality and Older People*. London: Centre for Policy on Ageing.

Hudson, B. (2000a) Adult care, in M. Hill (ed.) *Local Authority Social Services. An Introduction*. Oxford: Blackwell.

Hudson, B. (2000b) Social care: the vicious circle, *Health Service Journal*, 110 (5724), 28 September: 20–1.

Hugman, R. (1998) Social work and de-professionalization, in P. Abbot and L. Meerabeau, *The Sociology of the Caring Professions*, 2nd edn. London: UCL Press.

Hunt, L. (1997) The implications of practice, in L. Hunt, M. Marshall and C. Rowlings (eds) *Past Trauma in Late Life: European Perspectives on Therapeutic Work with Older People*. London: Jessica Kingsley.

Hunt, L., Marshall, M. and Rowlings, C. (eds) (1997) *Past Trauma in Late Life: European Perspectives on Therapeutic Work with Older People*. London: Jessica Kingsley.

Hunt, M. (1987) The process of translating research findings into nursing practice, *Journal of Advanced Nursing*, 12: 101–10.

Hunter, D.J. and Wistow, G. (1987) *Community Care in Britain. Variations on a Theme*. London: King Edward's Hospital Fund for London.

Hunter, D.J., McKeganey, N.P., MacPherson, I.A. with Cantley, C., Donald, S. and Dingwall-Fordyce, I. (1988) *Care of the Elderly. Policy and Practice*. Aberdeen: Aberdeen University Press.

Hutchinson, S.A., Leger-Krall, S. and Skodol Wilson, H. (1997) Early probable Alzheimer's disease and Awareness Context Theory, *Social Science and Medicine*, 45(9): 1399–409.

Ignatieff, M. (1993) *Scar Tissue*. London: Vintage.

Iliffe, S. (1997) Problems in recognising dementia in general practice: how can they be overcome?, in M. Marshall (ed.) *State of the Art in Dementia Care*. London: Centre for Policy on Ageing.

Iliffe, S. (1999) Commissioning dementia care – an emerging strategy?, *Journal of Dementia Care*, 7(3): 14–15.

Ineichen, B. (1998) Cultural concepts of care for the demented, in A. Wimo, B. Jönsson, G. Karlsson and B. Winblad (1998) *Health Economics of Dementia*. Chicester: John Wiley.

Innes, A. (1998) Behind labels: what makes behaviour 'difficult'?, *Journal of Dementia Care*, 6(5): 22–5.

Innes, A., Capstick, A. and Surr, C. (2000) Mapping out the framework, *Journal of Dementia Care*, 8(2): 20–1.

Jack, R. (ed.) (1998) *Residential Versus Community Care. The Role of Institutions in Welfare Provision*. Basingstoke: Macmillan.

Jacques A. and Jackson G. (2000) *Understanding Dementia*, 3rd edn. Edinburgh: Churchill Livingstone.

James, A., (1992) Quality and its social construction by managers in care service organisations, in D. Kelly and B. Warr, *Quality Counts: Achieving Quality in Social Care Services*. London: Whiting and Birch/Social Care Association.

James, P.D. (1994) *The Children of Men*. London: Penguin.

James, W. ([1892] 1960) *The Varieties of Religious Experience*. London: Collins.

Jenkins, C. (1998) Bridging the divide of culture and language, *Journal of Dementia Care*, 6(4): 22–4.

Jenkins, D. (1999) *Intimate Caring Skills: Urinary and Faecal Incontinence; A Heightened Problem when Dementia is a Factor*. Stirling: Dementia Services Development Centre.

Jensen, S.M. (1997) Multiple pathways to self: a multisensory art experience, *Art Therapy*, 14: 178–86.

Jerrom, B., Mian, I., Rukanyake, N.G. and Prattero, D. (1993) Stress on relative caregivers of dementia sufferers, and predictors of the breakdown of community care, *International Journal of Geriatric Psychiatry*, 8: 331–7.

Jewell, A. (1999a) Introduction, in A. Jewell (ed.) *Spirituality and Ageing*. London: Jessica Kingsley.

Jewell, A. (ed.) (1999b) *Spirituality and Ageing*. London: Jessica Kingsley.

Jivanjee, P. (1993) Enhancing the well-being of family caregivers to patients with dementia. Paper presented at International Mental Health Conference, Institute of Human Ageing, Liverpool, 24 June.

Johnson, A. (1998) All play and no work? Take a fresh look at activities, *Journal of Dementia Care*, 6(6): 25–7.

Johnson, G. and Scholes, K. (1993) *Exploring Corporate Strategy*. Hemel Hempstead: Prentice Hall.

Johnson, M. (1976) That was your life: a biographical approach to later life, in J.M.A. Munnichs and W.J.A. Van Den Heuvel (eds) *Dependency and Interdependency in Old Age*. The Hague: Martinus Nijhoff.

Johnson, M.L., Cullen, L. and Patsios, D. (1999) *Managers in Long-term Care. Their Quality and Qualities*. Bristol: The Policy Press.

Johnson, P. and Stears, G. (1997) *Why Are Older Pensioners Poorer?* London: Institute for Fiscal Studies.

Jolley, D. (1997) Old age psychiatry and dementia: somebody cares, in M. Marshall (ed.) *State of the Art in Dementia Care*. London: Centre for Policy on Ageing.

Jones, K. and Fowles, A.J. (1984) *Ideas on Institutions*. London: Routledge and Kegan Paul.

Jones, P. (ed.) (1989) *Management in Service Industries*. London: Pitmans.

Jones, P. (1992) An introduction to service organisations. Unpublished, University of Brighton.

Jones, S.N. (1995) An interpersonal approach to psychotherapy with older persons with dementia, *Professional Psychology – Research and Practice*, 26: 602–7.

Judd S., Marshall, M. and Phippen, P. (eds) (1997) *Design for Dementia*. London: Hawker Publications.

Kahana, E. and Kinney, J. (1991) Understanding caregiving interventions in the context of the stress model, in R.F. Young and E.A. Olsen (eds) *Health, Illness and Disability in Later Life – Practice, Issues and Interventions*. Newbury Park: Sage.

Kaplan, E.S. (1990) Facing the loss of what makes us uniquely human: working with dementia patients, in B. Genevay and R. Katz (eds) *Counter Transference and Older Adults*. Thousand Oaks, CA: Sage Publications.

Keady, J. (1996) The experience of dementia: a review of the literature and implications for nursing practice, *Journal of Clinical Nursing*, 5: 275–88.

Keady, J. (1997) Maintaining involvement: a meta concept to describe the dynamics of dementia, in M. Marshall (ed.) *State of the Art in Dementia Care*. London: Centre for Policy on Ageing.

Keady, J. (1999) The dynamics of dementia: a modified grounded theory study. Unpublished PhD thesis, University of Wales, Bangor.

Keady, J. and Adams, T. (2001) Community mental health nurses in dementia care: their role and future, *Journal of Dementia Care*, 9(2): 33–5.

Keady, J. and Gilliard, J. (1999) The early experience of Alzheimer's disease: implications for partnership and practice, in T. Adams and C. Clarke (eds) *Dementia Care: Developing Partnerships in Practice*. London: Ballière Tindall.

Keady, J. and Gilliard, J. (in press) Testing times: the experience of neuropsychological assessment for people with suspected Alzheimer's, in P. Harris (ed.) *Alzheimer's: Pathways to the Person*. Baltimore: John Hopkins University Press.

Keady, J. and Nolan, M.R. (1994a) Working with dementia sufferers and their carers in the community: exploring the nursing role. Paper presented at International Nursing Conference, University of Ulster, Coleraine.

Keady, J. and Nolan, M. (1994b) Younger-onset dementia: developing a longitudinal model as the basis for a research agenda and as a guide to interventions with sufferers and carers, *Journal of Advanced Nursing*, 19: 659–69.

Keady, J. and Nolan, M.R. (1995) A stitch in time: facilitating proactive interventions with dementia caregivers: the role of community practitioners, *Journal of Psychiatric and Mental Health Nursing*, 2: 33–40.

Keady, J., Nolan, M. and Gilliard, J. (1995) Listen to the voices of experience, *Journal of Dementia Care*, May/June: 15–17.

Kelly, A. (1998) Professionals and the changed environment, in A. Symonds and A. Kelly (eds) *The Social Construction of Community Care*. Basingstoke: Macmillan.

Kelly, D. and Warr, B. (1992) *Quality Counts: Achieving Quality in Social Care Services*. London: Whiting and Birch/Social Care Association.

Kendall, S. (1997) What do we mean by evidence? Implications for primary health care nursing, *Journal of Interprofessional Care*, 11(1): 23–34.

Kennedy, L. (1990) *Euthanasia: The Good Death*. London: Chatto and Windus.

Kerr, D. (1997) *Down's Syndrome and Dementia. Practitioner's Guide*. Birmingham: Venture Press.

Kiernan, C. and Alborz, A. (1995) *A Different Life. Final Report to the Mental Health Foundation on Project Factors Influencing the Ending of Informal Care of Adults with Learning Disabilities*. Manchester: Hester Adrian Research Centre, University of Manchester.

Killeen, J. (1996) *Advocacy and Dementia*. Edinburgh: Alzheimer Scotland Action on Dementia.

Killick, J. (1994) There is so much to hear when you stop and listen to individual voices, *Journal of Dementia Care*, 2: 16–17.

Killick, J. (1997) *You Are Words*. London: Hawker Publications.

Killick, J. and Allan, K. (1999) The arts in dementia care: touching the human spirit, *Journal of Dementia Care*, 7(5): 33–7.

Killick, J. and Cordonnier, C. (2000) *Openings: Dementia Poems and Photographs*. London: Hawker Publications.

King, M., Speck, P. and Thomas, A. (1994) Spiritual and religious beliefs in acute illness: is this a feasible area for study?, *Social Science and Medicine*, 38(4): 631–6.

King, M., Speck, P. and Thomas, A. (1995) The Royal Free Interview for religious and spiritual beliefs: development and standardization, *Psychological Medicine*, 25: 1125–34.

King's Fund Centre (1986) *Living Well into Old Age: Applying Principles of Good Practice to Services for People with Dementia*: London: King's Fund.

Kitchen, S.S. (1997) Research, the therapist and the patient, *Journal of Interprofessional Care*, 11(1): 49–55.

Kitson, A., Harvey, G. and McCormack, B. (1998) Enabling the implementation of evidence based practice: a conceptual framework, *Quality in Health Care*, 7: 149–58.

Kitwood, T. (1990) The dialectics of dementia: with particular reference to Alzheimer's disease, *Ageing and Society*, 10: 177–96.

Kitwood, T. (1993) Towards a theory of dementia care: the interpersonal process, *Ageing and Society*, 13: 51–67.

Kitwood, T. (1994) Care for the 'whole person' must start with nurturing ourselves, *Journal of Dementia Care*, July/August: 1.

Kitwood, T. (1995) Cultures of care: tradition and change, in T. Kitwood and S. Benson (eds) *The New Culture of Dementia Care*. London: Hawker.

Kitwood, T. (1996) A dialectical framework for dementia, in R.T. Woods (ed.) *Handbook of the Clinical Psychology of Ageing*. Chichester: Wiley.

Kitwood, T. (1997a) The concept of personhood in G.M. Jones and B.M. Miesen (eds) *Care Giving in Dementia: Research and Applications. Volume 2*. London: Routledge.

Kitwood, T. (1997b) *Dementia Reconsidered: The Person Comes First*. Buckingham: Open University Press.

Kitwood, T. (1997c) The experience of dementia, *Ageing and Mental Health*, 1: 13–22.

Kitwood, T. (1997d) Personhood maintained, in T. Kitwood, *Dementia Reconsidered: The Person Comes First*. Buckingham: Open University Press.

Kitwood, T. and Benson, S. (1995) *The New Culture of Dementia Care*. London: Hawker Publications.

Kitwood, T. and Bredin, K. (1992a) A new approach to the evaluation of dementia care, *Journal of Advances in Health and Nursing Care*, 1(5): 41–60.

Kitwood, T. and Bredin, K. (1992b) *Person to Person: A Guide to the Care of Those with Failing Mental Powers*. Essex: Gale Centre Publications.

Kitwood, T. and Bredin, K. (1992c) Towards a theory of dementia care: personhood and well-being, *Ageing and Society*, 12: 269–87.

Kitwood, T., Buckland, S. and Petre, T. (1995) *Brighter Futures*. Oxford: Anchor Housing Association.

Knapp, M. and Wigglesworth, R. (1998) Costing community care of people with dementia, in A. Wimo, B. Jönsson, G. Karlsson and B. Winblad (1998) *Health Economics of Dementia*. Chicester: John Wiley.

Knocker, S. (1998) Rich with meaning. *Alzheimer's Disease Society Newsletter*, November.

Kramer, T. (1995) *Completing the Jigsaw: The Integration of Assessment, Case Management and Education in Dementia Care*. Sydney, Australia: The Hammond Institute.

Kübler-Ross, E. (1970) *On Death and Dying*. London: Tavistock.

Kung, H. (1980) *Does God Exist?* London: Collins.

Lacey, E.A. (1994) Research utilization in nursing practice – a pilot study, *Journal of Advanced Nursing*, 19: 987–95.

Langan, M. and Means, R. (1995) *Personal Finances, Elderly People with Dementia and the 'New' Community Care*. London: Anchor Housing Association.

Law Commission (1995) *Mental Incapacity*. London: Law Commission, 231.

Law Commission (1997) *Who Decides? Making Decisions on Behalf of Mentally Incapacitated Adults*. London: The Stationery Office.

Lazarus, R.S. (1969) *Psychological Stress and the Coping Process*. New York, NY: McGraw Hill.

Lazarus, R.S. (1993) Coping theory and research: past, present and future, *Psychosomatic Medicine*, 55: 234–47.

Lee-Treweek, G. (1994) Bedroom abuse: the hidden work in a nursing home, *Generations Review*, 4(1): 2–4.

Lemert, E. (1964) Social structure, social control and deviation, in M.B. Clinard (ed.) *Anomie and Deviant Behaviour. A Discussion and Critique*. New York, NY: Free Press.

Lévesque, L., Cossette, J. and Laurin, L. (1995) A multidimensional examination of the psychological and social well-being of caregivers of a demented relative, *Research on Aging*, 17(3): 322–60.

Levin, E. (1997) Carers – Problems, strains and services, in R. Jacoby and C. Oppenheimer (eds) *Psychiatry in the Elderly*. Oxford: Oxford University Press.

Levin, E., Moriarity, J. and Gorbach, P. (1992) *Better for the Break*. London: HMSO.

Levin, E., Sinclair, I. and Gorbach, P. (1989) *Families, Services and Confusion in Old Age*. Aldershot: Gower.

Lewin, K. (1947) Frontiers in group dynamics: concept, method and reality in social science, *Human Relations, 1*.

Lewin, K. (1951) *Field Theory in Social Sciences*. Harper and Row.

Lewis, C.S. (1966) *A Grief Observed*. London: Faber and Faber.

Lewis, J. and Glennerster, H. (1996) *Implementing the New Community Care*. Buckingham: Open University Press.

Lindesay, J. and Jagger, C. (1997) Knowledge, uptake and availability of health and social services amongst Asian, Gujarati and white elderly persons. *Ethnicity and Health*, 2(1/2): 59–69.

Lintern, T., Woods, B. and Phair, L. (2000) Training is not enough to change care practice, *Journal of Dementia Care*, 6(2): 15–17.

Lipsky, M. (1980) *Street Level Bureaucracy*. New York, NY: Russell Sage Foundation.

Lowenstein, D.A., Arguelles, T., Arguelles, S. and Linn-Fuentes, P. (1994) Potential cultural bias in the neuro-psychological assessment of the older adult, *Journal of Clinical and Experimental Neuropsychology*. 16: 623–6.

Lyketos, C.G., Lindell Veiel, L., Baker, A. and Steele C. (1999) A randomized controlled trial of bright light therapy for agitated behaviours in dementia patients residing in long-term care, *International Journal of Geriatric Psychiatry*, 14: 520–5.

Lyman, K.A. (1989) Bringing the social back in: a critique of the biomedicalization of dementia, *Gerontologist*, 29(5): 597–605.

Lyman, K.A. (1998) Living with Alzheimer's disease: the creation of meaning among persons with dementia, *Journal of Clinical Ethics*, 9(1): 49–57.

Lyons, K.S. and Zarit, S.H. (1999) Formal and informal support: the great divide, *International Journal of Geriatric Psychiatry*, 14: 183–96.

McAdams, D.P. (1995) What do we know when we know a person?, *Journal of Personality*, 63: 365–96.

McAllister, C.L. and Silverman M.A. (1999) Community formation and community roles among persons with Alzheimer's disease: a comparative study of experiences in a residential Alzheimer's facility and a traditional nursing home, *Qualitative Health Research*, 9(1): 65–85.

McArthy, M., Addington-Hall, J. and Altmann, D. (1997) The experience of dying with dementia: a retrospective study, *International Journal of Geriatric Psychiatry*, 12: 404–40.

McCarty, E.F. (1996) Caring for a patient with Alzheimer's disease: process of daughter caregiver stress, *Journal of Advanced Nursing*, 23: 792–803.

McColman, C. (1997) *Spirituality: Where Body and Soul Encounter the Sacred.* Georgetown, MA: North Star Publications.

MacDonald, G. (1997) Social work research: the state we're in, *Journal of Interprofessional Care*, 11(1): 57–65.

McGowin, D. (1993) *Living in the Labyrinth.* Cambridge: Mainsail Press.

Mackay, L. (1989) *Nursing a Problem.* Milton Keynes: Open University Press.

McKee, K.J. (1994) Coping in family carers of elderly people with dementia. Paper presented at the Alzheimer's Disease International Tenth International Conference, Edinburgh.

McKee, K.J. (1999) This is your life: research paradigms in dementia care, in T. Adams and C.L. Clarke (eds) *Dementia Care: Developing Partnerships in Practice.* London: Ballière Tindall.

Mackie, J. (1997) Must something be done?, *Journal of Dementia Care*, 5(1): 21–2.

McNamara, C. and Kempenaar, L. (1998) The benefits of specific sensory stimulation, *Journal of Dementia Care*, 6(6): 14–15.

Macrae, H. (1999) Managing courtesy stigma: the case of Alzheimer's disease, *Sociology of Health and Illness*, 21(1): 54–70.

McShane, R., Gelding, K., Keene, J. *et al.* (1998) Getting lost in dementia: a longitudinal study of behavioural symptoms, *International Psychogeriatrics*, 10(3): 253–60.

McWalter, G., Toner H., Corser, A. *et al.* (1994) Needs and need assessment: their components and definitions with reference to dementia, *Health and Social Care*, 2: 213–19.

McWalter, G.J., Toner, H.L., Eastwood, J. *et al.* (1996) *CarenapD Manual: User Manual for the Care Needs Assessment Pack for Dementia (CarenapD).* Stirling: Dementia Services Development Centre.

Mace, N. and Rabins, P. (1985) *The 36-hour Day.* London: Age Concern.

Magni, E., Zanetti, O., Bianchetti, A., Binetti, G. and Trabucchi, M. (1995) Evaluation of an Italian education programme for dementia caregivers: results of a small-scale pilot study, *International Journal of Geriatric Psychiatry*, 10: 569–73.

Maguire, C., Kirby, M., Coen, R. *et al.* (1996) Family members' attitudes toward telling the patient with Alzheimer's disease their diagnosis, *British Medical Journal*, 313: 529–30.

Malin, N., Manthorpe, J., Race, D. and Wilmot, S. (1999) *Community Care for Nurses and the Caring Professions.* Buckingham: Open University Press.

Malin, V. (2000) From continuous to continuing long-term care, in G. Bradley and J. Manthorpe (eds) *Working on the Fault Line.* Birmingham: Venture Press.

Mandelstam, M. (1997) *Equipment for Older or Disabled People and the Law.* London: Jessica Kingsley.

Mandelstam, M. (1999) *Community Care Practice and the Law*, 2nd edn. London: Jessica Kingsley.

Manning, N. (ed.) (1985) *Social Problems and Welfare Ideology*. Aldershot: Gower.

Marcoen, A. (1994) Spirituality and personal well-being in old age, *Ageing and Society*, 14: 521–36.

Marshall, M. (1990) *Working with Dementia: Guidelines for Professionals*. Birmingham: Venture Press.

Marshall, M. (1997a) Design and technology for people with dementia, in R. Jacoby and C. Oppenheimer, *Psychiatry in the Elderly*, 2nd edn. Oxford: Oxford University Press.

Marshall, M. (1997b) Therapeutic buildings for people with dementia, in S. Judd, M. Marshall and P. Phippen (eds) *Design for Dementia*. London: Hawker Publications.

Marshall M. (2000) *ASTRID: A Guide to Using Technology within Dementia Care*. London: Hawker Publications.

Marshall, M. and Cox, S. (1998) Current and future trends in the development of dementia services, *The Mental Health Review*, 3(1): 16–21.

Maslow, A.H. (1970) *Motivation and Personality*, 2nd edn. London: Harper and Row.

Meacher, M. (1972) *Taken for a Ride*. London: Longman.

Mead, G.H. (1934) *Mind, Self and Society*. Chicago, IL: The University of Chicago Press.

Means, R. (1997) Personal finances and elderly people with dementia: a challenge for local authorities, in M. Marshall (ed.) *State of the Art in Dementia Care*. London: Centre for Policy on Ageing.

Means, R. and Smith, R. (1998a) *From Poor Law to Community Care. The Development of Welfare Services for Elderly People 1939–1971*, 2nd edn. Bristol: The Policy Press.

Means, R. and Smith, R. (1998b) *Community Care. Policy and Practice*, 2nd edn. Basingstoke: Macmillan.

Mechanic, D. (1962) The concept of illness behaviour, *Journal of Chronic Diseases*, 15: 189–94.

Mechanic, D. (1992) *Medical Sociology*, 2nd edn. New York, NY: Free Press.

Melzer D., Ely, M. and Brayne, C. (1997) Cognitive impairment in elderly people: population based estimate of the future in England, Scotland and Wales, *British Medical Journal*, 315(7106): 462.

Melzer, D., Hopkins, S., Pencheon, D., Brayne, C. and Williams, R. (1992) *Epidemiologically Based Needs Assessment: Dementia*. London: NHS Management Executive.

Mercken, C. (1998) Interaction between toddlers and elderly with dementia: a study from the Netherlands, *Registered Homes*, 2(9): 122.

Metropolitan Anthony of Sourozh (1999) The spirituality of old age, in A. Jewell (ed.) *Spirituality and Ageing*. London: Jessica Kingsley.

Meyer, J. and Batehup L. (1997) Action research in health-care practice: nature, present concerns and future possibilities, *Nursing Times Research*, 2(3): 175–86.

Midence, K. and Cunliffe, L. (1996) The impact of dementia on the sufferer and available treatment interventions: an overview, *Journal of Psychology*, 130: 589–602.

Miesen, B.L.M. (1992) Attachment theory and dementia, in G.M. Jones, and B.L.M. Miesen (eds) *Care Giving in Dementia, Research and Applications. Volume 1*. London: Routledge.

Miesen, B.L.M. (1993) Alzheimer's disease, the phenomenon of parent fixation and Bowlby's attachment theory, *International Journal of Geriatric Psychiatry*, 8: 147–53.

Miller, E. and Morris, R.G. (1993) *The Psychology of Dementia*. Chichester: Wiley.

Mills, M.A. (1997) 'The gift of her friendship'. Person-centred Care Series, 12, *Journal of Dementia Care*, 5(5): 24–5.

Mills, M.A. (1998) *Narrative Identity and Dementia: A Study of Autobiographical Memories and Emotions*. Aldershot: Ashgate Publishing.

Mills, M.A., Coleman, P.G., Jerrome, D. *et al.* (1999) Changing patterns of dementia care: the influence of attachment theory in staff training, in J. Bornat, P. Chamberlayne and L. Chant (eds) *Reminiscence: Practice, Skills and Settings*. Dagenham: Centre for Biography in Social Policy (BISP), University of East London.

Milne, D., Pitt, I. and Sabin, N. (1993) Evaluation of a carer support scheme for elderly people: the importance of coping, *British Journal of Social Work*, 23: 157–68.

Ministerial Task Force on Dementia Services in Victoria (1997) *Dementia Care in Victoria: Building a Pathway to Excellence*. Melbourne: Human Services Communication Unit.

Minuchin, S. (1974) *Families and Family Therapy*. Cambridge, MA: Harvard University Press.

Mittleman, M.S. and Ferris, S.H. (1996) A family intervention to delay nursing home placements of patients with Alzheimer's disease, *JAMA*, 267(26): 1725–57.

Moffat, L. (1996) Helping to re-create a personal sacred space, *Journal of Dementia Care*, 4 (May/June): 19–21.

Moniz-Cook, E. (1998) Research focus: psychosocial approaches to 'challenging behaviour' in care homes, *Journal of Dementia Care*, 6(5): 33–8.

Moniz-Cook, E. (1999) Interventions in challenging behaviour: functional analysis revisited. Paper presented at the PSIGE Annual Conference, University of Bath, July.

Moniz-Cook, E. and Woods, R. (1997) Editorial: The role of memory clinics and psychosocial interventions in the early stages of dementia, *International Journal of Geriatric Psychiatry*, 12: 1143–5.

Morgan, D.G. and Laing, G.P. (1991) The diagnosis of Alzheimer's disease: spouse's perspectives, *Qualitative Health Research*, 1 (August): 370–87.

Morgan, D.G. and Stewart, N.J. (1999) The physical environment of special care units: needs of residents with dementia from the perspective of staff and family caregivers, *Qualitative Health Research*, 9(1): 105–18.

Moriarty, J. and Webb, S. (1997) How do older people feel about assessment?, *Journal of Dementia Care*, 5(5): 20–22.

Moriarty, J. and Webb, S. (2000) *Part of their Lives: Community Care for Older People with Dementia*. Bristol: The Policy Press.

Morris, R.G. (1996) The neuropsychology of Alzheimer's disease and related dementias, in R.T. Woods (ed.) *Handbook of the Clinical Psychology of Ageing*. Chichester: Wiley.

Morris, R.G. and McKiernan, F. (1994) Neuropsychological investigation of dementia, in A. Burns and R. Levy (eds) *Dementia*. London: Chapman and Hall.

Motenko, A. (1987) The frustrations, gratifications and well-being of dementia caregivers, *The Gerontologist*, 29(2): 166–72.

Mozley, C.G., Huxley, P., Sutcliffe, C. *et al.* (1999) 'Not knowing where I am doesn't mean I don't know what I like': cognitive impairment and quality of life responses in elderly people, *International Journal of Geriatric Psychiatry*, 14(9): 776–83.

Mozley, C.G., Sutcliffe, C., Bagley, H. *et al.* (2000) *The Quality of Life Study: Outcomes for Older People in Nursing and Residential Homes. Report to the NHS Executive.* Manchester: PSSRU, University of Manchester.

Munnichs, J. and Miesen, B. (1986) *John Bowlby – Attachment, Life-span and Old-age.* The Netherlands: Van Loghum Slaterus, Deventer.

Murphy, C. (1994) *'It Started With a Seashell'. Life Story Work and People with Dementia.* Stirling: Dementia Services Development Centre.

Murphy, C. (1998) What's on the minds of people with dementia?, *Working with Older People,* 2: 25–7.

Murphy, E., Dingwall, R., Greatbatch, D., Parker, S. and Watson, P. (1998) Qualitative research methods in health technology assessment: a review of the literature, *Health Technol Assessment,* 2(16).

Myers, F. and MacDonald, C. (1990) 'I was given options, not choices'. Involving older users and carers in assessment and care planning, in R. Bland (ed.) *Developing Services for Older People and Their Families.* Research Highlights in Social Work No. 29. London: Jessica Kingsley.

Neidhardt, E.R. and Allen, J.A. (1993) *Family Therapy with the Elderly.* London: Sage.

Nelson, H. (1982) *National Adult Reading Test Manual.* Windsor, Berks: NFER–Nelson.

Nelson-Jones, R. (1982) *The Theory and Practice of Counselling Psychology.* London: Holt, Rinehart and Winston.

Netten, A. (1993) *A Positive Environment? Physical and Social Influences on People with Senile Dementia in Residential Care.* Aldershot: Ashgate Publishing in Association with PSSRU, University of Kent at Canterbury.

Nettleton, S. (1995) *The Sociology of Health and Illness.* Cambridge: Polity Press.

NICE (National Institute for Clinical Excellence) (2001) *Donepezil, Rivastigmine and Galantamine for the Treatment of Alzheimer's Disease. Technology Appraisal Guidance No. 19.* London: Department of Health.

Nocon, A. and Qureshi, H. (1996) *Outcomes of Community Care for Users and Carers: A Social Services Perspective.* Buckingham: Open University Press.

Nolan, M.R. and Grant, G. (1992) *Regular Respite: An Evaluation of a Hospital Rota Bed Scheme for Elderly People.* London: Age Concern.

Nolan, M.R., Grant, G. and Keady, J. (1996) *Understanding Family Care.* Buckingham: Open University Press.

Nolan, M., Grant, G. and Keady, J. (1998) *Assessing the Needs of Family Carers: A Guide for Practitioners.* Brighton: Pavilion Publishers.

Nolan, M., Keady, J. and Grant, G. (1995) CAMI: a basis for assessment and support with family carers, *British Journal of Nursing,* 4(14): 822–6.

Norman, A. (1985) *Triple Jeopardy: Growing Old in a Second Homeland.* London: Centre for Policy on Ageing.

Oakley, A. (1972) *Sex, Gender and Society.* London: Temple Smith.

O'Carroll, R.E., Baikie, E.M. and Whittick, J.E. (1987) Does the national adult test hold in dementia?, *British Journal of Clinical Psychology,* 26: 315–16.

O'Donovan, S. (1994) *Simon's Nursing Assessment Manual for the Care of Older People with Dementia.* Bicester: Winslow Press Ltd.

Ogg, J., Evans, J.G., Jeffreys, M. and MacMahon, D.G. (1998) Professional responses to the challenge of old age, in M. Bernard and J. Phillips (eds) *The Social Policy of Old Age.* London: Centre for Policy on Ageing.

Oliver, M. (1986) Social policy and disability: some theoretical issues, *Disability, Handicap and Society,* 1(1): 5–18.

Oliver, M. (1990) *The Politics of Disablement*. Basingstoke: Macmillan.

Oliver, M. (1996) A sociology of disability or a disablist sociology?, in L. Barton (ed.) *Disability and Society: Emerging Issues and Insights*. London: Longman.

Oliver, M. (1997) Emancipatory research: realistic goal or impossible dream?, in C. Barnes and G. Mercer (eds) *Doing Disability Research*. Leeds: The Disability Press.

O'Neill, D. (1992) Dementia and driving, *Journal of the Royal Society of Medicine*, 85(4): 199–202.

Opie, A. (1992) *There's Nobody There: Community Care of Confused Older People*. Auckland: Oxford University Press.

Opie, A. (1994) The instability of the caring body: gender and caregivers of confused older people, *Qualitative Health Research*, 4(1): 31–50.

Orell, M. and Sahakian, B.J. (1995) Education and dementia, *British Medical Journal*, 310: 951–2.

Øvretveit, J. (1993) *Coordinating Community Care. Multidisciplinary Teams and Care Management*. Buckingham: Open University Press.

Øvretveit, J. (1997) How patient power and client participation affects relations between professions, in J. Øvretveit, P. Mathias and T. Thompson (eds), *Interprofessional Working For Health and Social Care*. Basingstoke: Macmillan.

Øvretveit, J., Mathias, P. and Thompson, T. (eds) (1997) *Interprofessional Working For Health and Social Care*. Basingstoke: Macmillan.

Oxman, A.D., Thomson, M.A., Davis, D.A. and Haynes, R.B. (1995) No magic bullets: a systematic review of 102 trials of interventions to improve professional practice, *Canadian Medical Association Journal*, 153(10): 1423–31.

Oyebode, J., Evans, A., Foster, F., McDermott, P. and Pyke, P. (1996) Creating a new individualised service, *Journal of Dementia Care*, 4(5): 18–19.

Packer, T. (1999) Paper presented at the Journal of Dementia Care Conference, Bournemouth, 12–13 May.

Packer, T. (2000) Does person-centred care exist?, *Journal of Dementia Care*, 8(3): 19–21.

Pallett, P.J. (1990) A conceptual framework for studying family caregiver burden in Alzheimer's-type dementia, *Journal of Nursing Scholarship, IMAGE*: 22(1): 53–8.

Parker, G. (1993) *With This Body*. Buckingham: Open University Press.

Parker, G. and Lawton, D. (1990a) *Further Analysis of the 1985 General Household Survey Data on Informal Care. Report 1: A Typology of Caring*. Social Policy Research Unit, Working Paper DHSS 716, 12.90. York: University of York.

Parker, G. and Lawton, D. (1990b) *Further Analysis of the 1985 General Household Survey Data on Informal Care. Report 2: The Consequences of Caring*. Social Policy Research Unit, Working Paper DHSS 716, 12.90. York: University of York.

Parker, J. and Penhale, B. (1998) *Forgotten People: Forgotten Approaches to Dementia Care*. Aldershot: Arena.

Parsloe, P. (1999) Some spiritual and ethical issues in community care for frail elderly people: a social work view, in A. Jewell (ed.) *Spirituality and Ageing*. London: Jessica Kingsley.

Parsons, M. (1999) *The Clive Project: An Evaluation of a Home Based Service for Younger People with Dementia*. Oxford: Oxford Dementia Centre.

Parsons, T. (1951) *The Social System*. London: Routledge and Kegan Paul.

Patel, N., Mirza, N.R., Lindblad, P., Amstrup, K. and Samaoli, O. (1998) *Dementia and Minority Ethnic Older People. Managing Care in the UK, Denmark and France*. Lyme Regis: Russell House Publishing.

Payne, M. (2000) *Teamwork in Multiprofessional Care*. Basingstoke: Macmillan.

Peace, S. and Johnson, J. (1998) Living arrangements for older people, in M. Bernard and J. Phillips (eds) *The Social Policy of Old Age*. London: Centre for Policy on Ageing.

Peace, S., Kellaher, L. and Willcocks, D. (1997) *Re-evaluating Residential Care*. Buckingham: Open University Press.

Penhale, B. (1999) Researching elder abuse: lessons for practice, in P. Slater and M. Eastman (eds) *Elder Abuse: Critical Issues in Policy and Practice*. London: Age Concern England.

Peppard, N.R. (1991) *Special Needs Dementia Units: Design, Development and Operations*. New York, NY: Springer Publishing Company.

Perren, L. and Webber, T. (1998) *Organisational Health – Diagnosis and Treatment*. London: Financial Times Management.

Perrin, T. (1997a) Occupational need in severe dementia: a descriptive study, *Journal of Advanced Nursing*, 25: 934–41.

Perrin, T. (1997b) The positive response schedule for severe dementia, *Aging and Mental Health*, 1(2): 184–91.

Perrin, T. (1998) Lifted into a world of rhythm and melody, *Journal of Dementia Care*, 6(1): 22–24.

Perrin, T. and May, H. (1999) *Well-being in Dementia. An Occupational Approach for Therapists and Carers*. London: Churchill Livingstone.

Peters, T. and Waterman, R. (1982) *In Search of Excellence*. London: Harper Collins.

Petersen, A. (1999) Counselling the genetically 'at risk': the poetics and politics of 'non-directiveness', *Health, Risk and Society*, 1(3): 253–65.

Petre, T. (1995) People with dementia in sheltered housing, in T. Kitwood and S. Benson (eds) *The New Culture of Dementia Care*. London: Hawker Publications.

Petzsch, H.M.D. (1984) *'Does he Know How Frightening he is in his Strangeness?' A Study of Attitudes to Dementing People*. Edinburgh: Department of Christian Ethics and Practical Theology, University of Edinburgh.

Phair, L. (1990) *What the People Think. Homefield Place from the Clients' Point of View*. East Sussex: Eastbourne Health Authority.

Phillips, J. and Penhale, B. (eds) (1996) *Reviewing Care Management for Older People*. London: Jessica Kingsley.

Phillipson, C. (1982) *Capitalism and the Construction of Old Age*. London: Macmillan.

Phillipson, C. and Thompson, N. (1996) The social construction of old age. New perspectives on the theory and practice of social work with older people, in R. Bland (ed.) *Developing Services for Older People and Their Families*. Research Highlights in Social Work 29. London: Jessica Kingsley.

Philp, I., McKee, K.J., Meldrum, P. *et al.* (1995) Community care for demented and non-demented elderly people: a comparison study of financial burden, service use and unmet needs in family supporters, *British Medical Journal*, 310: 1503–6.

Pickles, V. (1997) Music's power, purpose and potential. *Journal of Dementia Care*, 5(3): 20–1.

Picot, S.J. (1995) Rewards, costs, and coping of African American caregivers, *Nursing Research*, 44(3): 147–52.

Pirsig, R.M. (1974) *Zen and the Art of Motorcycle Maintenance* (reprinted 1989). London: Black Swan.

Pollit, P.A. (1996) Dementia in old age: an anthropological perspective, *Psychological Medicine*, 26(5): 1061–74.

Pollitt, C. (1997) Business and professional approaches to quality improvement: a comparison of their suitability for the personal social services, in A. Evers, R.

Haverinen, K. Leichsenring and G. Wistow (eds) *Developing Quality in Personal Social Services: Concepts, Cases and Comments*. Aldershot: Ashgate Publishing.

Pool, J. (1999) *The Pool Activity Level Instrument*. London: Jessica Kingsley.

Post, S. (1995) *The Moral Challenge of Alzheimer's Disease*. Baltimore, MD and London: The Johns Hopkins University Press.

Public Concern at Work (1998) *Public Interest Whistleblowing*. London: Public Concern at Work.

Quinton, A. (1973) *The Nature of Things*. London: Routledge.

Qureshi, H., Patmore, C., Nicholas, E. and Bamford, C. (1998) *Overview: Outcomes of Social Care for Older People and Carers*. York: SPRU, University of York.

Rashid, S. (2000) Social work and professionalization: a legacy of ambivalence, in C. Davies, L. Finlay and A. Bullman (eds) *Changing Practice in Health and Social Care*. London: Sage.

Rawls, J. (1972) *A Theory of Justice*. Oxford: Oxford University Press.

Ray, M. (1999) Developing person-centred standards for care homes, *Journal of Dementia Care*, 7(6): 16–18.

RCP (Royal College of Physicians) (1998) *Enhancing the Health of Older People in Long-term Care*. London: Royal College of Physicians.

RCP/RCP (Royal College of Psychiatrists and Royal College of Physicians) (1998) *The Care of Older People with Mental Illness: Specialist Services and Medical Training*, Council Report CR69. London: Royal College of Psychiatrists and Royal College of Physicians of London.

Reason, J. (1997) *Managing the Risks of Organisational Accidents*. Aldershot: Ashgate Publishing Ltd.

Reed, J. and Biott, C. (1995) Evaluating and developing practitioner research, in J. Reed and S. Procter (eds) *Practitioner Research in Health Care: The Inside Story*. London: Chapman and Hall.

Reed, J. and Payton, V. (1997) Understanding the dynamics of life in care for older people: implications for deinstitutionalization practice. *Health and Social Care in the Community*, 5(40): 261–8.

Reed, J. and Procter, S. (1995) Practitioner research in context, in J. Reed and S. Procter (eds) *Practitioner Research in Health Care: The Inside Story*. London: Chapman and Hall.

Reed, J., Morgan, D. and Palmer, A. (1998) *Discharging Older People From Hospital to Care Homes: Implications for Nursing*. Centre for Care of Older People Occasional Paper. Newcastle-upon-Tyne: Faculty of Health, Social Work and Education, University of Northumbria.

Reed, J., Cantley, C., Stanley, D. *et al.* (2000) *An Evaluation of the Lewis Project: A Service for People with Early Onset Dementia*. Newcastle: Centre for Care of Older People, University of Northumbria and Dementia North.

Regan, D. and Smith, J. (1997) *The Fullness of Time: How Homes for Older People Can Respond to their Residents' Need for Wholeness and a Spiritual Dimension to Care*. London: Counsel and Care.

Riordan, J.M. and Bennett, A.V. (1998) An evaluation of an augmented domiciliary service to older people with dementia and their carers, *Aging and Mental Health*, 2(2): 137–43.

Riseborough, M. (ed.) (1998) *Setting the Quality Standard for Independent Living: A Discussion Paper*. Birmingham: The HOPE Network.

RIS MRC CFAS (Resource Implications Study Group of the Medical Research Council Cognitive Function and Ageing Study) (1999) Informal caregiving for frail older people at home and in long-term care institutions: who are the key supporters?, *Health and Social Care in the Community*, 7(6): 434–44.

Ritchie, R. (1995) Constructive action research: a perspective on the process of learning, *Educational Action Research*, 3(3): 305–23.

Robb, B. (1967) *Sans Everything: A Case to Answer*. London: Nelson.

Robbins, T.W., James, M., Owen, A.M. *et al.* (1994) Cambridge Neuropsychological Test Automated Battery (CANTAB): a factor analytical study of a large sample of normal elderly volunteers, *Dementia*, 5: 266–81.

Robertsson, B., Karlsson, I., Styrud, E. and Gottfries, C.G. (1997) Confusional State Evaluation (CSE): an instrument for measuring severity of delirium in the elderly, *British Journal of Psychiatry*, 170, June: 565–70.

Rogers, C. (1965) *Client Centred Therapy: Its Current Practice, Implications and Theory*. New York, NY: Houghton Mifflin.

Rolfe, G. (1998) The theory-practice gap in nursing: from research-based practice to practitioner-based research, *Journal of Advanced Nursing*, 28(3): 672–9.

Roper-Hall, A. (1987) Should you involve an older person about whom there is an issue of cognitive competence in family meetings? *PSIGE (Psychologists Special Interest Group in the Elderly) Newsletter*, 24: 8–11.

Ross, F. and Meerabeau, L. (1997) Editorial: Research and professional practice, *Journal of Interprofessional Care*, 11: 5.

Roth, M., Tym, C., Mountjoy, L.Q. *et al.* (1986) CAMDEX – a standardised instrument for the diagnosis of mental disorders in the elderly, *British Journal of Psychiatry*, 149: 698–709.

Royal Commission on Long Term Care (1999) *With Respect to Old Age: Long Term Care – Rights and Responsibilities*, Cm 4192-1. London: The Stationery Office.

Rummery, K. and Glendinning, C. (2000) *Primary Care and Social Services: Developing New Partnerships for Older People*. Abingdon: Radcliffe Medical Press.

Sabat, S. and Collins, M. (1999) Intact social, cognitive ability and selfhood: a case study of Alzheimer's disease. *American Journal of Alzheimer's Disease*, January/February: 11–19.

Sabat, S. and Harre, R. (1992) The construction and deconstruction of self in Alzheimer's disease, *Ageing and Society*, 12: 443–61.

Sackett, D.L., Rosenberg, W.M.C., Gray, J.A.M., Haynes R.B. and Richardson W.S. (1996) Evidence based medicine: what it is and what it isn't, *British Medical Journal*, 312: 71–2.

Sackett, D.L., Richardson, W.S., Rosenberg, W. and Haynes, R.B. (1997) *Evidence-based Medicine. How to Practise and Teach EBM*. Edinburgh: Churchill Livingstone.

Saks, M. (2000) Professionalism and health care, in C. Davies, L. Finlay and A. Bullman (eds) *Changing Practice in Health and Social Care*. London: Sage.

Sanderson, H., Kennedy, J., Ritchie, P. and Goodwin, G. (1997) *People, Plans and Possibilities: Exploring Person Centred Planning*. Edinburgh: Scottish Human Services.

Schmenner, R. (1986) How can service businesses survive and prosper?, *Sloan Management Review*, Spring: 21–32.

Schön, D.A. (1983) *The Reflective Practitioner*, reprinted 1996. Aldershot: Arena, Ashgate Publishing.

Schutz, A. (1972) *The Phenomenology of the Social World*. London: Heinemann.

Schutz, A. and Luckmann, T. (1974) *The Structures of the Life World*. London: Heinemann.

Schweitzer, P. (1999) Remembering yesterday, caring today, *Signpost*, 3: 23–5.

Scottish Office (1999) *Social Inclusion Strategy*. Edinburgh: Scottish Office.

Sears, D. (1998) *Compassion for Humanity in the Jewish Tradition*. Northvale, NJ and Jerusalem: Jason Aronson.

Seaton, M. (1995) Prevention and detection of abuse, *Elders: the Journal of Care and Practice*, 4(4): 5–27.

Selai, C. and Trimble, M.R. (1999) Assessing quality of life in dementia, *Aging and Mental Health*, 3(2): 101–11.

Seligman, M., Maier, S. and Geer, J. (1968) Alleviation of learned helplessness in the dog, *Journal of Abnormal Psychology*, 73(3): 256–62.

Selvini Palazzoli, M., Cecchin, G.O., Prata, G. and Boscolo, L. (1978) *Paradox and Counterparadox*. New York, NY: Jason Aronson.

Shamy, E. (1997) *More than Body, Brain or Breath: A Guide to Spiritual Care of People with Alzheimer's Disease*. Wellington, NZ: Colcom Press.

Sharkey, P. (2000) *The Essentials of Community Care: A Guide for Practitioners*. Basingstoke: Macmillan.

Shaw, F. and Kenny, A. (1998) Can falls in patients with dementia be prevented?, *Age and Ageing*, 27(1): 7–9.

Sheard, D. (1997) Demolishing the barriers: community dementia team development in Coventry, in M. Marshall (ed.) *State of the Art in Dementia Care*. London: Centre for Policy on Ageing.

Sheard, D. and Cox, S. (eds) (1998) *Teams, Multidisciplinary and Interprofessional Working and Dementia*. Stirling: Dementia Services Development Centre.

Sherman, B. (1999) *Sex, Intimacy and Aged Care*. London: Jessica Kingsley.

Sival, R.C., Vingerhoets, R.W., Haffmans, P.M.J. *et al.* (1997) Effect of a program of diverse activities on disturbed behavior in three severely demented patients, *International Psychogeriatrics*, 9: 423–30.

Skelton-Robinson, M. and Jones, S. (1984) Nominal dysphasia and the severity of senile dementia, *British Journal of Psychiatry*, 145: 168–71.

Sloan, R.P., Bagiella, E. and Powell, T. (1999) Religion, spirituality and medicine, *The Lancet*, 353: 664–7.

Smale, G. and Tuson, G. with Biehal, N. and Marsh, P. (1993) *Empowerment, Assessment, Care Management and the Skilled Worker*. National Institute for Social Work Practice and Development Exchange. London: HMSO.

Small, J.A., Geldart, K., Gutman, G. and Scott, M.A.C. (1998) The discourse of self in dementia, *Ageing and Society*, 18: 291–316.

Smith, G. (1980) *Social Need: Policy, Practice and Research*. London: Routledge and Kegan Paul.

Smith, G. and Cantley, C. (1985) *Assessing Health Care. A Study in Organisational Evaluation*. Milton Keynes: Open University Press.

Spaid, W.M. and Barusch, A.S. (1994) Emotional closeness and caregiver burden in the marital relationship, *Journal of Gerontological Social Work*, 21(3/4): 197–211.

Spector, A., Orrell, M., Davies, S. and Woods, R.T. (1999a) Reality Orientation for dementia (Cochrane Review), in *The Cochrane Library, Issue 3*. Oxford: Update Software.

Spector, A., Orrell, M., Davies, S. and Woods, R.T. (1999b) Reminiscence Therapy for dementia (Cochrane Review), in *The Cochrane Library, Issue 4*. Oxford: Update Software.

Sperlinger, D. and McAuslane, L. (1993) 'I don't want you to think I am ungrateful . . . but it does not satisfy what I want'. A Pilot Study of the Views of Users of

Services for People with Dementia in the London Borough of Sutton. Mimeo, Surrey: Department of Psychology, St Helier NHS Trust.

Spicker, P.P. and Gordon, D. with Ballinger, B., Gillies, B., McWilliam, N., Mutch, W. and Seed, P. (1997) *Planning for the Needs of People with Dementia: The Development of a Profile for Use in Local Services*. Aldershot: Avebury.

Stalker, K., Duckett, P. and Downs, M. (1999a) *Going with the Flow: Choice, Dementia and People with Learning Difficulties*. Brighton: Parillion Publishing.

Stalker, K., Gilliard, J. and Downes, M. (1999b) Eliciting user perspectives on what works, *International Journal of Geriatric Psychiatry*, 14: 120–34.

Stanley, D. and Reed, J. (1999) *Opening Up Care. Achieving Principled Practice in Health and Social Care Institutions*. London: Edward Arnold.

Stanley, D., Reed, J. and Brown, S. (1999) Older people, care management and interprofessional practice, *Journal of Interprofessional Care*, 13(3): 229–37.

Stern, D. (1985) *The Interpersonal World of the Infant*. New York, NY: Basic Books.

Stewart, A. (1998) Alzheimer's disease: a review of current economic perspectives, *Ageing and Society*, 18(5): 586–600.

Stokes, G. (1986a) *Shouting and Screaming*. London: Winslow Press.

Stokes, G. (1986b) *Wandering*. London: Winslow Press.

Stokes, G. (1987a) *Aggression*. London: Winslow Press.

Stokes, G. (1987b) *Incontinence and Inappropriate Urinating*. London: Winslow Press.

Stokes, G. (1996) Challenging behaviour in dementia; a psychological approach, in R.T. Woods (ed.) *Handbook of the Clinical Psychology of Ageing*. Chichester: Wiley.

Stokes, G. (2000) *Challenging Behaviour*. Bicester: Winslow Press.

Stokes, G. and Goudie, F. (1990) *Working with Dementia*. London: Winslow Press.

Stoller, E.P. and Pugliesi, K.L. (1989) Other roles of caregivers: competing responsibilities or supportive resources?, *Journal of Gerontology*, 44(5): 231–2.

Stoner, C. and Hartman, R. (1997) Organisational therapy: building survivor health and competitiveness, *SAM Advanced Management Journal*, Summer: 25–41.

Strauss, A., Schatzman, L., Ehrlich, D., Bucher, R. and Sabschin, M. (1973) The hospital and its negotiated order, in G. Salaman and K. Thompson (eds) *People and Organisations*. Harlow: Longman for The Open University.

Strauss, R.R. (1957) The nature and status of medical sociology, *American Sociological Review*, 22: 200–4.

Street, A. (1995) *Nursing Replay: Researching Nursing Culture Together*. Melbourne: Churchill Livingstone.

Stuart-Hamilton, I. (1996) Intellectual changes in late life, in R.T. Woods (ed.) *Handbook of the Clinical Psychology of Ageing*. Chichester: Wiley.

Sturges, P.J. (1997) Dementia care management: healing the split, in M. Marshall (ed.) *State of the Art in Dementia Care*. London: Centre for Policy on Ageing.

Sutton, L.J. and Cheston, R. (1997) Rewriting the story of dementia: a narrative approach to psychotherapy with people with dementia, in M. Marshall (ed.) *State of the Art in Dementia Care*. London: Centre for Policy on Ageing.

Svanberg, R., Livingston, M., Stephenson, C. and Fairbairn, A. (1999) Popular solution that can offer 'best value', *Journal of Dementia Care*, 7(1): 24–8.

Svanberg, R., Stirling, E. and Fairbairn, A. (1997) The process of care management with people with dementia, *Health and Social Care in the Community*, 5(2): 134–9.

Sweeting, H. (1997) Keynote address: Dying and dementia, in S. Cox, M. Gilhooly and J. McLennan, *Dying and Dementia Conference Report*. Stirling: Dementia Services Development Centre.

Taylor, B. (1987) The confused elderly: a living bereavement . . . Alzheimer's disease, *Nursing Times*, 83(30): 27–30.

Taylor, M., Langan, J. and Hoggett, P. (1995) *Encouraging Diversity: Voluntary and Private Organisations in Community Care*. Aldershot: Arena, Ashgate.

Teri, L. and Gallagher-Thompson, D. (1991) Cognitive-behavioral interventions for treatment of depression in Alzheimer's patients, *The Gerontologist*, 31: 413–16.

Tester, S. (1999) *The Quality Challenge: Caring for People with Dementia in Residential Institutions in Europe*. Edinburgh: Alzheimer Scotland Action on Dementia.

Thompson, E.H., Fellerman, A.M., Gallagher-Thompson, D., Rose, J.M. and Lovett, S.B. (1993) Social support and caregiving burden in family caregivers of frail elderly, *Journal of Gerontology*, 48(5): 245–54.

Thompson, J. (1967) *Organisations in Action*. New York, NY: McGraw-Hill Book Co.

Thompson, J. (1995) *Strategy in Action*. London: Chapman Hall.

Thornton, P. and Tozer, R. (1994) *Involving Older People in Planning and Evaluating Community Care – Review of Initiatives*. York: Social Policy Research Unit, University of York.

Tibbs, M.A. (1995) Steering a course over troubled waters, *Journal of Dementia Care*, Sept/Oct: 14–16.

Tibbs, M.A. (1996) 'Amos: A self lost and found', *Journal of Dementia Care*, March/April: 10–11.

Tindall, L. and Manthorpe, J. (1997) Early onset dementia: a case of ill-timing?, *Journal of Mental Health*, 6(3): 237–49.

Toates, F. (1996) The embodied self: a biological perspective, in R. Stevens (ed.) *Understanding the Self*. London: Sage.

Tobin, S.S. (1991) *Personhood in Advanced Old Age: Implications for Practice*. New York, NY: Springer.

Towell, D. (ed.) (1988) *An Ordinary Life in Practice*. London: King Edward's Hospital Fund.

Townsend, P. (1979) *Poverty in the United Kingdom: A Survey of Household Resources and Standards of Living*. Harmondsworth: Penguin.

Townsend, P. (1981) The structured dependency of the elderly: a creation of social policy in the twentieth century, *Ageing and Society*, 1: 5–28.

Townsend, P. (1991) The social and economic hardship of elderly people in London: new evidence from a survey and a discussion of the influence of social policy upon current trends, *Generations, Bulletin of the British Society of Gerontology*, 9: 10–30.

Treetops, J. (1992) *A Daisy among the Dandelions: The Church's Ministry with Older People*. Leeds: Leeds Faith in Elderly People, Leeds Church Institute.

Treetops, J. (1996) *Holy, Holy, Holy: The Church's Ministry with People with Dementia*. Leeds: Leeds Faith in Elderly People.

Treetops, J. (1999) The memory box, in A. Jewell (ed.) *Spirituality and Ageing*. London: Jessica Kingsley.

Trevarthen, C. (1979) Communication and co-operation in early infancy: a description of primary subjectivity, in M. Bullova and P. Elkman (eds) *Before Speech: The Beginning of Interpersonal Communication*. New York, NY: Cambridge University Press.

Turnbull, A.P. and Turnbull, H.R. (1993) Participatory research in cognitive coping: from concepts to research planning, in A.P. Turnbull, J.M. Patterson, S.K. Behr *et al.* (eds) *Cognitive Coping, Families and Disability*. Baltimore, MD: Paul H. Brookes.

Turner, S.A. and Street, U.P. (1999) Assessing carers' training needs: a pilot inquiry, *Aging and Mental Health*, 3(2): 173–8.

Twigg, J. (1998) Informal care of older people, in M. Bernard and J. Phillips (eds) *The Social Policy of Old Age*. London: Centre for Policy on Ageing.

Twigg, J. and Atkin, K. (1994) *Carers Perceived: Policy and Practice in Informal Care*. Buckingham: Open University Press.

UKCC (1992) *Code of Professional Conduct*, 3rd edn. London: United Kingdom Central Council for Nursing, Midwifery and Health Visiting.

Ungerson, C. (1983) *Women and Caring: Skills, Tasks and Taboos, The Public and the Private*. London: Heinemann.

Ungerson, C. (1987) *Policy Is Personal – Sex, Gender and Informal Care*. London: Tavistock Publications.

Valle, R. (1998) *Caregiving across Cultures: Working with Dementing Illness and Ethnically Diverse Populations*. Washington, DC: Taylor & Francis.

van den Bergh, M. (1997) *A Guide for the Care of Jewish Patients in Hospital and Nursing Homes*. London: The Visitation Committee.

Vitaliano, P.P., Young, H.M. and Russo, J. (1991) Burden: a review of measures used among caregivers of individuals with dementia, *The Gerontologist*, 31: 67–75.

VOICES (Voluntary Organisations Involved in Caring for Older People) (1998) *Eating Well for Older People with Dementia: A Good Practice Guide for Residential and Nursing Homes and Others involved in Caring for Older People with Dementia*. Potters Bar: VOICES.

Walker, A. (1981) Towards a political economy of old age, *Ageing and Society*, 1: 73–94.

Walker, A. (1995) Integrating the family in the mixed economy of care, in I. Allan and E. Perkins (eds) *The Future of Family Care for Older People*. London: HMSO.

Walker, A. and Warren, L. (1996) *Changing Services for Older People*. Buckingham: Open University Press.

Walsh, F. (ed.) (1982) *Normal Family Processes*. New York, NY: Guilford Press.

Ward, L. (1997) Funding for change: translating emancipatory disability research from theory to practice, in Barnes, C. and Mercer, G. (eds) *Doing Disability Research*. Leeds: The Disability Press.

Warner, C. and Wexler, S. (1998) *Eight Hours a Day and Taken for Granted?* London: The Princess Royal Trust for Carers.

Warnock, M. (1998) *An Intelligent Person's Guide to Ethics*. London: Duckworth.

Warrington, E. and James, M. (1991) *Visual Object and Space Perception Battery (VOSP)*. Bury St Edmunds: Thames Valley Test Company.

Warrington, J. (1996) *Depression and Dementia: Coexistence and Differentiation*. Stirling: Dementia Services Development Centre.

Waterman, H., Webb, C. and Williams, A. (1995) Parallels and contradictions in the theory and practice of action research and nursing, *Journal of Advanced Nursing*, 22: 779–84.

Wechsler, D. (1982) *The Wechsler Adult Intelligence Scale – Revised, Manual*. New York, NY: The Psychological Corporation.

Weiss, C.H. (1986) The many meanings of research utilisation, in M. Bulmer (ed.) *Social Science and Social Policy*. London: Allen & Unwin.

Wenger, C.G. (1994) Dementia sufferers living at home, *International Journal of Geriatric Psychiatry*, 9: 721–33.

Whitsted-Lipinska, D. (1999) Counselling for people with dementia. Paper presented at the Journal of Dementia Care Conference, Bournemouth, 12–13 May.

Whitworth, A., Perkins, L. and Lesser, R. (1999) Communication in dementia care: a partnership approach, in T. Adams and C.L. Clarke (eds) *Dementia Care: Developing Partnerships in Practice*. London: Baillière Tindall.

Wilding, P. (1982) *Professional Power and Social Welfare*. London: Routledge and Kegan Paul.

Wilkin, D. and Hughes, B. (1986) The elderly and the health services, in C. Phillipson and A. Walker (eds) *Ageing and Social Policy*. Aldershot: Gower.

Williams, A. and Norton, C. (1999) All the saints go marching in after St Tony. *The Sunday Times*, 7 February.

Williams, R., Barrett, K. and Muth, Z. (eds) (1997) *Heading for Better Care: Commissioning and Providing Mental Health Services for People with Huntington's Disease, Acquired Brain Injury and Early Onset Dementia*, NHS Health Advisory Service Thematic Review. London: HMSO.

Wilson, P.H. (1999) Memory, personhood and faith, in A. Jewell (ed.) *Spirituality and Ageing*. London: Jessica Kingsley.

Wimo, A., Jönsson, B., Karlsson, G. and Winblad, B. (1998) *Health Economics of Dementia*. Chicester: John Wiley.

Wolfensberger, W. (1972) *The Principle of Normalisation in Human Services*. Toronto: National Institute for Mental Retardation.

Woods, R. (1997) Talking point: Kitwood's 'The experience of dementia', *Ageing and Mental Health*, 4: 11–12.

Woods, R.T. (1996) Institutional care, in R.T. Woods (ed.) *Handbook of the Clinical Psychology of Ageing*. Chichester: Wiley.

Woods, R.T. and McKiernan, F. (1995) Evaluating the impact of reminiscence on older people with dementia, in B.K. Haight and J. Webster (eds) *The Art and Science of Reminiscing: Theory, Research, Methods and Applications*. Washington, DC: Taylor & Francis.

Wuest, J., Ericson, P.K. and Stern, P.N. (1994) Becoming strangers: the changing family caregiving relationship in Alzheimer's disease, *Journal of Advanced Nursing*, 20: 437–43.

Wye, L. and McClenahan, J. (2000) *Getting Better with Evidence. Experiences of Putting Evidence into Practice*. London: King's Fund Publishing.

Yeandle, S. (1984) *Women's Working Lives*. London: Tavistock Publications.

Yeo, G. and Gallagher-Thompson, D. (eds) (1996) *Ethnicity and the Dementias*. Washington, DC: Taylor & Francis.

Yin, R.K. (1994) *Case Study Research. Design and Methods*, 2nd edn. London: Sage.

Zarit, S. and Zarit, J. (1983) Cognitive impairment in older persons: etiology, evaluation with intervention, in P. Lewinsohn and L. Teri (eds) *Coping and Adaptation in the Elderly*. New York, NY: Pergamon.

Zarit, S.H. and Edwards, A.B. (1996) Family caregiving, in R.T. Woods (ed.) *Handbook of the Clinical Psychology of Ageing*. Chichester: Wiley.

Zizoulias, J.D. (1985) *Being as Communion: Studies in Personhood and the Church*. Crestwood, NY: St Vladimir's Seminary Press.

Zola, I.K. (1972) Medicine as an institution of social control, *Sociological Review*, 20(4): 487–504.

Author index

Subject index